INTERNATIONAL REVIEW OF CHILD NEUROLOGY SERIES

TUBEROUS SCLEROSIS COMPLEX

Edited by

Paolo Curatolo

© 2003 Mac Keith Press
High Holborn House, 52–54 High Holborn, London WC1V 6RL, England

Senior Editor: Martin CO Bax
Editor: Hilary Hart
Managing Editor: Michael Pountney
Sub Editor: Sarah Pearsall

Set in Garamond on QuarkXpress

First published in this edition 2003

British Library Cataloguing-in-Publication data:
A catalogue record for this book is available from the British Library

ISBN: 1 898683 39 5

Printed by The Lavenham Press Ltd, Water Street, Lavenham, Suffolk, England
Mac Keith Press is supported by Scope

Distributed to non-members of ICNA by Cambridge University Press

INTERNATIONAL REVIEW OF CHILD NEUROLOGY SERIES

TUBEROUS SCLEROSIS COMPLEX

From Basic Science to Clinical Phenotypes

Edited by

PAOLO CURATOLO

Professor of Child Neurology and Psychiatry
Director of Division of Child Neurology and Psychiatry
Department of Neurosciences
Tor Vergata University
Rome, Italy

2003
MAC KEITH PRESS
for the
INTERNATIONAL CHILD NEUROLOGY ASSOCIATION

INTERNATIONAL REVIEW OF CHILD NEUROLOGY SERIES

CONTENTS

AUTHORS' APPOINTMENTS

Eishi Asano	Departments of Pediatrics and Neurology, Children's Hospital of Michigan, Wayne State University, Detroit, MI, USA
Patrick F Bolton	Department of Child Psychiatry, Institute of Psychiatry, King's College, London
Nunzio Bottini	The Burnham Institute, La Jolla, CA, USA
Alessandro Bozzao	Department of Neuroradiology, La Sapienza University, Rome, Italy
Jeremy P Cheadle	Institute of Medical Genetics, University of Wales College of Medicine, Health Park, Cardiff, UK
Diane C Chugani	Departments of Pediatrics and Radiology, Children's Hospital of Michigan, Wayne State University, Detroit, MI, USA
Harry T Chugani	Departments of Pediatrics, Neurology and Radiology, Children's Hospital of Michigan, Wayne State University, Detroit, MI, USA
Peter B Crino	Department of Neurology, PENN Epilepsy Center, University of Pennsylvania Medical Center, Philadelphia, PA, USA
Paolo Curatolo	Department of Pediatric Neurology and Psychiatry, Tor Vergata University, Rome, Italy
Michael Dowling	Division of Paediatric Neurology, South Western Medical Centre, Dallas, TX, USA
Okio Hino	Department of Experimental Pathology, Cancer Institute, Japanese Foundation for Cancer Research, Tokyo, Japan
Sergiusz Jóźwiak	Department of Neurology, Children's Memorial Health Institute, Warsaw, Poland
David J Kwiatkowski	Genetics Laboratory, Hematology Division, Brigham and Women's Hospital, Harvard Medical School, Boston, MA, USA
Guglielmo Manenti	Department of Radiology, Tor Vergata University, Rome, Italy
Masashi Mizuguchi	Department of Pediatrics, Jichi Medical School, Tochigi, Japan
Mary Pat Reeve	Genetics Laboratory, Hematology Division, Brigham and Women's Hospital, Harvard Medical School, Boston, MA, USA

Julian R Sampson — Institute of Medical Genetics, University of Wales College of Medicine, Health Park, Cardiff, UK

Harvey B Sarnat — Department of Pediatric Neurology, Cedars-Sinai Medical Center, Los Angeles, CA, USA

Robert Schwartz — Department of Dermatology, New Jersey Medical School, Newark, NJ, USA

Stefano Seri — Department of Pediatric Neurology and Psychiatry, Tor Vergata University, Rome, Italy

Magda Verdecchia — Department of Pediatric Neurology and Psychiatry, Tor Vergata University, Rome, Italy

FOREWORD

The International Child Neurology Association (ICNA) was founded in 1973 with the aim of improving the quality of care of children with neurological disorders. One of the methods it uses to further this aim is the publishing of the International Review of Child Neurology, a series of books on specific child neurology subjects. The series has an international audience and has drawn its authors from many parts of the globe. This book is no exception, with a multinational authorship which is quite apt for a volume on tuberous sclerosis as the disorder was almost simultaneously described by Bourneville from France and Hartdegen from Germany.

ICNA is committed to continue publication of this series to fulfil its stated aim.

Peter G Procopis
Senior Editor

PREFACE

Harvey B Sarnat

Tuberous sclerosis complex (TSC) is the prototype of a category of malformations uniquely characterized by disturbances in cellular differentiation and growth. Other diseases are also now recognized under the rubric of "disturbances of cellular lineage" involving multiple organ systems and tissues, but particularly the nervous system. These include Proteus syndrome and hemimegalencephaly, both the isolated and the syndromic forms of the latter. TSC is the most frequent and the most studied amongst these cytological disorders. My own personal studies of both surgical and autopsy brain tissue in children with tuberous sclerosis are highly consistent with the concept of a primary disorder of cellular lineage and mixed expression of neuronal and glial proteins in the same cells, which I reported in a previous study and have corroborated in several additional patients I have subsequently studied. Other authors have published similar results, discussed in the excellent chapter on neuropathology by Mizuguchi and Hino in this monograph. These findings have resulted in a reclassification of tuberous sclerosis as a "disorder of cellular lineage" in new schemes of CNS malformations that integrate molecular genetic with morphological criteria.

Despite the classical text of Manuel Gomez, including the third edition published as recently as 1999, a fountainhead of new molecular and genetic data has emerged that alone justifies another monograph on the topic. Clinical advances in recognition, imaging, including functional imaging, and neuropsychological studies, as well as the genetic and the histopathological cell markers of maturation and of lineage, also require a review at this time to summarize the wealth of literature in diverse medical specialties on TSC and to update patient care. Professor Paolo Curatolo, a foremost world authority on TSC, with both experience and insight of patients with this disease, has met the challenge well in this new monograph. He has called upon colleagues in various disciplines most capable of assisting him with focused chapters that describe the most recent findings and interpretations; these are the very individuals whose original contributions other authors would almost certainly cite in writing a review. The scope ranges from highly clinical studies of cognitive and linguistic functions to the animal model of TSC, the Eker rat. Even the rich historical aspects of the disease are chronologically described in a highly interesting presentation.

TSC is an important disease not only because it is a relatively common hereditary neurological disease with great morbidity, but because it has conceptual implications in many areas in which it forms a borderland with other pathological processes: dysplasia and neoplasia; hamartoma formation and other disturbances in morphogenic processes such as neuroblast migration and synaptogenesis; relationships between neurons and glial cells. It also raises important issues about the timing of the formation of the hamartomas and cytological dysgenesis. Do cortical hamartomas in humans develop after the migration of normal or abnormal neuroblasts, and how do they arrive at the cortex if the radial glial cells in the same subventricular zone from which they arise are also abnormal? Why are cortical tubers so much rarer in the Eker rat than in the human, whereas subependymal hamartomatous nodules are frequent in both species? Can this difference be related to the shorter time during which neuroblast migration proceeds to completion in the rat?

This present monograph is clearly the most authoritative and contemporary statement of current knowledge about TSC yet published. It is the first monograph to make a meaningful correlation between the fountainhead of new genetic and basic science data and the clinical presentation of the disease. It provides, furthermore, a guide to future research strategies by discussing unresolved issues. Whereas one cannot speak of the first volume of any book as a "classic", at least not until much time has passed, it nevertheless has the potential to become a classic, which will be realized in multiple future updates. I regard it a great honour to be invited to write the Foreword to the first edition of *Tuberous Sclerosis Complex,* with many future editions anticipated for the digestion and interpretation of research yet to be done in this fascinating and complex disease.

EDITOR'S PREFACE

Paolo Curatolo

My interest in tuberous sclerosis began in the early 1980s. At that time I worked in the Department of Child Neurology and Psychiatry in the University of Rome, and I was dedicating my time to children with early-onset and intractable seizures in which tuberous sclerosis represented one of the most frequent aetiologies. As a child neurologist, I was particularly intrigued by the special association in these children of different neurological phenotypes caused by tuberous sclerosis, including seizures, cognitive impairments and autism, and the puzzling interrelation between these three symptoms. The arrival of the first MRI instrument in Rome in 1984 gave me the opportunity to study in detail the localization of the cortical tubers in different lobes, and allowed me to investigate the relationship between EEG foci, the MRI localization of cortical tubers, and the cognitive and behavioural phenotypes.

In those years I also had the opportunity to meet for the first time Manuel Gomez, who has dedicated his life to the study of TSC, and to discuss with him issues relating to this complex and fascinating disease, a meeting which has been of great stimulus for my future clinical research. Manuel Gomez's monograph appeared in three different editions, the last of which was published in 1999. It was widely regarded as a milestone by all clinicians and researchers in the field.

Recent advances in the field of tuberous sclerosis and new discoveries from molecular genetics and biology are actually progressing at a rate of about 500 papers published each year. This is the reason that our clinical practice necessitates a continuous upgrading. With this book I seek to encapsulate in a single text modern knowledge about current research, ideas and practice on tuberous sclerosis, from basic neuroscience to clinical phenotypes.

The first part of the book is designed to provide the reader with a review of the historical background and current criteria for diagnosis. The next part of the book is intended to provide readers with detailed descriptions of the clinical manifestations of this protean disease. Special emphasis has been placed on the neurological phenotypes of the cortical tubers, including seizures, cognitive impairments and autism. A large part of the book deals with the recent significant advances in the fields of neuropathology, molecular genetics and neurobiology, which allow a better understanding of the pathogenesis of the disease. To cover this vast and complex subject I have enlisted a panel of experts in their respective fields.

No book is an individual enterprise. This book has benefited greatly from the co-operation, assistance, wisdom and generosity of many people: my editor, academic mentor, researchers, colleagues and family. Important material for many chapters in this book was pulled together by my researchers Drs Magda Verdecchia and Roberta Bombardieri, whose assistance proved fundamental to my writing. I would also like to give a special thank you to all the people with TSC and their families who put their trust in me, giving me constant energy and motivation to continue my efforts and research in the field. Finally, I am indebted to Mac Keith Press for their great patience, understanding and professional assistance in producing the book.

Scientific books reflect the continuous and dynamic process of knowledge acquisition, and are therefore never complete. It is my hope that this book will consolidate what is known about TSC in a single source, making it easier to apply this new information to the cure of individual patients, and perhaps stimulating scientific research on some of the remaining questions about this devastating disease.

1
HISTORICAL BACKGROUND

Paolo Curatolo

DEFINITION

Tuberous sclerosis complex (TSC) is a genetically determined, variably expressed, multisystem disorder that may affect any human organ with well-circumscribed, benign, non-invasive lesions. The skin, brain, retina, heart, kidney and lung are the organs more often involved. The importance of central nervous system (CNS) involvement in TSC is emphasized by the fact that the condition has retained its name for over a century. "Tuberous sclerosis of the cerebral convolutions" is the term used by Bourneville (1880) to describe the unique and distinctive cerebral pathology he found in a patient with seizures and learning disability.* The cerebral lesion, called *cortical tuber*, is the hallmark of a protean autosomal dominant disease with variable expression in one or more organs or tissues. The different lesions are included under the term *tuberous sclerosis complex* (TSC) proposed in 1942 by the pathologist Moolten.

Derived from a single pathologic feature, namely potato-like firmness of segments of the cerebral cortex, the term tuberous sclerosis complex persists as a designation for all forms and variants of the disease. However, the majority of patients identified as having the disorder do experience symptoms referable to the CNS. Even in subjects without neurological symptoms, CNS lesions are present in all brains studied. In those rare instances in which the brain is said to be anatomically normal, an exhaustive histological research would be likely to reveal lesions. CNS abnormalities therefore remain the hallmark of TSC and underline its most common and clinically serious manifestations.

Historical contributions to the knowledge of TSC are summarized in Table 1.1.

HISTORY OF TUBEROUS SCLEROSIS COMPLEX

1. THE FIRST DESCRIPTIONS

In 1835, Pierre François Rayer completed an atlas displaying skin diseases. In this atlas a young man's face dotted with small, erythematous papules with a characteristic distribution and similar appearance is shown, resembling the facial angiofibroma often observed in patients with the tuberous sclerosis complex (see Fig. 9.1, p. 138). On March 25, 1862, Friederich Daniel von Recklinghausen presented to the

---

* The term "learning disability" corresponds to "mental retardation" in American usage.

TABLE 1.1
Progress in understanding tuberous sclerosis complex (from Gomez 1999, modified)

Year	Authors	Findings
1835	Rayer	Illustration of facial angiofibroma in atlas
1862	Von Recklinghausen	Cardiac "myomata" in newborns
1880	Désiré-Magloire Bourneville	Cortical "tuberosities"
1885	Balzer and Ménétrier, Hallopeau and Leredde	Report "adenoma sebaceum"
1901	Pellizzi	Dysplasia, heterotopia, myelination defect
1905	Perusini, Campbell	Pathology of brain, kidney, heart, skin
1908	Vogt	Diagnostic triad
1910	Kirpicznik	Genetic condition
1913	Berg	Hereditary nature
1914	Schuster	*Forme fruste* with normal intelligence
1918	Lutenbacher	Lung involvement
1920	Van der Hoeve	Retinal phakoma
1924	Marcus	Radiographic findings
1932	Critchley and Earl	Discover white spots, report "autistic" behaviour
1967	Lagos and Gomez	38% of patients have normal intelligence
1975	Pampiglione and Pugh	Infantile spasms as the presenting seizure
1979	Gomez	New criteria for diagnosis; decline of the Vogt's triad
1984	Dulac et al.	A cluster of spasms is preceded by a focal EEG discharge
1987	McMurdo et al.	Magnetic resonance imaging (MRI) demonstrates cortical tubers
1987	Roach et al.	Number of tubers
1987	Fryer et al.	Mapping of *TSC1* to chromosome 9q34.3
1988	Curatolo and Cusmai	Localization of tubers
1990	Chiron et al.	Vigabatrin as an effective antiepileptic treatment
1992	Kandt et al.	Mapping of *TSC2* to chromosome 16p13.3
1993	The European Chromosome 16 Tuberous Sclerosis Consortium	Cloning of *TSC2*; its product is called *tuberin*
1995	Maeda et al.	Introduction of MRI with fluid-attenuated inversion recovery
1997	Van Slegtenhorst et al.	Cloning of *TSC1*; its product is called *hamartin*
1997	Bolton and Griffiths	Autism and temporal lobe
2001	Dabora et al.	Genotype–phenotype relationship

Obstetrical Society of Berlin the pathological findings in a newborn infant who had "died after taking a few breaths". The heart had several tumours protruding on the cardiac surface, while others bulged into the cardiac chambers and still others were embedded in the ventricular walls. Von Recklinghausen labelled these cardiac tumours "myomata" and added briefly that the infant's brain contained a "great number of scleroses". Von Recklinghausen's brief report contains the first description of the two pathologic lesions more often observed in newborn infants with TSC: cardiac rhabdomyomas and cortical tubers (Gomez 1999).

In 1880 Bourneville gave the first detailed report of its neurological symptoms and gross cerebral pathology. In his paper, Bourneville described the pathological findings in the brains of three "idiots". Bourneville coined the term "tuberous sclerosis of the cerebral convolutions" for his third patient because its gross nodular appearance and induration resembled tubers. The patient was a 3-year-old girl admitted to *La Salpetriére* with convulsive seizures and learning disabilities. Her seizures had started in infancy and at first involved only the eyes. At the age of 2 years, they became more generalized so that both upper extremities would become "somewhat rigid and slightly rotated". Examination when she was 15 years old disclosed facial skin lesions. The patient also had many small "molluscum" lesions on the neck and a right spastic hemiplegia. Each day for several months the girl continued to have many seizures, and on May 7, 1879, she was found dead in her bed. On postmortem examination, Bourneville found that many cerebral convolutions had hard, raised, whitish areas of greater density than the surrounding cortex, and he wrote: "In one word, we are dealing with a hypertrophic sclerosis of portions of the circumvolutions." Bourneville concluded that the seizures had a focal origin and progressed to generalized attacks, and attributed their partial onset to the conspicuous sclerotic lesions in the ascending frontal and parietal convolutions of the left cerebral hemisphere.

One year later, Bourneville and Brissaud (1881) made a new clinicopathological observation. The patient was a 4-year-old boy admitted to *La Bicêtre*. He had had predominantly right-sided seizures since the age of 4 months, had learned to walk at 2 years of age, and could say only one syllable at age 4. Subsequently, his seizures became more frequent and prolonged. On auscultation he had a loud cardiac murmur. Later he developed cyanosis and crepitant pulmonary rales, stopped eating and drinking, and finally died on January 6, 1880. Pathological examination of the brain disclosed sclerotic, hypertrophic convolutions. Brain cuts demonstrated ventricles normal in size, but their lateral walls were covered with many small sclerotic tumours, 2 to 5 mm in diameter. The kidneys on sectioning disclosed small yellowish-white tumours. Bourneville and Brissaud proposed that the association of the cerebral lesions and the kidney tumours was significant. In 1890, Pringle reported in much detail the same type of facial lesion on a 25-year-old woman of subnormal intelligence. He called the lesion "congenital adenoma sebaceum".

2. CLINICAL PHENOTYPE

In 1908, Vogt described the association between the cerebral sclerosis of the circumvolutions reported by Bourneville and the facial adenoma sebaceum. Through Vogt's work, the syndrome consisting of seizures, learning disability and "adenoma sebaceum" was established as the classic clinical triad of features for the diagnosis of TSC. Vogt also stated that cardiac and renal tumours form part of the disease.

Noting the similarity between TSC, neurofibromatosis and von Hippel-Lindau disease in the spotty distribution of these lesions and their tendency to grow as benign tumours, in 1920, van der Hoeve developed the concept of phakomatoses, disorders characterized by the presence of circumscribed lesions or phakomas with the potential of getting larger and forming a real tumour by cellular proliferation. Van der Hoeve listed the varieties of phakomata found pathologically in patients with TSC: tumefactions in the cerebral cortex with proliferation of glia, tumours within the ventricles, heterotopical spots in the white substance, renal cysts, intestinal lipomas, thyroid adenomas, bone cysts, facial adenoma sebaceum, etc.

In 1932, Critchley and Earl reported on their observations in 29 patients with TSC. They were the first to emphasize the diagnostic value of white spots (hypomelanotic skin macules) in patients with TSC. Furthermore, they reported autistic behaviour 11 years before Kanner (1943) published his classic paper describing the paradoxical and bewildering disturbance of behaviour that he called "early infantile autism". These descriptions are quoted as an introduction to behaviour in TSC. Critchley and Earl noted that "often the family history shows no evidence of tuberous sclerosis but bears a strong psychopathic taint" (1932: 314). "The psychosis always resembles a primitive form of catatonic schizophrenia, though the exact form of the reaction varies with the level of mental development at which it occurs. . . . The depth of psychosis is independent of the degree of intellectual defect, although the two processes are so inextricably intertwined as to render impossible any accurate estimation of the part played by either in any given case. . . . All manner of bizarre attitudes and stereotyped movements occur, and these are most striking in the hands and fingers" (ibid.: 322).

In 1967, Lagos and Gomez documented a family in which five generations were affected by TSC. These authors reviewed the clinical features of 71 individuals with TSC seen at the Mayo Clinic during a 30-year period, and reported that 38% of the 69 patients with available intelligence data had average intelligence, while 62% had learning disabilities. All the patients with learning disability had previously had seizures, while of those with average intelligence, 69% had, or had previously had, seizures. These authors were unable to find any correlation between the presence of adenoma sebaceum, retinal phakoma or intracranial calcification and the mental status (Gomez 1979). These data determined a weakening of the classic triad of Vogt and gave rise to the revision of diagnostic criteria that followed.

The relationship between West syndrome and TSC has been known for many years (Gastaut et al. 1965). The high incidence of infantile spasms (IS) in TSC has long been emphasized. Pampiglione and Pugh in 1975 reported that infantile spasms were the presenting symptoms in up to 69% of patients with TSC. Conversely TSC has been found by Curatolo and Cusmai (1987) in 11% in a series of 164 infants affected by IS who underwent CT, suggesting the existence of an important association between TSC and IS. However, in recent years important advances in the understanding of seizures associated with TSC have indicated that infants with TSC exhibit some characteristic clinical and EEG features, distinguishing these infants from those with classical West syndrome including hypsarrhythmia. In particular, Dulac et al., in 1984, stressed the fact that occasionally a particular combination of focal and generalized seizures is present and that a cluster of spasms may be preceded by a focal EEG discharge.

3. PATHOLOGICAL FINDINGS

In 1905, Perusini reported a precise microscopic description of the cortical tubers, finely illustrated with ink drawings of atypical neurons, subcortical areas of hypomyelination, and subependymal nodules. He also reported the frequent association of the cerebral, renal and cardiac lesions with the "cutaneous adenomas" in TSC patients.

In 1942, Moolten proposed that the lesions of TSC belong to one of three types. In Moolten's own words, "the basic lesion is hamartial, becoming in turn tumour-like but benign (hamartoma) or truly neoplastic (hamartoblastoma)". Moolten, recognizing the complexity and "hamartial nature" of tuberous sclerosis, renamed it "the tuberous sclerosis complex". This is now the preferred name, although in a few European countries, where eponymic names of diseases are often used, it is called Bourneville disease.

Pathologically, TSC is a disorder of cell migration, proliferation and differentiation. Present evidence suggests that the CNS lesions of TSC are due to a developmental disorder of neurogenesis and neuronal migration. Two populations of neuroepithelial cells are generated by the germinal matrix in TSC. One is a population of normal neuroblasts which form normal neurons and astroglia and which migrate to the cortical plate where they form histologically normal cerebral cortex. The second is an abnormal cell population which forms primitive cells that often fail to show clear neuronal and glial differentiation. Some of these cells, named "neuroastrocytes", remain in the germinal matrix zone where they form subependymal nodules and giant cell tumours. Some neuroastrocytes show partial migration, forming heterotopias in the subcortical white matter. More differentiated cells migrate to the cortical plate where they form aggregates of dysplastic cortex, the cortical tubers. Cells in tubers share with those in subependymal nodules and giant cell tumours the frequent absence of clear neuronal and glial differentiation, showing features of primitive stellate neurons with few dendritic spines. Tuberin and hamartin are widely expressed in human fetal tissues. This evidence suggests a critical function of these two proteins in early development and maturation of the brain. Tuberin was undetectable in subependymal giant cell astrocytomas examined in three patients, suggesting that a complete inactivation of tuberin expression is associated with tumour development. It is likely that hamartin and tuberin participate in the same pathways of cellular growth control and share a common biochemical pathway. The proteins appear to co-localize at the cellular level, and recent evidence suggests that there is a direct binding between tuberin and hamartin. These two proteins form a cytosolic complex interacting at the N-terminal ends of both proteins. This interaction is abolished by some TSC-associated mutations.

4. IMAGING

In 1924, Marcus described roentgenographic intracranial calcifications as a sign of TSC. With the introduction of pneumoencephalography, the intraventricular subependymal nodules on the walls of the lateral ventricles could be demonstrated in a living patient for the first time. The image was called "candle guttering" because of its resemblance to the drippings of a burning candle. As a consequence of both these discoveries, the number of patients diagnosed increased dramatically.

Only occasionally were asymptomatic relatives of the severely affected patients recognized as having TSC, prior to the improvement of imaging methods, which began in the mid-1970s. The introduction of cranial computed tomography in 1974, followed by echocardiography, renal ultrasound and magnetic resonance imaging in 1982, provided new, reliable and non-invasive methods of diagnosis. These advances allowed new and more extensive criteria in establishing diagnosis and, as a consequence, the number of affected individuals with TSC rapidly increased.

McMurdo et al., in 1987, gave us the first pathologic demonstration that the signal changes on MRI corresponded with cortical tubers. At that time we believed that uncontrolled epileptic seizures were largely responsible for the learning disabilities of children with TSC. Roach et al. first reported in 1987 that children with a higher number of cortical tubers detected by MRI had poorer seizure control and more severe developmental delay. In 1988, Curatolo and Cusmai reported a topographic correspondence between EEG foci and the largest tubers detected by MRI, emphasizing the importance of cortical tubers as epileptogenic areas. In 1989, Nixon et al. demonstrated that MRI was unable to detect all the cortical tubers that can be identified pathologically. In 1990, Chiron et al. reported Vigabatrin as an effective drug treatment for infantile spasms associated with TSC. In 1995 Maeda et al. noted that fluid-attenuated inversion recovery was more sensitive than spin-echo sequences and may identify more and smaller cortical tubers than the standard T2-weighted images. Goodman et al. (1997) confirmed that the count of cortical tubers detected by MRI is a good biomarker in predicting the severity of cerebral dysfunction.

Positron emission tomography may reveal hypometabolic regions not predicted by MRI, demonstrating that the disturbance of cerebral function may be more extensive than indicated by morphological studies alone.

The use of multimodality imaging may improve detection of epileptogenic foci in children with TSC.

5. GENETICS

Since the earliest descriptions of TSC at the end of the nineteenth century, physicians and scientists have sought the underlying cause of the disease (von Recklinghausen 1862, Bourneville 1880).

TSC was first recognized as a genetic condition by Kirpicznik in 1910. He reported a family with affected individuals in three generations, and described the condition in identical and fraternal twins. Earlier studies had noted that the facial lesions of TSC, erroneously called "adenoma sebaceum", were inherited in families (Balzer and Ménétrier 1885, Pringle 1890).

The hereditary nature of TSC was first reported by Berg in 1913. Schuster (1914) confirmed it, and recognized as exceptional the patient with only the adenoma sebaceum component of the Vogt triad, that is, without learning disability. This phenotype has been named the *forme fruste* – a term derived from the French and used for any "incomplete" phenotype or to indicate reduced expression of the TSC gene (Gomez 1999).

Since then, the studies by Gunther and Penrose (1935) and Nevin and Pearce (1968) have demonstrated the dominant inheritance of TSC and its high mutation rate.

In 1951, Dickerson described three families with multiple members affected with TSC, and reviewed the literature concerning all that was known about familial cases.

Until the late 1980s, very little real progress was made toward uncovering the molecular basis of tuberous sclerosis. Fortunately, progress in the field of molecular genetics dramatically improved the ability to study this complex genetic disease.

The first report of genetic linkage analysis identifying a probable TSC gene on chromosome 9q34 appeared in 1987. This gene was denoted *TSC1* (van Slegtenhorst et al. 1997). Subsequent studies indicated that not all TSC families demonstrated linkage to the 9q34 region (indicating that there probably were other TSC genes).

Later, chromosome 16p13 was identified as the site of a second TSC locus denoted *TSC2* (Kandt et al. 1992, The European Chromosome 16 Tuberous Sclerosis Consortium 1993).

TSC results from mutations in *TSC1*, the gene on chromosome 9q34, and *TSC2*, the gene on chromosome 16p13. Frequent loss of heterozygosity for alleles in 16p13.3 and rare loss in 9q34 have been found in hamartomas from TSC patients, indicating that a second somatic mutation may be required to produce the TSC phenotype at the cellular level. These findings are consistent with *TSC1* and *TSC2* acting as growth suppressor genes. The *TSC2* gene maps to the gene-rich region of 16p13.3, approximately 2.25 Mb from the telomere and immediately adjacent to the *PKD1* gene. The 5.5 kb transcript spans an estimated 43 kb of the genomic sequence and comprises 42 known exons, of which 41 are coding, and encodes an 1807 aminoacid protein called tuberin. The *TSC1* gene consists of 23 exons of which the last 21 contain coding sequence. The *TSC1* protein, which is called hamartin, consists of 1164 aminoacids.

In a comprehensive neurological and molecular diagnostic evaluation, Dabora et al. (2001) reported that children with *TSC2* mutations tend to have more severe neurological manifestations than children with *TSC1* mutations, with a much higher rate of infantile spasms and learning disability, suggesting that the neurological outcome may be related to the TSC mutation itself.

REFERENCES

Asano E, Chugani DC, Muziko O, et al. (2000) Multimodality imaging for improved detection of epileptogenic foci in tuberous sclerosis complex. *Neurology* 54: 1976–84.

Balzer F, Ménétrier P (1885) Etude sur un cas d'adénomes sébacés de la face et du cuir chevelu. *Arch Physiol Norm Pathol* (série III) 6: 564–76.

Berg H (1913) Vererbung der Tuberòser Sklerose durch zweigzu drei Generationem. *Ges Neurol Psychiatr* 19: 528–39.

Bolton PF, Griffiths PD (1997) Association of tuberous sclerosis of temporal lobes with autism and atypical autism. *Lancet* 349: 392–5.

Bourneville DM (1880) Sclérose tubéreuse des circonvolutions cérébrales: idiotie et épilepsie hémiplégique. *Arch Neurol (Paris)* 1: 81–91.

Bourneville DM, Brissaud E (1881) Encéphalite ou sclérose tubéreuse des circonvolution cérébrales. *Arch Neurol (Paris)* 1: 390–410.

Campbell AW (1905) Cerebral sclerosis. *Brain* 28: 382–96.

Chiron C, Dulac O, Luna D (1990) Vigabatrin in infantile spasms. *Lancet* 335: 363–4.

Critchley M, Earl CJC (1932) Tuberose sclerosis and allied conditions. *Brain* 55: 311–46.

Curatolo P, Cusmai R (1987) Autism and infantile spasms in children with tuberous sclerosis. *Dev Med Child Neurol* 29: 550–1.

Curatolo P, Cusmai R (1988) MRI in Bourneville disease: relationship with EEG findings. *Neurophysiol Clin* 18: 149–57.

Dabora SL, Jóźwiak S, Franz DN, Roberts PS, Nieto AA, Chung J, Choy YS, Reeve MP, Thiele E, Egelhoff JC, Kasprzyk-Obara J, Domanska-Pakiela D, Kwiatkowski DJ (2001) Mutational analysis in a cohort of 224 tuberous sclerosis patients indicates increased severity of TSC2 compared with TSC1 disease in multiple organs. *Am J Hum Genet* 68(1): 64–80.

Dickerson WW (1951) Familial occurrence of tuberous sclerosis. *Arch Neurol Psychiatr* 65: 683–702.

Dulac O, Lemaitre A, Plouin P (1984) The Bourneville syndrome: clinical and EEG features of epilepsy in the first year of life. *Boll Lega Ital Epil* 45/46: 39–42.

The European Chromosome 16 Tuberous Sclerosis Consortium (1993) Identification and characterization of the tuberous sclerosis gene on chromosome 16. *Cell* 75: 1305–15.

Fryer AE, Chalmers AH, Connor JM, et al. (1987) Evidence that the gene for tuberous sclerosis is on chromosome 9. *Lancet* 1: 659–61.

Gastaut H, Roger J, Soulayrol R, Salomon G, Regis H, Lob H (1965) Encephalopathie myoclonique infantile avec hypsarythmie et sclerose tubereuse de Bourneville. *J Neurol Sci* 2: 140–60.

Gomez MR (1979) History. In: Gomez MR (ed) *Tuberous Sclerosis*. New York: Raven Press, pp 1–10.

Gomez MR (1999) History of tuberous sclerosis complex. In: Gomez MR (ed) *Tuberous Sclerosis, 3rd edn*. New York: Raven Press, pp 3–9.

Goodman M, Lamm SH, Engel A, Shepherd CW, Hourser OW, Gomez MR (1997) Cortical tuber count: a biomarker indicating neurologic severity of tuberous sclerosis complex. *J Child Neurol* 12: 85–90.

Gunther M, Penrose LS (1935) The genetics of epiloia. *J Genet* 31: 413–30.

Hallopeau H, Leredde M (1885) Sur un cas d'adenomes sébacés à forme sclereuse. *Ann Dermatol Syph* 6: 473–9.

Hartdegen A (1881) Eine Fall von multipler Verhartung des Grosshirns nebst histologisch eigenartigen harten Geschwusten der Seitenventriklel (Glioma gangliocellulare) bei eine Neugeboren. *Arch Psychiatr Nervenkr* 11: 117–31.

Jones AC, Shyamsundar MM, Thomas HW, Maynard J, Idziaszczyk S, Tomkins S, Sampson JR, Cheadle JP (1999) Comprehensive mutation analysis of TSC1 and TSC2 and phenotypic correlations in 150 families with tuberous sclerosis. *Am J Hum Genet* 64: 1305–15.

Kandt RS, Haines JL, Smith M, et al. (1992) Linkage of an important gene locus for tuberous sclerosis to a chromosome 16 marker for polycystic kidney disease. *Nature Genet* 2: 37–41.

Kanner L (1943) Autistic disturbances of affective contact. *J Ped* 2: 217–50.

Kirpicznik J (1910) Ein Fall von Tuberoser Sklerose und gleichzeitigen multiplen Nierengeschwülsten. *Virchow Arch Pathol Anat* 202(3): 358.

Lagos JC, Gomez MR (1967) Tuberous sclerosis: reappraisal of a clinical entity. *Mayo Clinic Proc* 42: 26–49.

Lutenbacher R (1918) Dysembryomes métatypique des reins. Carcinose submiliaire aigue du poumon avec emphysème généralisé et double pneumothorax. *Ann Med* 5: 435–50.

McMurdo SK, Moore SG, Brant-Zawadzki M, et al. (1987) MR imaging of intracranial tuberous sclerosis. *AJR Am J Roentgenol* 148: 791–6.

Maeda M, Tartaro A, Matsuda T, Ishii Y (1995) Cortical and subcortical tubers in tuberous sclerosis and FLAIR sequence. *J Comput Assist Tomogr* 19: 660–7.

Marcus H (1924) *Svenska Làk Sallsk Forth*, cited by Dickerson WW (1945) Characteristic roentgenographic changes associated with tuberous sclerosis. *Arch Neurol Psychiatry* 53: 199–204.

Moolten SE (1942) Hamartial nature of the tuberous sclerosis complex and its bearing on the tumour problem: report of one case with tumour anomaly of the kidney and adenoma sebaceum. *Arch Intern Med* 69: 589–623.

Nevin NC, Pearce WG (1968) Diagnostic and genetical aspects of tuberous sclerosis. *J Med Genet* 5: 273–80.

Nixon JR, Miller M, Okazari H, Gomez MR (1989) Cerebral tuberous sclerosis: postmortem magnetic resonance imaging and pathologic anatomy. *Mayo Clin Proc* 64: 305–11.

Pampiglione G, Pugh E (1975) Infantile spasms and subsequent appearance of tuberous sclerosis syndrome. *Lancet* 2: 1046.

Pellizzi GB (1901) Contributo allo studio dell'idiozia. *Riv Sperim Freniat* 27: 265–9.

Perusini G (1905) Uber einen Fall von Sclerosis tuberosa hypertrophica. *Monatsschr Psychiatr Neurol* 17: 69–255.

Pringle JJ (1890) A case of congenital adenoma sebaceum. *Br J Dermatol* 2: 1–14.

Rayer PFO (1835) *Traité theorique e pratique des maladies de la peau, 2nd edn.* Paris: JB Baillière.

Rintahaka PJ, Chugani HT (1997) Clinical role of positron emission tomography in children with tuberous sclerosis complex. *J Child Neurol* 12: 42–52.

Roach E, Williams DP, Laster DW (1987) Magnetic resonance imaging in tuberous sclerosis. *Arc Neurol* 44: 301–3.

Schuster P (1914) Beitrage zur Klinik der tuberosen Sklerose des Gehirns. *Dtsch Z Nervenheilkd* 50: 96–133.

Seri S., Cerquiglini A, Pisani F, Christoph MM, Pascual Marqui R., Curatolo P (1998) Frontal lobe epilepsy associated with tuberous sclerosis: electroencephalographic-magnetic resonance image fusioning. *J Child Neurol* 13: 33–8.

van der Hoeve J (1920) Eye symptoms in tuberous sclerosis of the brain. *Trans Ophthalmol Soc UK* 20: 329–34.

van Slegtenhorst M, de Hoogt R, Hermans C, et al. (1997) Identification of the tuberous sclerosis gene TSC1 on chromosome 9q34. *Science* 277: 805–8.

Vogt H (1908) Zur Pathologie und pathologischen Anatomie der verschiedenen Idiotieform. *Monatsschr Psychiatr Neurol* 24: 106–50.

von Recklinghausen F (1862) Ein Herz von einem Neugeborene welches mehrere theils nach aussen, theils nach den Hòhlen prominirende Tumoren (Myomen) trug. *Monatschr Geburtsheilkd* 20: 1–2.

2
DIAGNOSTIC CRITERIA

Paolo Curatolo

INTRODUCTION

Tuberous sclerosis complex is commonly defined as an autosomal-dominantly inherited multisystem disorder characterized by widespread hamartomas in a great number of organs in the human body, including the brain, heart, skin, eyes, kidney and liver.

Approximately 96% of the patients who suffer from TSC have one or more kinds of skin lesions, an estimated 90% have symptoms or signs of cerebral pathology, and 84% have seizures. Furthermore, over 60% have renal pathology, and nearly 50% suffer from retinal hamartomas (Gomez 1999). The phenotype of patients affected by TSC varies according to the number and size of the lesions, the organ or organs involved, and sometimes the exact location of the lesions. Similarly, the age of the patient is another important factor to be considered, as there are lesions that do not appear until a certain age (i.e. angiomyolipomas), while other hamartomas that appear during fetal life may disappear in infancy (i.e. rhabdomyomas). The random distribution, number, size and location of the lesions in the affected organs result in a great variety of clinical signs.

Hamartomas histologically identical to those found in TSC patients can also be detected in individuals who apparently are not affected by TSC, because they lack other diagnostic features of TSC. These isolated lesions are possibly the result of random somatic mutations.

The careful research for signs of TSC in a proband and in his/her family members is crucial when attempting to establish the diagnosis. The degree of expression in TSC can be extremely variable. This variable expression, with some gene carriers having only minimal signs or symptoms of the disease, can make genetic counselling and epidemiological studies very difficult. This is so since, in spite of recent advances at the molecular level, there is still no biochemical marker for the gene defect available on a clinical basis.

CRITERIA FOR DIAGNOSIS

It was in 1908 that Vogt pointed out the classic essential diagnostic triad of TSC: seizures, learning disability and adenoma sebaceum (angiofibromas). It was not until 1979 that a pediatric neurologist, Gomez, in the light of his past work based on the comprehensive medical records system of the Mayo Clinic in Rochester, Minnesota, succeeded in greatly improving the diagnosing method. Examining the large representative series, he observed that only 29% of all patients presented all three of Vogt's triad characteristics. Furthermore, in 6% of the patients none of the classic features could be diagnosed (Gomez 1979, Gomez 1988). Gomez believed that there were two different criteria for the primary and secondary diagnosis of TSC (Table 2.1). For the primary diagnosis to take place the patient must have one of the following three groups of clinical signs: (a) a characteristic skin lesion, either facial angiofibroma (adenoma sebaceum), or a periungual or subungual fibroma (Koenen's tumour); (b) cortical tubers or subependymal hamartomas demonstrable by pathologic examination; (c) multiple retinal hamartomas. Although we believe at present that radiologically verifiable subependymal lesions, displayed as areas of increased attenuation in the CT, can be accepted as a characteristic sign of TSC, they were not taken as sufficient evidence for the diagnosis of TSC when this study was first undertaken.

It sometimes happened that one of the previously mentioned characteristics was not present, making a primary diagnosis of TSC impossible. When this happened, two of the following clinical features were accepted for a secondary diagnosis: (a) infantile spasms; (b) hypomelanotic macules or depigmented ash-leaf-shaped lesions of the skin; (c) shagreen patch; (d) a single retinal hamartoma; (e) intraventricular tubers or subependymal nodular calcifications in brain CT; (f) bilateral, renal angiomyolipomas found by pathological examination or by excretory urography (intravenous pyelogram) or CT; (g) pathologically confirmed cardiac rhabdomyomas; (h) an immediate relative (parents, sibling or child) in whom the primary diagnosis of TSC has been made by the previously defined criteria.

The 1992 tuberous sclerosis complex diagnostic criteria classified the clinical features according to the likely specificity of each TSC feature. Signs regarded as highly specific were considered more seriously than signs believed to be less specific (Roach et al. 1992). Therefore, the clinical features of TSC were classified according

TABLE 2.1
Criteria for primary and secondary diagnosis of TSC according to Gomez (1979)

Primary diagnosis	Secondary diagnosis
Cortical tubers	Infantile spasms
Subependymal hamartomas	Hypomelanotic macules
Retinal hamartomas	Shagreen patch
Angiofibroma (adenoma sebaceum)	Single retinal hamartoma
Ungual fibroma (Koenen's tumour)	Subependymal or cortical calcifications (CT)
	Multiple renal tumours
	Cardiac rhabdomyoma
	Immediate relative with tuberous sclerosis

to their diagnostic importance as primary (pathognomonic), secondary or tertiary (Roach et al. 1992). By following such a scheme, the diagnosis of TSC could be definite when one primary criterion, or two secondary ones, or one secondary and two tertiary ones, were present. However, these criteria have been regarded as too complicated, and difficult to apply in clinical practice.

Subsequently, a group of clinicians and geneticists at the Tuberous Sclerosis Complex Consensus Conference held in 1998 reassessed the clinical diagnostic criteria, bearing in mind all the new knowledge about TSC gained since the original criteria were established. The specificity of some clinical signs once regarded as pathognomonic for TSC was questioned. There is now more information about the incidence of hypomelanotic macules in normal individuals, and there is evidence that renal angiomyolipomas and lymphangiomyomatosis can occur simultaneously in people in whom TSC is apparently absent (Smolarek et al. 1998, Roach et al. 1998). In addition, focal cortical dysplasia and ungual fibromas have been noticed to occur in individuals without other evidence of TSC.

The new criteria were divided into two groups, major and minor, and are listed in Table 2.2. The final diagnosis of TSC is established when two major features or one major plus two minor features can be demonstrated.

Despite such a copious list of diagnostic criteria, the diagnosis of TSC in infants and children may still prove challenging. This is due to the fact that most of the findings traditionally regarded as among the most specific for tuberous sclerosis become apparent only in late childhood or adulthood, limiting their usefulness for early diagnosis. Jóźwiak et al. (2000) investigated the frequency of clinical findings

TABLE 2.2
Revised clinical diagnostic criteria for tuberous sclerosis complex (modified from Roach et al. 1998)

Major features	Minor features
Facial angiofibromas or forehead plaques	Multiple, randomly distributed pits in dental enamel
Non-traumatic ungula or periungual fibroma	Hamartomatous rectal polyps
Hypomelanotic macules (three or more)	Bone cysts
Shagreen patch (connective tissue nevus)	Cerebral white matter radial migration lines
Multiple retinal nodular hamartomas	Gingival fibromas
Cortical tuber	Non-renal hamartoma
Subependymal nodule	Retinal achromic patch
Subependymal giant cell astrocytoma	"Confetti" skin lesions
Cardiac rhabdomyoma, single or multiple angiomyolipoma	Multiple renal cysts

in a series of 106 children stratified into five age groups (0 to 2 years of age, 2 to 5 years, 5 to 9 years, 9 to 14 years, and 14 to 18 years).

Hypomelanotic macules were the most frequent feature of TSC in the youngest children (Table 2.3). They were observed in 89.6%, and preceded the appearance of other signs and symptoms such as seizures or facial angiofibromas. Three other features of TSC (cardiac rhabdomyoma, infantile spasms and subependymal nodules) were observed with similar frequency. In children aged 2 to 5 years, subependymal nodules were the most frequent feature, being present in 97.3% of patients. A history of seizures was seen in 91.5% of these children. It should be stressed that the diagnosis of TSC is not easy in newborns and infants where the majority of visceral and skin lesions are still undetectable. The onset of infantile spasms or partial seizures in infants with hypomelanotic macules strongly suggests the diagnosis of TSC.

RECOMMENDATIONS FOR DIAGNOSTIC EVALUATION

As previously mentioned, TSC can affect any part of the body, and the clinical manifestations are highly variable, even among affected members of the same family. Some features of TSC can be present at birth, while other symptoms tend to appear later in life. Although many of these problems are easily detected by today's diagnostic techniques, a rational use of these studies is prevented by the lack of a standardized approach. To deal with this issue, a subcommittee at the Tuberous Sclerosis Consensus Conference held in June 1998 in Annapolis, Maryland developed recommendations regarding diagnostic studies in three different categories: (1) patients with a new diagnosis; (2) established patients in order to detect late complications; (3) potentially affected family members of children who suffer from tuberous sclerosis complex.

1. EVALUATION OF NEWLY DIAGNOSED PATIENTS

At the time of initial diagnosis, diagnostic studies are commonly performed either to confirm the presence of tuberous sclerosis complex, or to evaluate presenting symptoms such as seizures or cardiac dysfunction. In addition, it is often useful to establish a baseline assessment in areas that could develop complications later. Unless specific areas of concern are identified with these initial studies, further investigations should focus on areas with a high risk of dysfunction and on lesions that can possibly be treated.

Moreover, at the time of initial presentation, the majority of patients with TSC undergo magnetic resonance imaging (MRI) to search for additional evidence of TSC, already suspected on the basis of other signs (Roach et al. 1998). The number, size and perhaps the location of the dysplastic cortical lesions detected by MRI tend to correlate with the severity of the clinical neurological dysfunction (Curatolo et al. 1991, Shepherd et al. 1995, Goodman et al. 1997).

TABLE 2.3
Frequency of clinical signs in children with definite tuberous sclerosis in different age groups (modified from Józwiak et al. 2000)

Below 2 years		From 2 to 5 years		From 5 to 9 years		From 9 to 14 years		From 14 to 18 years	
Criteria	%	Criteria	%	Criteria	%	Criteria	%	Criteria	%
Hypomelanotic macules	89.6	Subependymal nodules	97.3	Hypomelanotic macules	97.2	Subependymal nodules	100.0	Subependymal nodules	100.0
Cardiac rhabdomyoma	83.3	Hypomelanotic macules	95.3	Subependymal nodules	96.6	Hypomelanotic macules	97.2	Cortical/subcortical tubers	100.0*
Epilepsy, usually IS	83.0	Epilepsy	91.5	Epilepsy	94.3	Epilepsy	96.2	Hypomelanotic macules	97.2
Subependymal nodules	82.9	Facial angiofibromas	63.2	Facial angiofibromas	73.6	Facial angiofibromas	77.4	Epilepsy	96.2
Renal AMLs	16.7	Renal AMLs	41.7	Renal AMLs	63.9	Renal AMLs	64.7	Renal AMLs	92.3
Facial angiofibromas	10.4	Cardiac rhabdomyoma	21.4	Shagreen patch	34.9	Shagreen patch	47.2	Facial angiofibromas	77.4
Retinal hamartoma	8.2	Shagreen patch	20.8	Cardiac rhabdomyoma	21.1	Cardiac rhabdomyoma	41.2	Cardiac rhabdomyoma	75.0*
		Retinal hamartoma	17.1	Retinal hamartoma	20.6	Liver AMLs	23.5	Shagreen patch	48.1
		Forehead plaque	9.3	Forehead plaque	16.0	Forehead plaque	18.9	Liver AMLs	46.2
				Liver AMLs	11.1	Retinal hamartoma	17.2	Retinal hamartoma	31.3
						Periungual fibromas	11.3	Forehead plaque	18.9
								Periungual fibromas	15.1

*Small group examined

Electroencephalography (EEG) is useful when the initial presentation includes epileptic seizures (Seri et al. 1991). Nevertheless, children who have never manifested seizures and are not suspected of having epileptic seizures generally do not need to undergo baseline EEGs.

Usually adolescents and adults have a greater chance of developing symptomatic renal angiomyolipomas than children, but it sometimes happens in childhood (Jóźwiak et al. 1998). For each patient, renal ultrasonography is carried out at the time of diagnosis. Furthermore, cardiac arrhythmias occasionally occur even in patients with TSC who do not have a demonstrable cardiac rhabdomyoma. An arrhythmia can be present at birth or develop later. Wolff–Parkinson–White syndrome appears to be the most commonly noted arrhythmia in patients with TSC. Therefore, a baseline study must be performed at the time of diagnosis. Echocardiography may reveal one or more cardiac rhabdomyomas in more than half of the younger individuals with TSC (Gibbs 1985, Jóźwiak et al. 1994). However, these cardiac tumours are more innocuous than they might seem, as they tend to involute over the years, often disappearing completely by adulthood. Moreover, the most rapid reduction in lesion size occurs during the first three years of life, after which rhabdomyomas tend to change less dramatically (Di Mario et al. 1996).

Each patient affected by TSC should have an accurate ophthalmic examination at the time of diagnosis. Multiple retinal hamartomas are an unquestionable sign of TSC (see also Chapter 10).

Children usually do not suffer from facial angiofibromas or ungual fibromas at the time of initial diagnosis, and typical hypomelanotic macules can be recognized early on by most clinicians who are knowledgeable about TSC. A dermatological examination is important when the skin lesions are atypical or when the diagnosis of TSC is uncertain.

The panel of experts recommends a scrupulous age-appropriate screening for behavioural, cognitive and neurodevelopmental dysfunction at the time of diagnosis. Unfortunately, children with apparently normal initial testing and developmental milestones can still suffer milder deficits that interfere with their learning. It is advisable that each child is reassessed around the time school begins, even if no abnormalities were detected by the previous screenings.

Children with abnormal behaviour or cognitive function should be periodically retested, and re-evaluation is also appropriate when there is a significant change in behavioural or cognitive function. Newly diagnosed adolescents or young adults with a well-established pattern of completely normal social and cognitive function, as determined by educational achievement, sometimes do not require formal testing.

Gene characterization could ultimately identify patients at a greater or lesser risk of particular complications. Moreover, further diagnostic studies could be performed selectively on individuals at greatest risk for certain specific complications, thereby decreasing the number of useless investigations. It is possible that, in the near future, gene typing at the time of initial diagnosis will reveal its usefulness, once molecular testing becomes readily available and there are sufficient data to determine which clinical phenotypes correlate with which gene defects.

2. Ongoing Evaluation of Established Patients

According to Roach et al. (1998), long-term surveillance testing should be directed toward lesions which are frequent, lesions which can be treated if identified early, and lesions which have a significant risk of dysfunction or death. A surveillance protocol based on the natural history of TSC provides some practical basis for driving follow-up tests. Every effort should be made to minimize costly testing of asymptomatic patients and to maximize the likelihood of early identification of a treatable lesion. The guidelines that follow are designed for long-term clinical management of an asymptomatic patient whose diagnosis is perfectly assured.

Central nervous system

Subependymal giant cell astrocytomas occur in 6 to 14% of patients affected by TSC. Although these tumours are histologically benign, they are locally invasive, and they can cause hydrocephalus because of their typical occurrence in the anterior lateral ventricle. Enlarging giant cell tumours can be removed through early identification, before symptoms develop and before they become locally invasive.

The panel recommended that children undergo periodic cranial imaging with either CT or MRI every one to three years, depending on the level of clinical suspicion in each child. In general, there is a greater likelihood for children to develop subependymal giant cell astrocytomas than for adults. Usually the need for EEG is dictated by the clinical features and response of seizures to antiepileptic drugs. As a rule, EEG is not required for adults with TSC who do not have epileptic seizures. However, since seizures are not always clinically obvious, EEG should always be considered in the evaluation of a patient with an unexplained decline of cognitive or behavioural function in whom epileptic seizures are suspected. During early infancy, the seizure pattern can change rapidly, and sometimes it might be necessary to repeat the studies at frequent intervals.

A number of neurodevelopmental and behavioural dysfunction patterns occur as a result of TSC. In contrast to learning disability, which is a classic and common feature of TSC, autism, attentional deficits and other difficulties are probably under-recognized (Hunt and Dennis 1987, Curatolo et al. 1991). The children who suffer such problems can benefit from early recognition and specific education and treatment plans. Formal cognitive testing is not necessary for adolescents and adults with well-established patterns of normal social and cognitive function. When a patient is diagnosed with TSC in infancy or early childhood, testing should be repeated around the time the child enters school. Older children should be reassessed periodically in response to educational or behavioural concerns.

18 TUBEROUS SCLEROSIS COMPLEX

Kidney

By the age of 10 years, almost 75% of children with TSC have sonographic evidence of one or more renal angiomyolipomas (Ewalt et al. 1998, Weiner et al. 1998). During the first decade of life, the number and size of the renal angomyolipomas tend to increase, but large renal angiomyolipomas are more likely to cause symptoms than smaller lesions (Steiner et al. 1993). It is therefore wise to monitor more closely patients with large tumours. According to the panel, renal ultrasonography should be undertaken every one to three years. How frequently the patient is tested depends mostly on the degree of concern and on the results of previous examinations. Regardless of age, patients who have large renal lesions or lesions that seem to have grown substantially should have more frequent follow-up examinations. MRI might be necessary for these patients to define with greater precision the extent of the kidney disease.

Heart

Although about two-thirds of infants with TSC have echocardiographic evidence of one or more cardiac rhabdomyomas, these tumours tend to regress over time and can disappear altogether by adulthood (Alkalay et al. 1987, Smythe et al. 1990, Webb et al. 1993). The majority of patients with TSC who have a cardiac rhabdomyoma remain asymptomatic (Jóźwiak et al. 1994). Continuous cardiac evaluations are unnecessary for most asymptomatic TSC patients. However, some patients may occasionally develop arrhythmias during adolescence or adulthood. Those patients who have new symptoms that might indicate cardiac dysfunction, and those with previous symptoms, will benefit from periodic studies to evaluate heart function.

Lungs

Pulmonary disease (lymphangiomyomatosis) due to TSC is uncommon, especially in children and in men. In the rare cases in which it occurs, it is suffered almost exclusively by women (Smolarek et al. 1998). The average age of onset is 32 to 34 years. The best method to use to understand pulmonary abnormalities of TSC is the chest CT. The panel recommended no routine testing in either asymptomatic children or adolescents. Women should undergo chest CT at least once on reaching adulthood. If pulmonary symptoms develop, this test should be repeated.

Retina

Around 75% of patients with TSC have retinal lesions (Kiribuchi et al. 1986). In a severely impaired child, ophthalmic examinations are sometimes difficult to perform without sedation, and are unlikely to identify impending visual loss from a treatable lesion. Repeated ophthalmologic evaluations are usually unnecessary, unless there is some specific reason for concern. Retinal hamartomas are rare in children below

3 years of age. When present they tend to grow slowly over an extended period of time (see also Chapter 10).

Skin
Facial angiofibromas are benign skin tumours that can have major consequences for some patients. Laser therapy is one way in which skin tumour growth can be limited, even though the treatments often need to be repeated periodically as the lesions tend to re-grow gradually after the treatment is over. Ungual fibromas sometimes cause severe problems, which can be effectively treated.

3. EVALUATION OF FAMILY MEMBERS
Since a number of affected individuals show only subtle clinical features of TSC, diagnosis of family members may be difficult. Such a problem is crucial for accurate genetic counselling in this autosomal dominant disorder. Most affected individuals who are subject to a thorough physical examination, including a skin examination with ultraviolet light and a retinal examination through dilated pupils, have at least subtle physical findings of TSC. Furthermore, a completely normal physical examination and extensive radiographic testing, including high-definition MRI, still cannot definitely exclude TSC, since there is always a chance of germline mosaicism.

In 1991, Roach et al. evaluated the ability of cranial MRI to identify minimally affected parents with TSC. Physical examinations and cranial MRI were undergone by 60 couples (120 parents). Eight parents had TSC diagnosed by physical examination, family history or various diagnostic procedures including MRI. However, MRI confirmed the diagnosis of TSC in only one parent, who had no definitive physical findings of the disorder (Roach et al. 1991). Thus, MRI may be helpful only occasionally in parents with few physical findings and other normal diagnostic studies. The usefulness of MRI often lies in its ability to help confirm a diagnosis that is already suspected.

No systematic studies have addressed the advantage of renal ultrasonography in identifying minimally affected individuals with TSC. Nonetheless, ultrasonography clearly demonstrates renal angiomyolipomas, and is broadly available and certainly cheaper than other studies. These are the reasons why renal ultrasonography is recommended where diagnostic studies are done on potentially affected family members.

In the future, molecular diagnosis will be used increasingly to differentiate TSC patients from clinically normal family members. Although molecular testing for TSC is not yet commercially available, it should soon be possible to identify certain individuals with TSC who do not satisfy the clinical diagnostic criteria (Roach et al. 1998). Occasionally, couples have more than one child with TSC, in spite of the fact that neither parent has either physical or radiological evidence of the disease. In these families TSC may result from germline mosaicism. Unfortunately, neither routine diagnostic studies nor DNA-based testing are likely to detect germline mosaicism in these individuals, because the parent who carries the mutation will not have a detectable mutation in DNA extracted from leukocytes (Yates et al. 1997, Rose et al. 1999). Therefore, genetic counselling for families with one affected child should include a small (1 to 2%) possibility of recurrence, even in parents who have no evidence of TSC after a thorough diagnostic evaluation (Roach et al. 1998).

Testing recommendations at the time of diagnosis and recommended frequency of follow-up investigation are summarized in Tables 2.4 and 2.5.

IMPACT OF THE DIAGNOSIS ON THE FAMILY

TSC diagnosis can have an extremely severe impact on the patient's family. Parents commonly feel anger, guilt and frustration, and the siblings' lives may be totally disrupted during the arduous process of looking after the child with severe disabilities. It is therefore vital that the physicians who interact with the patient's relatives

TABLE 2.4
Summary of testing recommendations (modified from Roach et al. 1999)

Assessment	Initial testing
Neurodevelopmental testing	At diagnosis and at school entry
Ophthalmic examination	At diagnosis
Electroencephalography	At diagnosis
Electrocardiography	At diagnosis
Echocardiography	If cardiac symptoms occur
Renal ultrasonography	At diagnosis
Chest computed tomography	At adulthood (women only)
Cranial magnetic resonance imaging	At diagnosis

TABLE 2.5
Recommended frequency of follow-up investigations

Assessment	Repeat testing
Neurodevelopmental testing	As clinically indicated
Ophthalmic examination	As clinically indicated
Electroencephalography	As indicated for seizure management
Electrocardiography	As clinically indicated
Echocardiography	If cardiac dysfunction occurs
Renal ultrasonography	Every 1 to 3 years
Chest computed tomography	If pulmonary dysfunction occurs
Cranial magnetic resonance imaging	Children/adolescent: every 1 to 3 years

provide accurate information at the time of diagnosis, giving a clearly understandable explanation regarding the fundamental genetic aspects of TSC.

The wide clinical spectrum of the disease, the various organs that may be affected, and the tests that will be done both at the time of diagnosis and at screening and follow-up should be explained. Due to the extreme variability of the disease, it is difficult for child neurologists to provide parents with a prediction of the long-term outcomes concerning epilepsy and learning disability. Parents may greatly benefit from contact with TSC organizations and support groups. In particular, the experience of other families with children affected by TSC can be of great help.

GENETIC COUNSELLING

Genetic counselling should be provided for all patients affected by TSC and their relatives at risk. Here the role of the physician should be to advise and provide support for family planning and other personal decisions. Any person with TSC has a 50% chance of transmitting this gene to his/her children. In the case of a new mutation, the chance of having another affected child is very small, perhaps less than 2%. Estimations regarding the proportion of patients affected by new mutations display high variations in reported series, ranging from 50 to 75% (Fleury et al. 1980, Sampson et al. 1989).

EPIDEMIOLOGY

Early studies of the prevalence and incidence of TSC tended to focus on hospital populations instead of looking at the general population. These hospital-based studies lacked accuracy because TSC was believed to occur, and was therefore looked for, only in patients who suffered learning disability, had seizures and had facial angiofibroma. Contemporary studies aimed at ascertaining the prevalence of TSC in defined populations have been more accurate because investigators now appreciate the different phenotypes of TSC. These studies have searched for patients suffering from lung, skin and renal diseases suggestive of TSC, even if there is no evidence of learning disability or seizures. It is clear that, for an accurate population study, a knowledge of all the different phenotypes of TSC is essential.

POPULATION-BASED STUDIES

Population-based studies are considered today the most accurate method of determining the true prevalence of TSC. In Table 2.6 the different population studies that have been undertaken are shown. The basis of each survey was the reported clinical cases and, in some studies, the detection of TSC in asymptomatic relatives of the proband.

Previous studies conducted between 1950 and 1970 by Stevenson and Fischer, Nevin and Pearce, and Singer reported very low figures. These studies were done before the introduction of computed tomography in 1974, which made the detection of subependymal nodules possible. As with previous hospital-based studies, these surveys did not take all the different phenotypes into consideration.

In 1984, Hunt and Lindenbaum updated the Oxford study of Nevin and Pearce. With the help of computed tomography and ultrasound scanning used for diagnosis, they were able to detect 68 cases in a population of 2,328,100. In this study total prevalence was estimated at 1:34,200; for people under 45 years of age it was 1:24,600, while for people under 15 it was 1:17,300, and for people under 5 it was 1:15,400. The scientists believed that the birth prevalence might be even higher than it is now considered to be. In the west of Scotland a further population study was undertaken. In this study 101 cases were identified, giving a total prevalence of 1:27,000, and a prevalence of 1:10,000 for children under 10 years of age. Similar results were obtained by Webb et al., who found 131 cases of TSC among 3.4 million people in the south of England. The prevalence in the population was 1:26,500.

Two studies were done as part of the Olmsted County Epidemiological Project, a project in which medical records of nearly all the population of Rochester, Minnesota permitted the identification of all TSC cases.

When investigating the prevalence of genetic disease by means of a population study, there is a chance that large family clusters might provide a higher figure for the prevalence of the condition. The probability of this happening increases if the population is small. This is not the case in the Olmsted County study, since the total

TABLE 2.6
Prevalence of TSC according to population studies (modified from Shepherd 1999)

Authors	Year	Population sampled	Prevalence
Stevenson and Fischer	1956	Population of Northern Ireland	1:150,000*
Nevin and Pearce	1968	Population of Oxford Regional Health Authority	1:100,000*
Singer	1971	Chinese population of Hong Kong	1:70,000*
Hunt and Lindenbaum	1984	Population of Oxford Regional Health Authority	1:34,200
Wiederholt et al.	1985	Population of Rochester, Minnesota	1:9704
Sampson et al.	1989	Population of the west of Scotland	1:27,000
Shepherd et al.	1991	Population of Olmsted County, Minnesota (includes Rochester)	1:14,492
Webb et al.	1996	Population of part of the south of England	1:26,500
O'Callaghan et al.	1998	Population of Wessex, UK	1:12,500

* Studies in 1956, 1968 and 1971 did not use neuroimaging. Hence the estimated prevalence is much lower.

population studied included 100,000 people. Therefore it is believed that this study is the most accurate, due to the comprehensive medical record system used.

The rate of occurrence of tuberous sclerosis at birth is unknown. Recent epidemiological studies report a prevalence of 1:12,000 to 1:15,000 in children aged under 10 years. When viewing this statistic, one has to take into consideration the fact that mildly affected cases are rarely diagnosed in childhood, so there is a selection bias towards those with learning disability. Therefore, the real frequency of learning disability may be lower than previously thought. A recent study in an unbiased population of patients with tuberous sclerosis showed a prevalence of 38% (95% confidence interval 19 to 56%). This indicates that the real incidence at birth may be as high as 1:6000 (Webb et al. 1993).

In the past few years, improved testing methods have led to the identification of individuals with less severe manifestations of TSC, therefore increasing dramatically the estimates of the disorder's frequency. According to the National Tuberous Sclerosis Association, approximately 50,000 Americans and 1 million individuals worldwide are affected by TSC.

The correct way to calculate the disorder's rate of occurrence in autosomal dominant diseases is to carry out a thorough survey, maximizing contacts with clinicians, family doctors, patients' support groups, and other health professionals.

O'Callaghan et al. (1998) estimate the prevalence of TSC in Wessex, UK by capture-recapture analysis; 131 cases of tuberous sclerosis were originally identified by the Wessex survey, in a population of 3–4 million. The results of the capture-recapture analysis illustrate that, in spite of the efforts of the investigators to locate all cases, more than half remained undetected. A further estimate of prevalence, which took unascertained cases into consideration, is 8 per 100,000 population (95% confidence interval 6.8–12.4%).

Therefore, traditional methods of ascertaining the disorder's frequency, however rigorously applied, fail to identify all cases, and many people with TSC do not receive either genetic counselling or specialist medical supervision.

REFERENCES

Alkalay AL, Ferry DA, Lin B, et al. (1987) Spontaneous regression of cardiac rhabdomyoma in tuberous sclerosis. *Clin Pediatr (Phila)* 26: 532–5.

Curatolo P, Cusmai R, Cortesi F, et al. (1991) Neuropsychiatric aspects of tuberous sclerosis. *Ann NY Acad Sci* 615: 8–16.

Di Mario FJ, Diana D, Leopold H, Chameides L (1996) Evolution of cardiac rhabdomyoma in tuberous sclerosis complex. *Clin Pediatr (Phila)* 12: 615–19.

Ewalt DE, Sheffield E, Sparagana SP, et al. (1998) Renal lesion growth in children with tuberous sclerosis complex. *J Urol* 160: 141–5.

Fleury P, de Groot WP, Delleman JW, Verbeeten B Jr, Frankenmolen-Witkiezwicz IM (1980) Tuberous sclerosis: the incidence of sporadic cases versus familial cases. *Brain Dev* 2(2): 107–17.

Gibbs JL (1985) The heart and tuberous sclerosis. An echocardiographic and electrocardiographic study. *Br Heart J* 54: 596–9.

Gomez MR (1979) *Tuberous Sclerosis*. New York: Raven Press.

Gomez MR (1988) Criteria for diagnosis. In: Gomez MR (ed) *Tuberous Sclerosis, 2nd edn*. New York, Raven Press, pp 9–19.

Gomez MR (1999) Definition and criteria for diagnosis. In: Gomez MR (ed) *Tuberous Sclerosis Complex, 3rd edn*. New York: Raven Press, pp 10–23.

Goodman M, Lamm SH, Engel A, et al. (1997) Cortical tuber count: a biomarker indicating cerebral severity of tuberous sclerosis complex. *J Child Neurol* 12: 85–90.

Hunt A, Dennis J (1987) Psychiatric disorders among children with tuberous sclerosis. *Dev Med Child Neurol* 29: 190–8.

Hunt A, Lindenbaum RH (1984) Tuberous sclerosis: a new estimate of prevalence within the Oxford region. *J Med Genet* 21: 272–7.

Jóźwiak S, Kawalec W, Dluzewska J, et al. (1994) Cardiac tumors in tuberous sclerosis: their incidence and course. *Eur J Pediatr* 153: 155–7.

Jóźwiak S, Goodman M, Lamm SH (1998) Poor mental development in patients with tuberous sclerosis complex. Clinical risk factors. *Arch Neurol* 55: 379–84.

Jóźwiak S, Schwartz RA, Janniger CK, Bielicka-Cymerman J (2000) Usefulness of diagnostic criteria of tuberous sclerosis complex in pediatric patients. *J Child Neurol* 15: 652–9.

Kiribuchi K, Uchida Y, Fukuyama Y, Maruyama H (1986) High incidence of fundus hamartomas and clinical significance of a fundus score in tuberous sclerosis. *Brain Dev* 8: 509–17.

Nevin NC, Pearce WG (1968) Diagnostic and genetical aspects of tuberous sclerosis. *J Med Genet* 5(4): 273–80.

O'Callaghan JK, Shiell AW, Osborne JP, Martyn CN (1998) Prevalence of tuberous sclerosis in UK. *Lancet* 392; 23: 318–19.

Roach ES, Kerr J, Mendelsohn D, et al. (1991) Detection of tuberous sclerosis in parents by magnetic resonance imaging. *Neurology* 41: 262–5.

Roach ES, Smith M, Huttenlocher P, Bhat M, Alcorn D, Hawlry L (1992) Report of the diagnostic criteria committee of the National Tuberous Sclerosis Association. *J Child Neurol* 7: 221–4.

Roach ES, Gomez MR, Northrup H (1998) Tuberous Sclerosis Complex Consensus Conference: revised clinical diagnostic criteria. *J Child Neurol* 13: 624–8.

Roach ES, DiMario FJ, Kandt RS, Horthrup H (1999) Tuberous Sclerosis Consensus Conference: recommendations for diagnostic evaluation. *J Child Neurol* 14: 401–7.

Rose VM, Au K-S, Pollon G, et al. (1999) Germline mosaicism in tuberous sclerosis: how common? *Am J Hum Genet* 64: 986–92.

Sampson JR, Yates JR, Pirrit LA, Fleury P, Winship I, Beighton P, Connor JM (1989) Evidence for genetic heterogeneity in tuberous sclerosis. *J Med Genet* 26(8): 511–16.

Seri S, Cerquiglini A, Cusmai R, Curatolo P (1991) Tuberous sclerosis: relationships between topographic mapping EEG, VEPs and MRI findings. *Neurophysiol Clin* 21: 161–72.

Shepherd CW (1999) The epidemiology of the tuberous sclerosis complex. In: Gomez MR, Sampson JR, Whittemore VH (eds) *Tuberous Sclerosis Complex*. Oxford: Oxford University Press.

Shepherd CW, Beard CM, Gomez MR, Kurland JT, Whisnaut JP (1991) Tuberous sclerosis complex in Olmsted County, Minnesota, 1950–1989. *Arch Neurol* 48: 400–1.

Shepherd CW, Houser OW, Gomez MR (1995) MR findings in tuberous sclerosis complex and correlation with seizure development and mental impairment. *Am J Neuroradiol* 16: 149–55.

Singer K (1971) Genetic aspects of tuberous sclerosis in a Chinese population. *Am J Hum Genet* 23: 33–40.

Smolarek TA, Wessner LL, McCormack FX, et al. (1998) Evidence that lymphangiomyomatosis is caused by TSC2 mutations: chromosome 16p13 loss of heterozygosity in angiomyolipomas and lymphonodes from women with lymphangiomyomatosis. *Am J Hum Genet* 62: 810–15.

Smythe JF, Dyck JD, Smallhorn JF, Freedom RM (1990) Natural history of cardiac rhabdomyoma in infancy and childhood. *Am J Cardiol* 66: 1247–9.

Steiner MS, Goldman SM, Fishman EK, Marshall FF (1993) The natural history of renal angiomyolipoma. *J Urol* 150: 1783–6.

Stevenson AC, Fischer OD (1956) Frequency of epiloia in Northern Ireland. *Br J Prev Soc Med* 10: 134–5.

Vogt H (1908) Zur Diagnostik der tuberosen Sklerose. *Z Erforsch Behandl Jugeudl Schwachsinns* 2: 1–16.

Webb DW, Thomas RD, Osborne JP (1993) Cardiac rhabdomyomas and their association with tuberous sclerosis. *Arch Dis Child* 68: 367–70.

Webb DW, Fryer AE, Osborne JP (1996) Morbidity associated with tuberous sclerosis: a population study. *Dev Med Child Neurol* 38: 146–55.

Weiner DM, Ewalt DE, Roach ES, Hensle TW (1998) The tuberous sclerosis complex: a comprehensive review. *J Am Coll Surg* 187: 548–61.

Wiederholt WC, Gomez MR, Kurland LT (1985) Incidence and prevalence of tuberous sclerosis in Rochester, Minnesota, 1950 through 1982. *Neurology* 35: 600–3.

Yates JRW, van Bakel I, Sepp T, et al. (1997) Female germline mosaicism in tuberous sclerosis confirmed by molecular genetic analysis. *Hum Mol Genet* 6: 2265–9.

3

NEUROLOGICAL MANIFESTATIONS

Paolo Curatolo and Magda Verdecchia

Neurological aspects of tuberous sclerosis complex (TSC) have long been studied. In his first report in 1880 Bourneville described a girl, with seizures, learning disability and right hemiplegia. Her seizures started in early infancy and at first involved only the eyes, becoming generalized at the age of 2 years. On postmortem examination Bourneville found that many cerebral circumvolutions had areas of greater intensity than the surrounding cortex, with a gross nodular appearance. He concluded that the seizures had a focal origin and later progressed to generalized attacks. He attributed their partial onset to the large sclerotic lesions involving the ascending frontal and parietal circumvolutions of the left cerebral hemisphere (Fig. 3.1).

Abnormalities of neuronal migration, cellular differentiation and excessive cell proliferation contribute to the formation of the various brain lesions and to the production of different neurological manifestations, including seizures, learning disability and autism. It is now becoming apparent that most of the neurobehavioural phenotypes exhibited by children with TSC are also organically determined and may reflect a direct effect of the abnormal genetic program.

Recently, progress in understanding the molecular pathogenesis of TSC, identification of mutations, and new genotype–phenotype correlation studies have brought significant improvement in our knowledge of the neurological phenotypes associated with TSC. TSC, a genetic disease with multiple localized several lesions, seems a good model for the investigation of the relationship between the genotype and the different neurological phenotypes. Due to its cognitive and behavioural changes that correlate with demonstrable lesions, TSC could be a prototype to understand complex human behaviours and to elucidate in a fundamental manner how the brain works. In this chapter we will take a general overview of the neurological manifestations, which will be explained in depth in the following chapters.

CHARACTERIZATION OF THE TSC GENES

TSC results from mutations in *TSC1*, the gene on chromosome 9q34, and *TSC2*, the gene on chromosome 16p13 (European Chromosome 16 Tuberous Sclerosis Consortium 1993, van Slegtenhorst et al. 1997). Frequent loss of heterozygosity for alleles in 16p13.3 and rare loss in 9q34 have been found in hamartomas from TSC patients, indicating that a second somatic mutation may be required to produce the TSC phenotype at the cellular level (Green et al. 1994a, 1994b). These findings are consistent with the *TSC1* and the *TSC2* acting as growth suppressor genes (Carbonara et al. 1994).

The *TSC2* gene maps to a gene-rich region of 16p13.3, approximately 2.25 Mb from the telomere and immediately adjacent to the *PKD1* gene. The 5.5 kb transcript spans an estimated 43 kb of genomic sequence and comprises 42 known exons, of which 41 are coding, and encodes an 1807 aminoacid protein, called tuberin, with little similarity to other known genes. 163 aminoacids near the COOH terminus are homologous to the catalytic domain of a guanosin triphosphatase (GTPase) activating protein GAP3 (rap1GAP). GAPs are regulators of the GTP binding and hydrolysing activity of the Ras superfamily of proteins that help to regulate cell growth, proliferation and differentiation.

The *TSC1* gene consists of 23 exons of which the last 21 contain coding sequence. The *TSC1* protein, which is called hamartin, consists of 1164 aminoacids with a calculated mass of 130 kilodaltons. The protein is generally hydrophilic and has a single potential transmembrane domain at aminoacids 127 to 144, as well as a probable 266-aminoacid coiled-coil region beginning at position 730 (van Slegtenhorst et al. 1997, Vinters et al. 1998).

The mutations observed in *TSC1* consist of small deletions, small insertions and point mutations. The majority of mutations are likely to inactivate protein function, and these findings support the hypothesis that *TSC1* functions as a tumour suppressor gene. At the moment, 424 different mutations in both TSC genes are known. There is an equal distribution of mutations between *TSC1* and *TSC2* among familial cases, while among sporadic cases *TSC2* mutations are much more frequent than *TSC1* mutations. The wide range of tissues in which TSC-associated hamartomas develop implies a fundamental role for both TSC genes in regulating cell proliferation and differentiation.

The characterization of the *TSC1* and *TSC2* genes is summarized in Table 3.1.

The complex relationships between the *TSC1* and *TSC2* gene products are currently under investigation. Several lines of evidence support a direct interaction between hamartin and tuberin, suggesting that these two proteins participate in some common cellular functions.

Sporadic patients with *TSC1* mutations had, on average, milder disease in comparison with patients with *TSC2* mutations. They had a lower frequency of seizures and moderate/severe learning disability, fewer subependymal nodules and cortical tubers, less severe kidney involvement, no retinal hamartomas, and less severe facial angiofibroma (Dabora et al. 2001). Moreover, *TSC2* mutations are associated with a significantly earlier epilepsy presentation than *TSC1* mutations, which results in frequent infantile spasms (Jóźwiak et al. 2001).

TABLE 3.1
Characterization of the *TSC1* and *TSC2* genes

	TSC1	*TSC2*
Localization	9q34	16p13.3
Structure	23 exons – 8.6 kb transcript alternate splicing in the 5\rquote UTR	41 exons – 5.5 kb transcript exons 25, 26 and 31 alternately spliced
Mutations	Small truncating mutations	Large deletions/rearrangements Small truncating mutations Missense mutations
Occurrence	10–15% of sporadic cases	70% of sporadic cases
Phenotype	? less mental impairment	? more likely to be mentally retarded Contiguous gene deletion syndrome with *PKD1*
LOH in hamartomas	Rare	Frequent
Product	Hamartin	Tuberin
Function(s)	? regulates cell adhesion through interaction with ezrin and rho Regulator/modulator of tuberin activity	? GTPase activating protein Role in the cell cycle
Subcellular localization	Cytoplasmic, ? cortical	Cytoplasmic, ? Golgi-associated
Animal models	Knockout mice under development	Eker rat Knockout mice *Drosophila (gigas)*

PATHOLOGICAL FINDINGS

Pathologically, TSC is a disorder of cell migration, proliferation and differentiation (Crino and Henske 1999). Present evidence suggests that the central nervous system lesions of TSC are due to a developmental disorder of neurogenesis and neuronal migration. Two populations of neuroepithelial cells are generated by the germinal matrix in TSC. One is a population of normal neuroblasts which form normal neurons and astroglia, and which migrate to the cortical plate where they form histologically normal cerebral cortex. The second is an abnormal cell population, which forms primitive cells which often fail to show clear neuronal and glial differentiation. Some of these cells, named "neuroastrocytes", remain in the germinal matrix zone where they form subependymal nodules and giant cell tumours. Some neuroastrocytes show partial migration, forming heterotopias in the subcortical

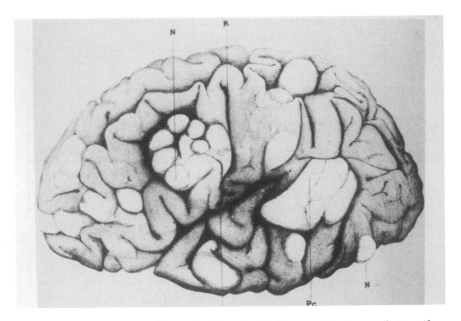

Fig. 3.1. Cerebral tuberous sclerosis showing sclerotic, hypertrophic circumvolutions (from Bourneville and Brissaud 1881).

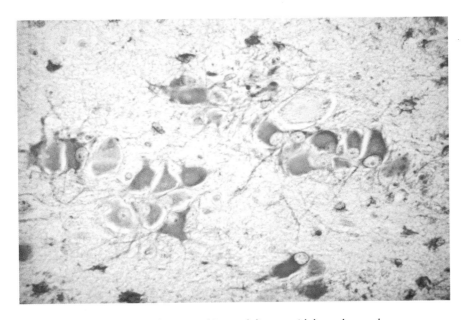

Fig. 3.2. Cortical tuber showing architectural disarray with large abnormal neurons.

white matter. More differentiated cells migrate to the cortical plate where they form aggregates of dysplastic cortex, the cortical tubers. Cells in tubers share with those in subependymal nodules and in giant cell tumours the frequent absence of clear neuronal and glial differentiation, showing features of primitive stellate neurons with few dendritic spines (Hirose et al. 1995, Crino and Henske 1999) (Fig. 3.2).

Tuberin and hamartin are widely expressed in human fetal tissues. This suggests a critical function of these two proteins in early development and maturation of the brain. Tuberin was undetectable from subependymal giant cell astrocytomas examined in three patients, suggesting a possible relationship between the degree of loss of tuberin and the severity of neurological disturbance (Mizuguchi et al. 1996). It remains still unknown how a deficiency of GAP activity for Rap1 or rab5, if that is the critical function of tuberin, leads to hamartoma development. The mechanism by which loss of hamartin expression produces TSC lesions is also unclear. Recently it has been reported that hamartin regulates cell adhesion, interacting with the Ezrin-Radixin-Moesin (ERM) family of actin-binding proteins. This interaction is essential for activation of the small GTP-binding protein Rho. These data suggest that a loss of hamartin causes the disruption of cell-matrix adhesion which in turn may induce initial development of TSC hamartomas. Therefore, in this case, Rho-mediated signalling pathway regulating cell adhesion may constitute a rate-limiting step in tumour formation (Lamb et al. 2000).

It is likely that hamartin and tuberin participate in the same pathway of cellular growth control and share a common biochemical pathway. The proteins appear to co-localize at the cellular level, and recent evidence suggests that there is a direct binding between tuberin and hamartin. These two proteins form a cytosolic complex interacting at the N-terminal ends of both proteins. This interaction is abolished by some TSC-associated mutations (Nellist et al. 1999). A mutation of either protein would therefore be sufficient to inactivate the complex and lead to the pathology seen in patients with TSC. The tuberin aminoacid substitutions N525S, K599M and R905Q do not affect the interaction with hamartin. In contrast, the tuberin missense changes R611Q, R611W, A614D, F615S, C696Y and V769E prevent the interaction with hamartin. These data suggest that the central region of tuberin, containing the aminoacids R611, A614, F615, C696 and V769, is important for maintaining the correct interaction with hamartin and in regulating the post-translational modification status of tuberin (Nellist et al. 2001).

BRAIN IMAGING

MRI studies provide excellent in vivo demonstration of the various pathological lesions, including cortical tubers, subependymal nodules or giant cell astrocytomas, and radial migration lines in cerebral white matter (Fig. 3.3). An especially inter-esting finding is the frequent demonstration of abnormal wedges of tissue extending from the subependymal zone to the cerebral cortex, and including cortical tubers,

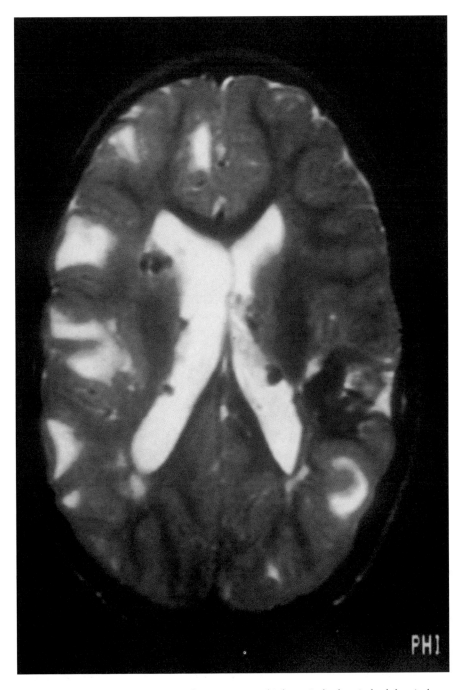

Fig. 3.3. Magnetic resonance imaging demonstrates multiple cortical tubers in both hemispheres and SENs in a 7-year-old girl with intractable seizures and severe learning disability.

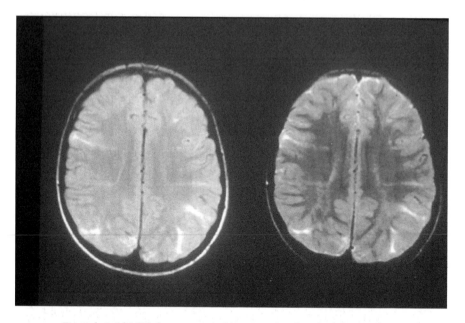

Fig. 3.4. Axial MRI demonstrates white matter bands in both hemispheres.

subependymal nodules, and radial hypomyelinated tracts extending from the subependymal area to the cortex (Fig 3.4).

Cortical tubers constitute the hallmark of the disease and are pathognomonic of cerebral TSC. The number and localization of cortical tubers may account for the variability of the neurological phenotype observed in TSC patients. It is the unpredictable distribution of these lesions that is thought to result in the broad range of neurological phenotypes observed in TSC, even within the same family. Symptoms of cortical tubers include seizures, learning disabilities, attention deficit disorders with hyperactivity, and autism.

Cortical and subcortical tubers are hamartias that are located mainly in the cerebral cortex and in the underlying white matter. Several imaging descriptions have been used in literature to define tubers, including sulcal islands, gyral cores, spindles and wedges (Houser et al. 1991, Shepherd et al. 1995). Presumably, all these different definitions reflect the dynamic profile of myelination, and are related to the question of whether a tuber is located in an unmyelinated, myelinating or myelinated brain.

Spin-echo MRI sequences reveal that cortical tubers generally enlarge the gyri, and appear as regions of low T1 and high T2 signal unless they calcify. Spin-echo MRI seems so sensitive that several authors have tried to study the relationship between the number and localization of the tubers and the clinical symptoms (Roach et al. 1987, Curatolo et al. 1991, Shepherd et al. 1995, Goodman et al. 1996). These

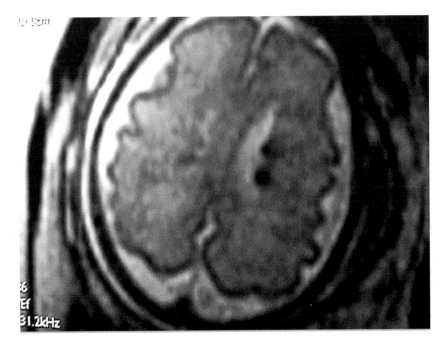

Fig. 3.5. Axial fetal MRI at 27 weeks of gestation showing multiple SENs and tubers.

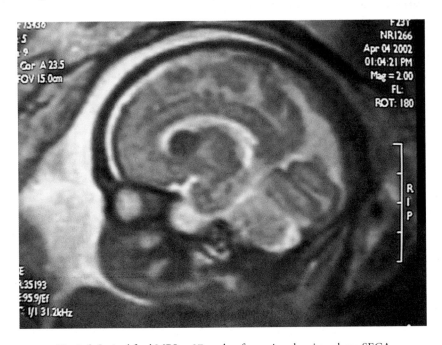

Fig. 3.6. Sagittal fetal MRI at 27 weeks of gestation showing a large SEGA.

studies show that the cortical tuber count is a good biomarker of the cerebral dysfunction, which can reasonably predict the neurological outcome. In addition, the localization of cortical tubers is important in determining the epileptic and the cognitive phenotype associated with the disease. However, FLAIR sequences are more sensitive than spin-echo sequences in detecting small tubers (Maeda et al. 1995). MRI is not able to identify all the tubers in a very young child with immature white matter. Recognition of tubers is particularly difficult in the first three months of life. Baron and Barkovich (1999) described the MRI findings in seven neonates and infants of less than 3 months of age. In these young patients the nodular subependymal and parenchimal lesions tend to be hyperintense in T1-weighted images and hypointense in T2-weighted images, just the opposite of what is seen in older children.

Subependymal nodules (SENs) are hamartomas that are typically seen in the subependymal wall of the lateral ventricles, mainly at the foramina of Monro. Some nodules protrude into the ventricular cavity. They are often multiple and small, ranging from 2 to 10 mm, and are partially or completely calcified (Hosoya et al. 1999). SENs develop during fetal life, are found in the great majority of patients with TSC, and are usually asymptomatic (Figs 3.5, 3.6). However, growth of these lesions at the foramen of Monro may determine a blockage of the CSF circulation, resulting in progressive lateral ventricular dilatation and intracranial hypertension. After contrast medium, SENs do not enhance.

The progressive growth of enhancing lesions at the foramen of Monro in a patient with TSC strongly suggests it is a subependymal giant cell astrocytoma (SEGA). A SEGA is usually defined as a subependymal lesion greater than 1 cm in diameter which enhances after administration of intravenous gadolinium. The histological distinction between SENs and SEGAs is not clear (Nixon et al. 1989, Shepherd et al. 1991). Up to 59% of patients recently studied by O'Callaghan et al. (2001) had at least one nodule that enhanced with intravenous gadolinium, and 17% had radiological evidence of a SEGA. Although all the lesions with enhancement characteristics should be closely monitored by sequential neuroimaging studies, it is unlikely that enhancement of a nodule with gadolinium carries a high risk of developing a clinically significant SEGA. Lateral ventricular enlargement, usually mild to moderate, occurs in 30 to 50% of individuals with TSC (Houser et al. 1991). Such dilatation is almost always associated with SENs. Occasionally the dilatation is secondary to an obstructing SEGA at the foramen of Monro, but in the great majority of patients the cause is not apparent.

SEGAs are typically reported between 4 and 10 years of age. Congenital SEGAs are rare. Mirkin et al. (1999) described in utero sonographic identification of an intraventricular brain mass at 27 weeks of gestation. The mass was further characterized by MRI in the first days after birth, and a SEGA was resected at 11 days of age. Early detection of SEGAs by periodic neuroimaging and prompt surgical resection may reduce morbidity and the risk of tumour recurrence.

Torres et al. (1998) investigated the utility of early diagnosis of SEGAs by means of a surveillance program. The patients whose SEGA was detected by periodic surveillance scanning before the onset of symptoms seemed to do better than those whose tumour was found because of symptoms. Criteria for surgery include the progressive increase in tumour size, the presence of hydrocephalus and/or symptoms of increased intracranial pressure, and new focal neurological deficits due to the tumour (Torres et al. 1998).

White matter lesions, including radial curvilinear bands and straight or wedge-shaped bands, are frequently observed (Canapicchi et al. 1996). White matter abnormalities were present in 95% of the cases reported by Griffiths and were most frequently found in relation to cortical tubers (Griffiths et al. 1998). The site, shape and histological findings of white matter lesions suggest that TSC is a disorder of both histogenesis and cell migration. In fact, the arrest of cell migration at different stages may explain the different sites of the various anomalies detected by MRI. Therefore, it is possible to hypothesize that subependymal nodules represent a failure of migration, white matter lesions an interruption of migration, and cortical tubers an abnormal completion of the migration process associated with a disorder of the cortical architecture.

SEIZURES

Seizures are the most common neurological symptom of TSC, occurring in 92% of patients referred at the Mayo Clinic (Gomez 1988). In 1984, Roger et al. reported a large series of 126 children with TSC and epilepsy; 63 infants presented West syndrome, a 50% rate. In this series Lennox–Gastaut syndrome was also common. We now believe that epilepsy associated with TSC shows mainly the characteristics of a partial epilepsy, with partial seizure followed by a cluster of spasms or by a secondary bilateral synchrony. Cortical tubers detected by MRI as high-intensity signal areas represent the epileptogenic foci of TSC, and a topographic relationship exists between EEG abnormalities and the largest MRI high-signal lesions (Curatolo and Cusmai 1988). MRI lesions in the occipital lobes show the best correlation with the EEG foci, whereas the weakest correlation is with frontal lesions.

Fluid-attenuated inversion recovery images have been shown to be more sensitive for the detection of small subcortical and cortical tubers, most of which were overlooked or misdiagnosed as the partial volume effect of the CSF on conventional T2-weighted images (Takanashi et al. 1995). MRI is not as yet able to detect all the cortical tubers that may be identified pathologically (Nixon et al. 1989). PET may reveal hypometabolic regions not predicted by MRI, demonstrating that the disturbance of cerebral function may be more extensive than indicated by morphological studies alone (Rintahaka and Chugani 1997).

The histologic abnormalities of cortical tubers, including dysmorphic and ectopic neurons, giant cells, disorganized cortical lamination, and abnormal connections, as

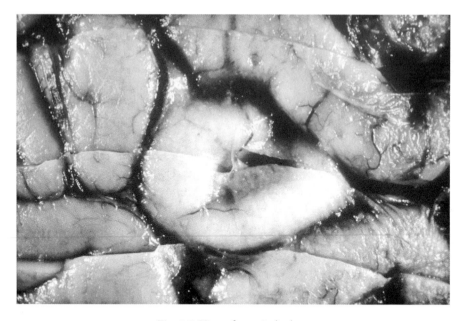

Fig. 3.7. View of a cortical tuber.

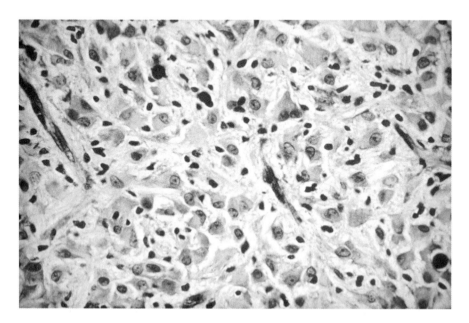

Fig. 3.8. Cerebral cortex showing disorganization of the normal cortical pattern. Abnormal neurons have lost their normal orientation.

well as the neurochemical abnormalities (diminished gabaergic synaptic activity, decreased number of GABA-A receptors), can explain the intrinsic epileptogenicity of the tubers (Figs 3.7, 3.8). Immunohistochemical and molecular analyses have indicated that the neuronal population of cortical tubers actively participates in the generation of partial seizures through the release of neurotransmitter-producing enzymes, neurotransmitter receptors and neuromodulators in the adjacent brain tissue (Crino and Henske 1999).

Epilepsy in TSC often begins in the very first months of life. The high incidence of infantile spasms and hypsarrhythmia has long been emphasized, but it is now clear that infants with TSC are clinically and electroencephalographically different from those with classical infantile spasms and hypsarrhythmia (Curatolo et al. 1991). In the same child, partial seizures may precede, coexist with, or evolve into infantile spasms. Many forms of subtle partial seizures, such as unilateral tonic or clonic phenomena, mainly localized in the face or limbs, and other seizures with subtle lateralizing features, such as tonic eye deviation, head turning, and unilateral grimacing, can occur frequently but may be missed by the parents until the third or fourth month of life when infantile spasms occur. Although the pathophysiological mechanisms responsible for the coexistence of infantile spasms and partial motor seizures are still uncertain, infantile spasms associated with TSC may be of focal nature, suggesting a rapid secondary generalization of partial seizures. Patients who have suffered from prolonged partial motor seizures, with or without secondary generalization, may present a post-ictal hemiparesis. In our experience, in these individuals an epileptogenic tuber is present in the motor cortex.

According to our studies, the age at which seizures and epileptiform activity become apparent depends on the location of the cortical tubers detected by MRI, and may coincide with functional maturation of the cortex, with an earlier expression for temporo-occipital regions than for frontal ones (Curatolo et al. 1991). An epileptogenic tuber may cause different clinical seizures in the same child as the child matures. Different seizures phenotype can also be due to different spread originating from the same epileptogenic area (Curatolo et al. 2001b, 2002). The EEG can help to better define the type of epilepsy and the epileptic syndrome associated with TSC.

A number of young children with TSC who present with partial seizures or infantile spasms at onset, later develop intractable seizures with multifocal EEG abnormalities associated with bilateral and more synchronous slow spike–wave complexes and an electroclinical pattern that resembles Lennox–Gastaut syndrome (LGS). At this stage it is difficult to recognize a focal origin of these apparently generalized abnormalities on visual inspection of the tracings, due to the presence of apparently bisynchronous EEG abnormalities. This phenomenon is particularly frequent for discharges originating in the frontal regions and followed by secondary bilateral synchrony. Frontal seizures are often characterized by apparently bilateral

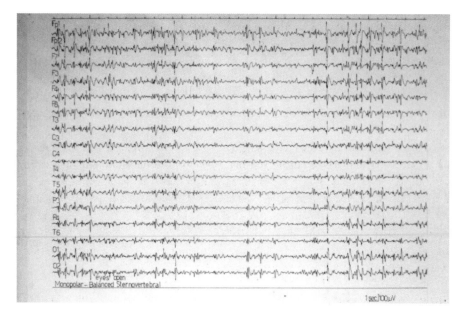

Fig. 3.9. Interictal EEG showing apparently generalized spike and wave discharges in a 12-year-old boy with intractable seizures, severe developmental delay, and autism. MRI reveals tubers in both frontal lobes. A lateralized onset from the left frontal tuber was detected by EEG mapping (see also Chapter 4).

clinical manifestations corresponding to a rapid electrographic generalization suggestive of bilateral cortico-cortical interactions (Fig. 3.9).

In patients with TSC, the differential diagnosis between LGS and localization-related symptomatic epilepsy originating in the frontal lobe may be extremely difficult, and only in a few cases can long-term video-EEG monitoring reveal subtle electroclinical manifestations suggestive of a focal seizure onset (Seri et al. 1998). In these patients, high time-resolution topographic EEG analysis and dipole localization methods may detect secondary bilateral synchrony (SBS), often originating in frontal regions and corresponding to prominent cortical tubers detected by MRI in the mesial surface of the frontal or anterotemporal lobes.

The natural history of epilepsy in patients with TSC, from infancy to childhood, tends to be one of increasing seizure frequency and severity, with poor response to antiepileptic drugs (AEDs) and a diminished quality of life because of the seizures and adverse medication effects. Unfavourable prognostic factors include onset earlier than 1 year of age, presence of several seizure types (infantile spasms and partial motor or complex partial seizures, drop attacks and atypical absences), multifocal discharges and/or SBS, and occurrence of new EEG foci during the evolution (Curatolo and Cusmai 1988, Curatolo et al. 1991).

Several new antiepileptic drugs have become available over the last few years, making the choice of the right AED even more difficult in children with TSC. The major achievement has been the observation that Vigabatrin is especially effective in controlling infantile spasms and partial seizures associated with TSC (Chiron et al. 1991, Curatolo 1994). Unfortunately, in recent years there have been several reports of the appearance of visual field defects after long-term treatment with Vigabatrin (see also Chapter 4).

At the moment there are inadequate data to assess whether the rapid suppression of seizures, particularly infantile spasms, prevents the development of learning disabilities and behavioural disorders, but, if it does, it again emphasizes the importance of early and prompt seizure control (Jambaqué et al. 2000). In a small proportion of selected patients, surgical removal of the cortical tuber causing the partial seizures may be a therapeutic possibility. In a child with intractable epilepsy, surgery can be considered if video-EEG monitoring reveals seizure onset from only one anatomic area. See Chapter 4 for further details.

LEARNING DISABILITY

Patients with TSC range from intellectually normal to severely impaired. The prevalence of learning disability varies from 38 to 80%, and the learning disability tends to be moderate or severe in degree. Children with infantile spasms and hypsarrhythmia are reported to be more severely affected than those with any other form of epilepsy (Gomez 1988). The question arises as to whether seizures cause learning disability or whether learning disability and epilepsy in children with TSC are two different aspects of the same underlying brain dysfunction.

The relationship between mental function and number of cortical lesions detected by MRI has been investigated. Although there was considerable variation in the mental function of patients with five or fewer cortical lesions, the development of all patients with ten or more cortical lesions was severely impaired (Goodman et al. 1996, Roach 1997). By contrast, no correlation has been found between the severity of learning disability and the number and size of tubers, including small subcortical and gyral core tubers, detected only on fluid-attenuated inversion recovery images (Takanashi et al. 1995).

Curatolo et al. (1991) have suggested that both number and localization of cortical tubers play an important role in cognitive outcome, and that epilepsy and learning disability probably reflect the underlying brain dysfunction caused by the cortical tubers. Late-onset partial seizures or transient infantile spasms were the only seizure types observed in the non-impaired individuals. All the patients with favourable evolution of their epilepsy had normal psychomotor development before the onset of the first seizure and usually had only one seizure type. Children with normal intelligence had small, isolated cortical tubers, mainly localized in the parietal and rolandic regions, and less severe epilepsy. They may have had different specific neuropsychological deficits related to the location of the cortical tubers, even when they were seizure-free. By contrast, patients with stable learning disability suffered from frequent partial seizures, developing multifocal or secondary generalized epilepsy, and showed multiple bilateral, strategically localized cortical tubers on MRI. Progressive intellectual deterioration observed in TSC children with intractable seizures may also be due to a heightened epileptogenicity of parasagittal frontal tubers.

Shepherd et al. (1995) reported that fewer tubers in the frontal regions might be a favourable predictor for cognitive development. The number of cortical tubers detected by MRI has been proven to be a good biomarker for the degree of cognitive disability (Goodman et al. 1996, Hosoya et al. 1999). Since the number of tubers is determined very early in the gestational period, it is likely that extensive brain disruption may predetermine which individuals will have poor cognitive outcome (Roach 1997).

However, normal cognitive function is still possible despite the presence of many tubers and an extensive brain involvement Although about half of children with TSC are of normal intelligence they are still prone to specific cognitive impairment related to the strategical location of the cortical tubers (Curatolo et al. 1991, Harrison et al. 1999). In our series (Jambaqué et al. 1991) of 23 patients aged from 3.5 to 16 years, only seven exhibited normal IQ scores. In this normally intelligent group we noted a variety of specific cognitive dysfunction including dyspraxia, dyscalculia and visuo-motor disturbance. We observed one child with an IQ of 107 and constructive apraxia, in whom a single tuberous lesion in the left parietal lobe was identified. See Chapter 5 for further details.

BEHAVIOURAL PHENOTYPES
In addition to learning disability, multiple behavioural problems, including sleep disorders, hyperactivity, attention deficit, aggressiveness and autism, have been found in children with TSC and are considered among the most pressing problems for parents (Curatolo et al. 1991, Gillberg et al. 1994). Repetitive and rhythmic head movements, rocking, bizarre and purposeless movements, and, more rarely, self-induced injuries are some of the behaviours usually displayed in severely impaired patients, who often are also unable to speak.

In a recent study on behavioural problems, by means of a postal questionnaire, on a series of 112 children, Hunt noted hyperactivity in 61%, peer problems in 59%, emotional problems in 38%, and conduct disorder in 37%. In these series there was no significant correlation between epilepsy and behavioural problems, suggesting that seizures are not likely to be the only cause of this behaviour in TSC. In our series the great majority of people with behavioural problems had learning disabilities and suffered from seizures (Curatolo et al. 1991, Jambaqué et al. 1991).

Attention deficit hyperactivity disorder is one of the major behaviour disorders in children with TSC, being reported in about 20% of children (Smalley et al. 1992, Hunt and Dennis 1987). Although the behavioural difficulties can be aggravated by underlying epilepsy, it is likely that in many individuals behavioural problems reflect a primary manifestation of cerebral involvement. Specific pharmacotherapy, with serotonin reuptake inhibitors, stimulants, clonidine and neuroleptics, can be of benefit for the management of problematic behaviours in TSC.

An association of TSC with autism is based on the joint occurrence of these two relatively rare disorders. The cause of this association remains unknown. The majority of reported TSC children with autistic-like behaviour had experienced infantile spasms and had learning disabilities, raising the question of cognitive defects as a primary cause of autism and behaviour problems (Curatolo and Cusmai 1987). Transient autistic behaviour seen in some children in association with infantile spasms or frontal lobe epilepsy may be a good example of behavioural disorders closely related to the epileptic dysfunction. Although the pathogenesis of autism in individuals with seizures and learning disability still remains a puzzle, it is possible that autism, epilepsy and learning disability are all different symptoms of the same underlying brain dysfunction.

Autism appears to be more common in infants with frontal and temporal tubers, and it has been suggested that an early dysfunction in the associative areas, owing to the location of cortical tubers, may be responsible for the autistic features (Curatolo et al. 1991). At the moment two pathways to autism and related pervasive developmental disorders could be envisaged, one involving the temporal lobes, the other the frontal lobes, perhaps each having similar but distinctive phenotypic profiles (Curatolo and Cusmai 1987, Bolton and Griffiths 1997, Seri et al. 1999).

An alternative explanation is that the behavioural phenotype seen in TSC reflects more direct effects of an abnormal genetic program. The *TSC2* gene product tuberin is highly expressed in brain regions involved in the behavioural phenotypes of the autistic disorder. A couple of genome scans in autism suggested that a potential susceptibility gene may be located on chromosome 16p13. The genetic dissection of the short arm of chromosome 16 in autism will help to localize this candidate gene and clarify its position with respect to the *TSC2* locus. Positional cloning of susceptibility genes in autism may provide important clues in the understanding of autistic behaviour associated with TSC (Curatolo et al. 2001a). See Chapter 6 for further details

SLEEP DISTURBANCES
Sleep disorders, such as night waking, waking early, seizure-related sleep problems, and excessive daytime sleepiness, are considered one of the most common behavioural manifestations in children with TSC (Hunt and Stores 1994). Only recently has attention been drawn to the prevalence of sleep disorders in children with TSC, and

data have been collected from questionnaires and family interviews (Hunt and Stores 1994). The main sleep-related problems that patients with TSC experience are settling (60%) and night waking (62%), and these can be exacerbated by parental stress and family problems.

The only study on sleep structure in TSC patients showed significant abnormalities in the polysomnographic recordings. The main features were a shorter total sleep time, a reduced sleep efficiency, a high number of awakenings and stage transitions, an increased wake after sleep onset, and a decrease in REM sleep (Bruni et al. 1995). Although the sample was relatively small (10 subjects), there was a clear tendency for children with seizures to show a more disturbed sleep architecture. A similar correlation was not evident for paroxysmal epileptiform activity density. By contrast, shorter awakenings not related to epileptic seizures were not detected by the families, suggesting that the prevalence of sleep disorders in TSC patients is probably underestimated.

Frequent awakenings are not specific to TSC patients and have been previously reported both in patients with learning disabilities (Petre-Quadens and Jouvet 1967) and in autistic patients without TSC (Taira et al. 1998). The high prevalence of seizures in this population requires the clinician to first rule out the possible epileptic nature of the episodes occurring during the night. Epilepsy is by far the most frequent cause of multiple awakenings in TSC patients, and careful history taking, associated with the use of home videos to record episodes, has proven to be very helpful. In selected cases, when a correct classification cannot be made or when the semiology of the ictal phenomena and of the associated EEG features is needed, polygraphic video-EEG recordings can be used. In the vast majority of cases, seizures occurring at night in TSC patients originate from the frontal lobe structures and are associated with complex motor phenomena (tonic posturing, clonic movement of one limb promptly bilateralizing), and require a careful clinico-neurophysiological assessment. This will result in more appropriate management of the epileptic condition and in choice of the correct drug regimen.

Melatonin given 20 minutes before bedtime has shown some promising results in children with TSC, drastically reducing sleep problems (O'Callaghan et al. 1999). Such an improvement in sleep also positively affects the daytime behaviour of the child. The mechanisms underlying this effect are not fully understood. The fact that melatonin does not exert any effect on sleep fragmentation leads us to believe that the main positive effect is in shortening sleep-onset latency and that it is more likely to be successful in those patients in whom frequent awakenings are not the main reported symptom. Prolonged sleep latency and frequent awakenings due to epileptic seizures need to be differentiated using polysomnography.

REFERENCES

Baron Y, Barkovich A (1999) MR imaging of tuberous sclerosis in neonates and young infants. *Am J Neuroradiol* 20: 907–16.

Bolton PF, Griffiths PD (1997) Association of tuberous sclerosis of temporal lobes with autism and atypical autism. *Lancet* 349: 392–5.

Bourneville DM, Brissaud E (1881) Encéphalite ou sclérose tubéreuse des circonvolutions cérébrales. *Arch Neurol (Paris)* 1: 390–410.

Bruni O, Cortesi F, Giannotti F, Curatolo P (1995) Sleep disorders in tuberous sclerosis: a polysomnographic study. *Brain and Dev* 17: 52–6.

Canapicchi R, Abbruzzese A, Guerrini R, Bianchi MC, Montanaro D, Cioni G (1996) Neuroimaging of tuberous sclerosis. In: Guerrini R, Andermann F, Canapicchi R, Roger J, Zifkin BG, Pfanner P (eds) *Dysplasias of Cerebral Cortex*. Philadelphia: Lippincott Raven, pp. 151–62.

Carbonara C, Longa L, Grosso E, et al. (1994) 9q34 loss of heterozygosity in a tuberous sclerosis astrocytoma suggests a growth suppressor-like activity also for the TSC1 gene. *Human Mol Gene* 3: 1829–32.

Chiron C, Dulac O, Beaumont D, Palacios L, Pajot N, Mumford J (1991) Therapeutic trial of Vigabatrin in refractory infantile spasms. *J Child Neurol* 6(2): 2552–9.

Crino PB, Henske EP (1999) New development in neurobiology of tuberous sclerosis complex. *Neurology* 53: 1384–90.

Curatolo P (1994) Vigabatrin for refractory partial seizures in children with tuberous sclerosis. *Neuropediatrics* 25: 55–6.

Curatolo P, Cusmai R (1987) Autism and infantile spasms in children with tuberous sclerosis. *Dev Med Child Neurol* 29: 550–1.

Curatolo P, Cusmai R (1988) MRI in Bourneville disease: relationships with EEG findings. *Neurophysiol Clin* 18: 149–57.

Curatolo P, Cusmai R, Cortesi F, et al. (1991) Neurologic and psychiatric aspects of tuberous sclerosis. *Ann NY Acad Sci* 615: 8–16.

Curatolo P, De Luca D, Bottini N, Dowling MM, Lucarelli P (2001a) Autism in tuberous sclerosis complex. *J Child Neurol* 16: 679.

Curatolo P, Seri S, Verdecchia M, Bombardieri R (2001b) Infantile spasms in tuberous sclerosis complex. *Brain Dev* 173: 502–7.

Curatolo P, Verdecchia M, Bombardieri R (2002) Tuberous sclerosis complex: a review of neurological aspects. *Eur J Ped Neurol* 6: 15–23.

Dabora SL, Józwiak S, Franz DN, et al. (2001) Mutational analysis in a cohort of 224 tuberous sclerosis patients indicates increased severity of TSC2, compared with TSC1, disease in multiple organs. *Am J Hum Genet* 68(1): 64–80.

European Chromosome 16 Tuberous Sclerosis Consortium (1993) Identification and characterization of the tuberous sclerosis gene on chromosome 16. *Cell* 75: 1–11.

Gillberg IC, Gillberg C, Ahlsen G (1994) Autistic behaviour and attention deficits in tuberous sclerosis: a population-based study. *Dev Med Child Neurol* 36: 50–6.

Gomez MR (1988) Neurologic and psychiatric features. In: Gomez MR (ed) *Tuberous Sclerosis*. New York: Raven Press, pp 21–36.

Goodman M, Lamm SH, Engel A, et al. (1996) Cortical tuber count: a biomarker indicating neurologic severity of tuberous sclerosis complex. *J Child Neurol* 12: 85–90.

Green AJ, Smith M, Yates JRW (1994a) Loss of heterozygosity on chromosome 16p13.3 in hamartomas from tuberous sclerosis patients. *Nature Genet* 6: 193–6.

Green AJ, Johnson PH, Yates JRW (1994b) The tuberous sclerosis gene on chromosome 9q34 acts as a growth suppressor. *Hum Mol Genet* 3: 1833–4.

Griffiths PD, Bolton P, Verity C (1998) White matter abnormalities in tuberous sclerosis complex. *Acta Radiol* 39; 59: 482–6.

Harrison JE, O'Callaghan FJ, Hancock E, Osborne JP, Bolton P (1999) Cognitive deficits in normally intelligent patients with tuberous sclerosis. *Am J Med Genet* 88: 642–6.

Hirose T, Scheithauer BW, Lopes MBS (1995) Tuber and subependymal giant cell astrocytoma associated with tuberous sclerosis: an immunohistochemical, ultrastructural, and immuno-electron microscopic study. *Acta Neuropathol* 90: 387–99.

Hosoya M, Naito H, Nihei K (1999) Neurological prognosis correlated with variations over time in the number of subependymal nodules in tuberous sclerosis. *Brain and Dev* 21: 544–7.

Houser OW, Shepherd CW, Gomez MR (1991) Imaging of intracranial tuberous sclerosis. *Ann NY Acad Sci* 615: 81–93.

Hunt A, Dennis J (1987) Psychiatric disorder among children with tuberous sclerosis. *Dev Med Child Neurol* 29: 190–8.

Hunt A, Stores G (1994) Sleep disorders and epilepsy in children with tuberous sclerosis: a questionnaire based study. *Dev Med Child Neurol* 36: 108–15.

Jambaqué I, Cusmai R, Curatolo P, Cortesi F, Perrot C, Dulac O (1991) Neuropsychological aspects of tuberous sclerosis in relation to epilepsy and MRI findings. *Dev Med Child Neurol* 33: 698–705.

Jambaqué I, Chiron C, Dumas C, Mumford J, Dulac O (2000) Mental and behavioural outcome of infantile epilepsy treated by Vigabatrin in tuberous sclerosis patients. *Epilepsy Res* 38: 151–60.

Jóźwiak S, Kwiatkowski DJ, Kasprzyk-Obara J, et al. (2001) Epilepsy and especially infantile spasms are more frequent among patients with TSC2 mutations. *J Child Neurol* 16: 675.

Lamb RF, Roy C, Diefenbach TJ, et al. (2000) The TSC1 tumour suppressor hamartin regulates cell adhesion through ERM proteins and the GTPase Rho. *Nat Cell Biol* 2(5): E76–8.

Maeda M, Tartaro A, Matsuda T, Ishii Y (1995) Cortical and subcortical tubers in tuberous sclerosis and FLAIR sequence. *J Comput Assist Tomogr* 19: 660–7.

Mirkin LD, Ey EH, Chaparro M (1999) Congenital subependymal giant-cell astrocytoma: case report with prenatal ultrasonogram. *Pediatr Radiol* 29: 776–80.

Mizuguchi M, Kato M, Yamanouchi H, Ikeda K, Takashima S (1996) Loss of tuberin from cerebral tissues with tuberous sclerosis and astrocytoma. *Ann Neurol* 40: 941–4.

Nellist M, van Slegtenhorst MA, Goedbloed M, et al. (1999) Characterization of the cytosolic tuberin-hamartin complex. Tuberin is a cytosolic chaperone for hamartin. *J Biol Chem* 274(50): 35647.

Nellist M, Goedbloed MA, Verhaaf B, et al. (2001) Tuberin amino acid substitutions interfere with the interaction between tuberin and hamartin. *J Child Neurol* 16: 674.

Nixon JR, Houser OW, Gomez MR, Okazaki H (1989) Cerebral tuberous sclerosis: MRI imaging. *Radiology* 170: 869–73.

O'Callaghan FJK, Clarke AA, Hancock E, Hunt A, Osborne JP (1999) Use of melatonin to treat sleep disorders in tuberous sclerosis. *Dev Med Child Neurol* 41: 123–6.

O'Callaghan FJK, Renowden S, Noakes M, Martyn CN, Osborne J (2001) Prevalence of subependymal giant cell astrocytomas in patients with tuberous sclerosis in the Wessex region. *J Child Neurol* 16: 678. Abstract.

Petre-Quadens O, Jouvet M (1967) Sleep in the mentally retarded. *J Neurol Sci* 4: 354–7.

Rintahaka PJ, Chugani HT (1997) Clinical role of positron emission tomography in children with tuberous sclerosis complex. *J Child Neurol* 12: 42–52.

Roach ES (1997) Tuberous sclerosis: function follows form. *J Child Neurol* 12: 75–6.

Roach ES, Williams DP, Laster DW (1987) Magnetic resonance imaging in tuberous sclerosis. *Arch Neurol* 44: 301–3.

Roger J, Dravet C, Bonivier C, Magaudda A, Bureau M, Fernandez-Alvarez E, Sanmarti FX, Fabregues I, Cenraud B, Larrieu JL (1984) L'épilepsie dans la sclérose tubéreuse de Bourneville. *Boll Lega It Epil* 45: 33–8.

Seri S, Cerquiglini A, Pascual Marqui M, Michel C, Pisani F, Curatolo P (1998) Frontal lobe epilepsy: EEG-MRI fusioning. *J Child Neurol* 13: 34–8.

Seri S, Cerquiglini A, Pisani F, Curatolo P (1999) Autism in tuberous sclerosis: evoked potential evidence for a deficit in auditory sensory processing. *Clin Neurophys* 110: 1825–30.

Shepherd CW, Scheithauer BW, Gomez MR, et al. (1991) Subependymal giant cell astrocytoma: a clinical, pathological, and flow cytometric study. *Neurosurgery* 28: 864–8.

Shepherd CW, Houser OW, Gomez MR (1995) MR findings in tuberous sclerosis complex and correlation with seizure development and mental impairment. *Am J Neuroradiol* 16:149–55.

Smalley SL, Tanguay PE, Smith M, Gutierrez G (1992) Autism and tuberous sclerosis. *J Autism Dev Disord* 22: 339–55.

Taira M, Takase M, Sasaki H (1998) Sleep disorders in children with autism. *Psychiatry Clin Neurosci* 52: 182–3.

Takanashi J, Sugita K, Fujii K, Niimi H (1995) MR evaluation of tuberous sclerosis: increased sensitivity with fluid-attenuated inversion recovery and relation to severity of seizures and mental retardation. *Am J Neuroradiol* 16: 1923–8.

Torres OA, Roach ES, Delgado MR, et al. (1998) Early diagnosis of subependymal giant cell astrocytoma in patients with tuberous sclerosis. *J Child Neurol* 13: 173–7.

van Slegtenhorst M, de Hoogt R, Hermas C, et al. (1997) Identification of the tuberous sclerosis gene TSC1 on chromosome 9q34. *Science* 277: 805–8.

Vinters HV, Kerfoot C, Catania M, et al. (1998) Tuberous sclerosis-related gene expressions in normal and dysplastic brain. *Epilepsy Res* 32: 12–23.

4
SEIZURES

Paolo Curatolo and Stefano Seri

EARLY EPILEPTIC MANIFESTATIONS

In patients with TSC, epilepsy often begins in the first year of life and in most cases as early as the first few months of life. Seizures beginning in the first days of life have been reported in seven patients with TSC. These seizures are resistant to initial medications and often medically intractable (Miller et al. 1998). In infancy, partial motor and epileptic spasms (ES) are the most common seizure types. Although ictal video-EEG recordings have been rarely reported, it has been documented that a sizeable proportion of spasms are preceded by partial seizures (Stephenson 1988). Furthermore, in the same child, partial seizures may precede, coexist with or evolve into ES.

One of the most commonly observed patterns in early-onset ES associated with TSC is the presence of apparently bilateral and symmetrical flexor tonic contraction of the limbs lasting for a few seconds, preceded by eye deviation. A vast number of subtle partial seizures, such as unilateral tonic or clonic phenomena, mainly localized to the face or limbs, can be under-recognized by the parents until the third or fourth month of life, when ES occur (Dulac et al. 1984). Isolated attacks develop within weeks into a typical cluster, especially upon awakening. The three main types of spasms (flexor, extensor, mixed) may occur in infants with TSC. Typical ES associated with TSC are rare. Lateralizing features such as tonic eye deviation, nystagmus, head turning, unilateral grimacing and asymmetrical involvement of the limbs may be observed. The tonic or atonic components displayed in ES are often asymmetrical. In some cases, the spasms may be unilateral, often with an adversive component (Dulac et al. 1984). Almost all cases of ES associated with TSC have their onset between the third and the eleventh month of life, with the highest incidence between 4 and 5 months (Dulac et al. 1984). Familial cases of ES reported in children with TSC are the expression of the autosomal dominant transmission of the disease.

At the age of occurrence of the spasms, TSC can be recognized by the presence of cutaneous hypopigmented maculae. Associated neurological abnormalities can include hemiparesis and subtle asymmetric motor deficits. The incidence of abnormal cognitive and motor development prior to the onset of the ES is lower than in other groups of symptomatic ES possibly because, at this age, a mild degree of cognitive delay can be overlooked.

INTERICTAL EEG FINDINGS

Focal or multifocal epileptiform abnormalities may be found when an EEG is performed between the neonatal period and the development of the ES. Infants with ES due to TSC exhibit a particular awake interictal EEG characterized by a multifocal asynchronous pattern of spike discharges and irregular slow activity of 2–3 hertz (Curatolo et al. 1991). Reducing the gain and increasing the spatial sampling can help in better visualizing focal or multifocal abnormalities (Figs 4.1, 4.2). Although the EEG foci can be located in any region of the brain, the most common location for ES is the posterior temporal and occipital regions (Cusmai et al. 1990). High time resolution topographic analysis of EEG has shown that, despite the presence of a multifocal pattern, EEG abnormalities may arise from a single dominant focus (Seri et al. 1991). The focal interictal EEG activity is related to a prominent neuroimaging abnormality in the temporo-occipital region, detected by magnetic resonance imaging (MRI) or by positron emission tomography (PET) (Cusmai et al. 1990) (Figs 4.3, 4.4).

Non-REM sleep is associated with increased epileptiform activity. Multifocal and focal abnormalities tend to generalize, and bursts of more synchronous polyspikes and waves separated by sudden voltage attenuation become evident, resembling a hypsarrhythmia (Dulac et al. 1984). Sleep spindles may or may not be recorded in these patients, due to the amount of epileptiform abnormalities. In REM

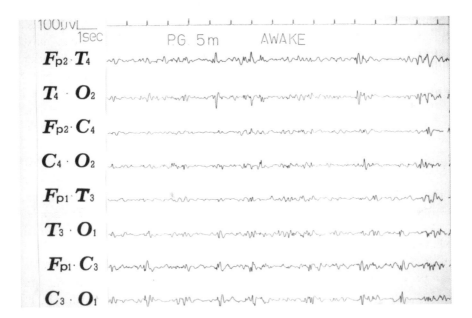

Fig. 4.1. Interictal awake EEG in a 5-month-old girl. Independent multifocal spikes can be identified, mainly in the left occipital region.

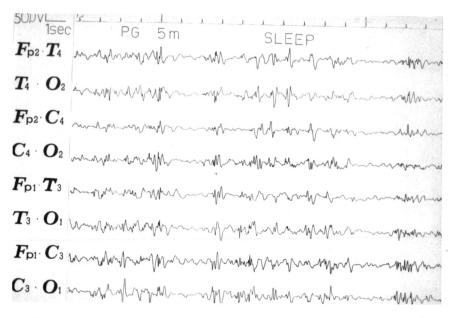

Fig. 4.2. Same patient and same recording as in Fig. 4.1. During NREM sleep the EEG abnormalities generalize. Note the lack of spindles.

sleep, on the contrary, epileptiform activity is less prominent, generalized discharges are usually suppressed, and there is a definite tendency for the EEG foci to become spatially very restricted. Severe sleep problems are frequent after the onset of ES and are mainly due to sleep-related epileptic events. All-night polysomnographic recordings in children with TSC who presented with ES have shown an increased number and duration of awakenings after sleep onset, and a marked reduction in total sleep time and in REM sleep time (Bruni et al. 1995) (Figs 4.5, 4.6). These interictal EEG abnormalities are reproducible in terms of topography and tend to persist in serial EEG records.

ICTAL EEG DATA

Video-EEG and polygraphic recordings of the spasms, as well as 24-hour EEG monitoring, have shown that a cluster of spasms can be regarded as a single seizure. Each one consists of a combination of both focal and bilateral manifestations, i.e. hemiclonic or motor adversive phenomena followed by a cluster of spasms. The involvement of the limbs is bilateral, but often asymmetrical (Dulac et al. 1984, Plouin et al. 1993). The typical ictal EEG is characterized at onset by a focal discharge of spikes and polyspikes, usually originating from the temporal, rolandic or occipital regions, followed by a generalized irregular slow-wave transient and an abrupt and diffuse desynchronization of background activity. In other instances, the

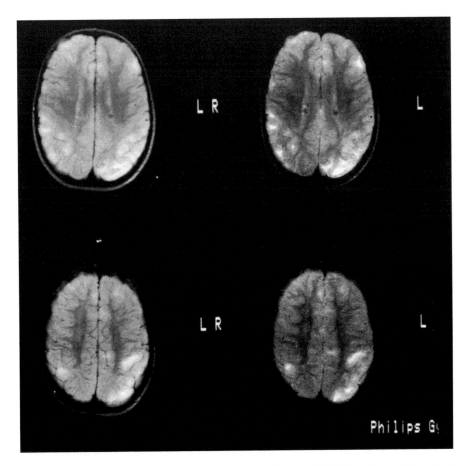

Fig. 4.3. Same patient as in Figs 4.1 and 4.2. Axial MRI shows multifocal hyperintensities in both hemispheres, mainly in the left parieto-occipital region.

first spasm coincides with the disappearance of interictal activity throughout the cluster, with the interictal activity only recurring at the end of it.

EVOLUTION OF CLINICAL AND EEG FEATURES
Although the mechanisms underlying the coexistence of ES and partial motor seizures are still uncertain, there is converging clinical evidence that ES associated with TSC may be of a focal nature. One possible explanation is that of a secondary generalization from a localized onset.

The age of onset of seizures and the age when epileptiform activity becomes apparent on the EEG are a function of the location and the intrinsic epileptogenicity of cortical tubers detected by MRI, and may coincide with functional maturation of the cortex, with an earlier expression for the temporo-occipital regions than for the

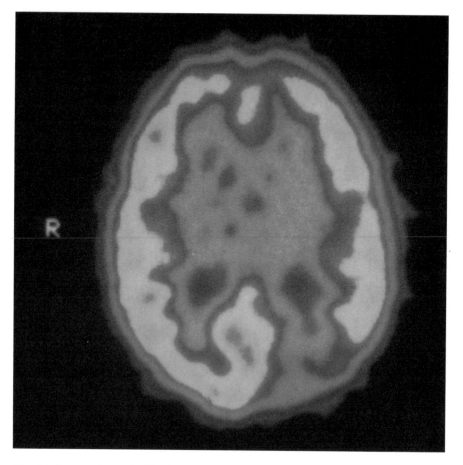

Fig. 4.4. Same patient as in Figs 4.1–3. Positron emission tomography reveals hypometabolic region in the left occipital region.

frontal ones. This can account for the observation that posterior cortical lesions are frequently associated with ES and a marked epileptogenicity during the first year of life. Furthermore, in the same child, complex partial seizures originating from a more anterior cortical tuber may not begin for a number of years.

The vast majority of children with TSC who had ES at onset eventually develop either partial motor, complex partial, or apparently generalized tonic, atonic or tonic-clonic seizures. In older children who suffered from ES, a video-EEG study has shown that almost all the epileptic seizures associated with the TSC can be described as partial (partial motor, complex partial) or having some form of secondary generalization (Stephenson 1988).

As maturation progresses, the modified hypsarrhythmic pattern tends to disappear and interictal EEG recordings tend to exhibit focal spikes or slowing, with

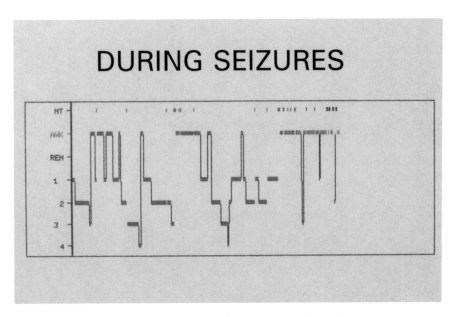

Fig. 4.5. Hypnogram showing extreme sleep fragmentation, evidenced by frequent sleep stage shiftings, and an increased number of awakenings (AWK) in a child with frequent nocturnal seizures.

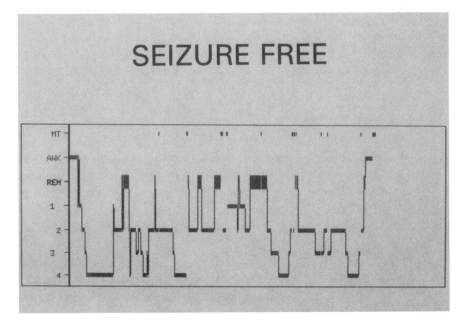

Fig. 4.6. Same patient as in Fig. 4.5. Seizures are now well controlled by Vigabatrin. Polysomnography reveals no awakenings during sleep. REM sleep is now present.

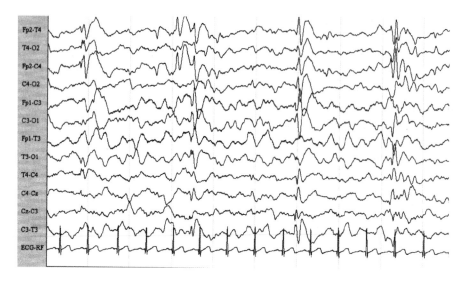

Fig. 4.7. Interictal EEG showing apparently generalized abnormalities in a 4-year-old child with intractable frontal lobe seizures.

transitional stages from discrete foci to multifocal discharges. Although the occipital and posterior temporal spikes prevailing at the onset tend to persist in morphology and location in serial EEG-records, after 2 years of age additional foci with a frontal localization become progressively evident. During sleep, the EEG is characterized by multifocal abnormalities associated with bursts of bilateral and more synchronous slow spike-waves, with a pattern similar to that seen in Lennox–Gastaut syndrome. At this stage, the recognition of focal origin of these apparently generalized abnormalities on standard EEG is difficult, but high time resolution topographic analysis of EEG and dipole localization methods may detect the presence of a secondary bilateral synchrony (SBS), often originating in the frontal regions and corresponding to prominent tubers detected by MRI (Seri et al. 1998). Computerized analysis of the EEG may allow prompt recognition of the focal onset of apparently generalized bursts, revealing small interchannel time differences. We suggested that the Lennox-like pattern seen in some TSC patients following ES is in fact due to frontal lobe seizures with a rapid secondary generalization (Seri et al. 1998) (Fig. 4.7).

EPILEPTOGENESIS IN TSC

In TSC, seizures have a focal or multifocal origin and a topographic correspondence exists between EEG foci and MRI high signal lesions, demonstrating the preponderant role of cortical tubers as epileptogenic foci (Curatolo and Cusmai 1988). Immunohistochemical and molecular analysis have indicated that the neuronal populations of cortical tubers might have intrinsic epileptogenicity and actively participate in the generation of partial seizures, through the release of neurotransmitters or neuromodulators into the adjacent brain tissue (Wolf et al. 1995).

Giant cells in tubers express neurotransmitter-producing enzymes and neurotransmitter receptors, such as NMDA receptor subunit 1 and $GABA_A$ receptor subunits (Crino and Henske 1999). Recently, it has been suggested that changes in the properties of $GABA_A$ receptors, possibly related to plastic changes in subunit combinations, may result in an altered regulation of inhibitory function (Olsen and Avoli 1997). Based on these findings, a decrease in GABAergic inhibition in cortical tubers can be postulated. In the near future, this could represent a fertile field for further investigation. The idea that epileptogenesis in TSC may be related to an impairment of GABAergic transmission is supported by the effectiveness of drugs with affinity with $GABA_A$-benzodiazepine receptors in the treatment of epilepsy. In a recent study, elevated GABA levels have been reported in brain biopsies of subjects with intractable epilepsy and TSC, and not from other causes. Furthermore, several studies have indicated that Vigabatrin (VGB), a specific and irreversible inhibitor of gamma-amino-butyric acid aminotransferase, has a higher efficacy in infantile spasms and partial seizures due to TSC than in those related to other aetiologies. It is possible to suppose that epilepsy in TSC may result from "aberrant plasticity" that may involve a subunit switch of $GABA_A$ receptors and changes in a regulatory system.

Concas et al. (1999) reported that the changes in the plasticity of $GABA_A$ receptors are related to the physiological changes in plasma and brain concentration of neurosteroids, which may act as endogenous modulators of $GABA_A$ receptors. Particularly, the 3α-reduced metabolites of progesterone (PROG) (3α, 5α-tetrahydroprogesterone and 3α, 5β-THP) are positive $GABA_A$ receptor modulators with a 20-fold higher potency than benzodiazepines, while their 3β-enantiomers (3β, 5α-THP, and 3β, 5β-THP) inhibit the ability of 3α-THP to potentiate $GABA_A$ receptor function. There is recent evidence that the magnitude of the steroid potentiation by GABA may be influenced by the α subunit, with chimeras containing the $α_1$ subunit being the most effective (Maitra and Reynolds 1998). Moreover, it has been reported that cortical tubers exhibit an alteration in glutamate and GABA receptor subunit mRNA expression, with decreased levels of $GABA_AR$ $α_1$ and $α_2$ subunit (White et al. 2001). The change in relative levels of different receptor isoform has been suggested to result in a decreased sensitivity of $GABA_A$ receptors by 3α-THP which in turn may modify neuroactive steroids synthesis (Smith et al. 1998).

In a recent study we have measured the plasma concentration of 3α-THP, 3β-THP and PROG in 18 TSC patients with or without seizures by gas chromatographic-mass spectrometric (GC-MS) method. We have found that the plasma levels of 3β-THP were increased in epileptic TSC patients, independently from the seizure frequency, compared to seizure-free subjects and a control group. The concentration of 3α-THP decreased significantly in TSC patients who presented seizures daily, compared to seizure-free TSC patients and control subjects (Verdecchia et al. 1998). These results suggest that in TSC epileptic patients there may be a disregulation of enzymes deputed to the synthesis of these neuroactive steroids, possibly resulting in a decreased GABAergic transmission. These modifications could be related to a genetically determined mechanism that regulates 3β-THP synthesis or metabolism, and/or to a functional regulation linked to the expression of receptors to which these neuroactive steroids bind.

MEDICAL TREATMENT

The medical treatment of seizures in TSC can often prove frustrating, due to the limited response to the conventional AEDs. The advent of the new molecules has certainly had a positive impact on short-term seizure control. Difficulties are related to the limited understanding of epileptogenesis in TSC and the paucity of definite knowledge of the mode of action of most AEDs in humans (Meldrum 1996).

One major mode of action of AEDs at the cellular level is through the Na^{++} channels, by preventing repetitive discharges and opposing the diffusion, rather than the initiation, of the epileptic discharge. Several AEDs are known to exert an activity on synaptic transmission. This is especially the case of VGB and TGB which increase the concentration of GABA in the CNS. Other agents probably act on glutamatergic transmission. In most cases, however, mechanisms of action are multiple and remain largely unknown. Even for AEDs synthesized after a precise hypothesis, the actual mode of action does not always seem to be univocally related to their known properties.

The supposed mechanisms of action of antiepileptic drugs are summarized in Table 4.1.

The exact role and clinical indications of new AEDs are not yet definitively established. In general, the new AEDs should not be used as first-choice drugs for the treatment of most patients with epilepsy until more data on their safety profile are available. This is particularly relevant as far as cognitive and behavioural effects are concerned. Some (Tiagabine, VGB, LTG) have been reported to aggravate certain generalized seizure types (Guerrini et al. 1998, Genton 2000). Interactions between conventional and new AEDs are summarized in Tables 4.2 and 4.3.

With the only possible exception of VGB, the same indications and limitations apply to TSC patients and to subjects with epileptic seizures and syndromes with other aetiologies. As a rule, the use of more than two AEDs should not be encouraged. In most cases, seizure control will not significantly improve, while the risk of adverse effects will dramatically increase. However, selected patients have been shown to benefit from the use of polytherapy. It is good practice to use AEDs with different sites and mechanisms of action (i.e. drugs acting mainly on GABAergic synaptic transmission with drugs acting on Na channels).

Adrenocorticotropic hormone and steroids have been the most popular treatment for ES. At high doses and when used for a protracted time, side effects can

TABLE 4.1
Supposed mechanisms of action of antiepileptic drugs

AEDs	Inactivation of Na channels	Inhibition of Ca T channels	Other Ca channels	Increase of GABA activity	Antagonism to NMDA receptors
PTH	+++		+	+	
PB	++		+	++	++
CBZ	+++			+	
VPA	++	+			+
ETS		+++			
BZD	+		+	+++	
LTG	+++		+		
VGB				+++	
TGB				+++	
GBP	+			++	
FBM	+		+	+	++
TPM	++			++	++

TABLE 4.2
Interactions between conventional and new AEDs

	FBM	GBP	LTG	Oxcarbazepine	Tiagabine	TPM	VGB
VPA	none	none	↑	↓	none	↓	none
CBZ	↓	none	↓	↓	↓	↓	none
PTH	↓	none	↓	↓	↓	↓	none
PB	↓	none	↓	↓	↓	↓	none
Primidone	↓	none	↓	↓	↓	↓	none

TABLE 4.3
Interactions between new and conventional AEDs

	VPA	CBZ	PTH	PB	Primidone
PB	↑ 10–30%	↓	↑ 10–30%	↑	unknown
GBP	none	none	none	none	none
LTG	↓ 25%	none	none	none	none
Oxcarbazepine	none	none	↑	↑	none
Tiagabine	none	none	none	none	none
TPM	↓ 10%	none	↑ 25%	none	none
VGB	None	none	↓	none	none

be frequent and serious. Although data from appropriately controlled trials are still insufficient for a consensus statement, there is some evidence that steroids may not be the drug of choice when ES are associated with TSC.

VIGABATRIN

Chiron et al. (1991) reported for the first time the efficacy of Vigabatrin (VGB) in refractory infantile spasms. The best results were obtained in patients with tuberous sclerosis, who had a sustained and complete disappearance of infantile spasms for follow-up periods of 8–33 months. In contrast, in the group with cryptogenetic infantile spasms only 50% maintained a good response to the treatment.

In 1996, Aicardi et al. published the results of a European multicentre retrospective survey regarding the use of Vigabatrin as add-on therapy in 192 infants diagnosed with infantile spasms. Complete cessation of spasms was obtained in 131 patients (68.2%); a decrease in cluster frequency was observed in 37 (19.3%). The better response was shown in the 28 children with tuberous sclerosis; 27 of these (96%) had a complete suppression of spasms. Aicardi et al. (1996) and Chiron et al. (1991) both reported an average of four days for control of seizures in those infants who responded to VGB. However, Chiron et al. (1991) observed that after cessation

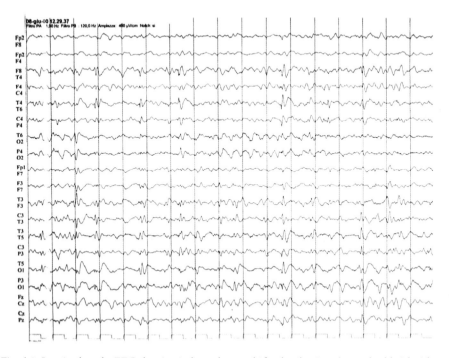

Fig. 4.8. Interictal awake EEG showing independent multifocal spikes in a 4-month-old girl with TSC and epileptic spasms.

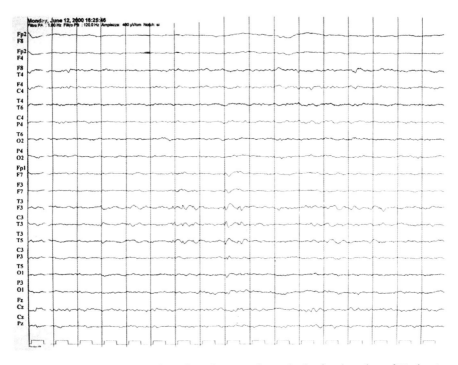

Fig. 4.9. Same patient as in Fig. 4.8. The girl recovered completely after three days of Vigabatrin treatment.

of infantile spasms children with tuberous sclerosis experienced partial seizures. It is possible to suppose, then, that infantile spasms in tuberous sclerosis represent a secondary generalization of partial seizures and that VGB treatment is able to control this secondary generalization (Figs 4.8, 4.9). Recently, Jambaqué et al. (2000) hypothesized that significant improvement of cognition and behaviour observed in infants with TSC after VGB treatment may be due to the control of the secondary generalization induced by infantile spasms; this control seems to be a key factor for cognitive outcome.

Hancock and Osborne (1999) reviewed 15 studies published in the English language literature investigating the use of VGB in the treatment of infantile spasms, and reported the efficacy of VGB in the treatment of spasms in infants suffering from TSC. Overall there were 390 patients treated, with complete cessation of seizures occurring in 242 (62%). The group of children with TSC who were treated with VGB had a 95% response rate, in spite of resistance to other therapies and delay in starting treatment. The effect was observed within one week in the vast majority of patients, a much quicker response than that observed with steroids, benzodiazepines or sodium valproate, which can take weeks to show efficacy (Fig. 4.4).

Mitchell and Shah (2000) reported their experience of the use of VGB in the treatment of infantile spasms, with or without TSC. Parents were instructed to begin VGB at the lowest practical dose. If a response occurred at the lower dose, they were instructed to continue it. Twelve out of 20 responded with complete cessation of infantile spasms and resolution of hypsarrhythmia, at doses ranging from 25 to 135 mg/kg/day. A clinical response was often observed after 1–2 doses. Mitchell et al. concluded that, in epileptic spasms, response to VGB is dose-independent and that spasms responded to VGB both as initial treatment and after other compounds had failed.

Although VGB is a very promising alternative to steroids, in some patients focal seizures may persist. A large majority of patients with epileptic spasms at onset later experience either simple partial motor or complex partial seizures, or apparently generalized seizures, often originating from more anterior cortical tubers. Preliminary data (Curatolo 1994) suggest that, in children with TSC, Vigabatrin could be effective in reducing frequency of focal seizures in up to 74% of patients. However, localization-related effectiveness of VGB shows better results on partial seizures originating from parieto-occipital lobes.

VGB is generally well tolerated. Hancock and Osborne (1999) in their review showed that, in total, 87 side effects were observed, including drowsiness, behavioural problems, hypotonia, insomnia and weight gain. The majority of these effects were transitory and none were reported to continue after the cessation of the VGB treatment; only seven infants were reported as having stopped treatment because of intolerance. The main reasons for stopping VGB treatment were hyperactivity, irritability, hypotonia and myoclonus.

In recent years converging evidence has been produced on the association between concentric narrowing of the visual field and VGB treatment. This can affect up to 40–50% of cases (Eke et al. 1997). This narrowing can be severe and irreversible, and continuation of the drug can be associated with progressive visual field loss (van Veelen et al. 2000). Clinical ophthalmologic signs are not usually seen until advanced stages and are obviously under-reported in patients with learning difficulty. For this reason, serial visual field studies should be performed when possible for early detection of such alterations (Mauri-Llerda et al. 2000).

However, current techniques for visual field testing require some degree of compliance. This poses a serious limitation to their use in infants and children, particularly in those with neuropsychiatric disorders. In these patients, electroretinography (ERG) could be of some help. The ERG abnormalities observed in children treated by VGB could reflect electrophysiological impairment of photoreceptors and pigment epithelium function related to GABA-induced ion transport changes in the outer retinal layer (Arndt et al. 1999). Currently, the minimum duration and doses of VGB treatment that can produce this side effect are unknown, and the feasibility of using low dosages and short treatment periods (2–3 months) should be investigated. However, reversibility of the visual field constriction after discontinuation of VGB has been reported in children (Versino and Veggiotti 1999). The young age of a patient could act as a favourable factor in reversing the complications of VGB (Giordano et al. 2000), although this finding needs to be replicated on large samples.

OTHER DRUGS

In the last 10 years, several new antiepileptic drugs have become available. Topiramate (TPM) is emerging as an effective drug in partial seizures, with or without secondary generalization, and in Lennox–Gastaut syndrome. Among 14 children with refractory epilepsy and TSC treated for six months with TPM as add-on therapy, seizures were reduced by more than 50% in nine patients; three patients had no seizures for six months (Franz et al. 2000). The mechanisms of action of TPM, apart from state-dependent blockade of sodium and calcium channels and inhibitory effect on carbon-anhydrase, include the enhancement of GABA activity on GABA-A receptors with elevation of cerebral GABA levels, and antagonism of glutamate receptors. For these reasons and given the good preliminary results obtained with TPM, this can be reported as a promising new agent for the treatment of partial seizures in TSC patients. In children, the usual starting dose is 0.5–1 mg/kg per day; the steady state dosage range varies from 2 to 15 mg/kg daily. The most common side effects include weight loss, dizziness, sleepiness, headache, tremor and cognitive dysfunction (Uldall and Bucholt 1999). Clinical experience suggests that titration has to be slow, with increments every second week, in order to permit the greatest possible number of children to benefit from its efficacy.

Lamotrigine (LTG) is more effective than TPM on some generalized seizures. Recently, Franz et al. (2001a) presented their experience with LTG add-on therapy in 57 patients with TSC. Twenty-four patients (42%) were seizure-free, and 21 (37%) had a greater than 50% reduction in seizure frequency. Eighteen (32%) had subjectively improved behaviour and/or alertness with daily activities. Thirty-eight (67%) had no change in this regard, and one (2%) became worse. Responders were more likely not to have a history of infantile spasms, and to have experienced only partial seizures. Improved alertness and behaviour were apparent in many patients, and the incidence of side effects was similar to that reported for other paediatric populations with symptomatic partial epilepsy. Although LTG is well tolerated, a skin rash can occur in 5 to 10% of subjects and concern has been raised that the incidence may be higher in children. The rash usually begins within the first 8 to 10 weeks of exposure. To minimize the risk of rash, LTG should be titrated slowly, with increments over a period of 6 to 8 weeks (Schmidt and Bourgeois 2000).

Levetiracetam is a novel antiepileptic drug for partial epilepsy. Its specific mechanism of action is unknown. Franz et al. (2001b) presented their experience with Levetiracetam treatment in nine individuals with TSC. All had medically intractable partial epilepsy. Treatment was initiated at 10 mg/kg/day in two or three daily doses and titrated until either a clinical response or intolerable side effects were observed. Two individuals became seizure-free. Four individuals experienced a greater than 50% reduction. Three individuals had a less than 50% reduction or no change in seizure frequency. Levetiracetam was withdrawn in one individual who had a greater than 50% reduction, due to intolerable hyperkinesis and agitation. Therapy was withdrawn in three other individuals due to lack of efficacy.

Oxcarbazepine has a lower incidence of cognitive side effects than its parent compound carbamazepine. Its primary side effect relates to the idiosyncratic development of hyponatremia, which is increased in individuals with pre-existing renal disease. Franz et al. (2001c) presented their clinical experience with the treatment of epilepsy in 16 individuals with tuberous sclerosis using oxcarbazepine. Six individuals became seizure-free. Five individuals experienced a greater than 50% reduction in seizure frequency. Treatment was initiated at 10 mg/kg/day in two or three daily doses. The dose was escalated by 5–10 mg/kg at 3–7 day intervals until seizure control was noted, clinical toxicity occurred, or dosage of 60 mg/kg/day was achieved without significant reduction in seizures. Patients who experienced at least a 50% reduction in seizure frequency continued titration until optimal efficacy was achieved. Oxcarbazepine was withdrawn in one individual due to cognitive slowing greater than that previously noted on carbamazepine. Therapy was withdrawn in four other individuals owing to a lack of efficacy.

Felbamate has been effective in partial seizures in patients with TSC, but it has not been properly tested because of the high risk of causing aplastic anaemia, leucopoenia and thrombocytopoenia, or hepatic damage. In patients with Lennox–Gastaut syndrome its use is acceptable when all other AEDs have failed to control seizures. A blood count and liver function tests should be performed every 15 days in patients treated with this drug.

In most of the patients with early-onset seizures, total control may be an unreasonable aim. In these cases, treatment should be focused on the suppression of the more dangerous seizures (i.e. drop attacks) without producing unacceptable adverse effects and inability to participate in daily living activities. When severely disabling seizures are present or when consistent electroclinical and imaging data suggest a confined area of seizure onset, alternative treatment to AEDs should be considered (Thiele 2000).

SURGICAL TREATMENT

Despite therapeutic trials with first-line and new AEDs, some children and adolescents with TSC will continue to present with seizures. When seizure activity proves intractable to medication the possibility of surgical treatment should be explored. The frequent presence in the same patient of multiple lesions on neuro-imaging poses a serious challenge in defining surgical amenability. This process involves the identification of converging electroclinical, morphological and functional

TABLE 4.4

Morphological data	
Epileptogenic lesion:	Structural brain abnormality responsible for the epileptic seizures
Epileptogenic area:	Brain area that is necessary and sufficient for initiating seizures and whose disconnection is necessary for abolition of seizures
Functional data	
Irritative zone:	Area of cortex that generates interictal spikes
Epileptogenic zone:	Area of cortex that generates the seizure, and area of early propagation
Symptomatogenic zone:	Area of cortex that generates the initial clinical symptomatology

imaging data, and requires a common operational framework between epileptologists, neuroradiologists and clinical neurophysiologists. In Table 4.4 we have summarized some of the terminology currently used in this context.

Evidence from multiple imaging modalities suggests that not all lesions in TSC patients are epileptogenic. Whenever possible, the identification of a single epileptogenic area and its selective surgical removal could significantly improve the quality of life of patients with TSC. The success rate is high when the patients are screened carefully.

PRESURGICAL ASSESSMENT
Electrophysiological findings
The value of long-term video-EEG monitoring in the presurgical assessment of epileptic patients is well established. In a review of 230 children who underwent video-EEG monitoring, in 64% of the cases results were critical in planning the surgical approach (Chen et al. 1995). The advent of digital equipment has made the high temporal resolution of EEG more readily available for more advanced analysis. A further significant improvement is related to the increasing spatial resolution of EEG, with many centres now being able to record from 64 to 256 channels. High-resolution EEG and MEG have shown a very high degree of accuracy in localizing interictal activity as well as early seizure EEG patterns, both in the time and frequency domains (Blanke et al. 2000, Michel et al. 1999). Invasive recordings (subdural strips/grids, stereo-EEG and intraoperative corticography) remain important in guiding surgical resection. Their limited spatial sampling can, however, fail to give account of the more complex activation patterns seen in some neocortical epilepsies.

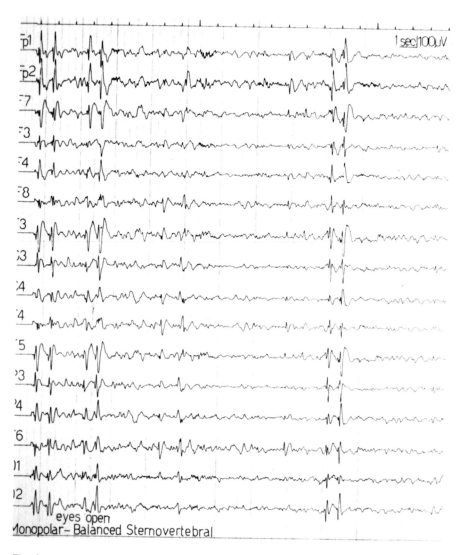

Fig. 4.10. Interictal EEG showing apparently generalized discharges in a boy with intractable complex partial seizures and drop attacks, and severe learning disability.

Although little data on patients with TSC is available, non-invasive techniques will play a greater role in the near future, particularly if their interpretation will supplement findings from the visual analysis of electro-clinical seizure patterns. In a recent study we have shown that source localization techniques and short time-lag estimation can be a valuable tool in the identification of the lateralized onset of bilateral discharges (Seri et al. 1998). Fig. 4.10 shows the extracranial localization

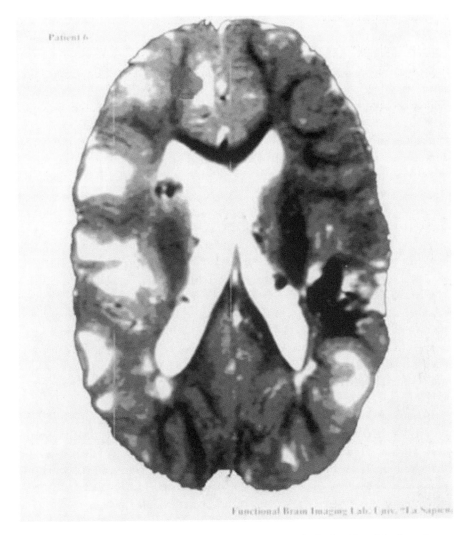

Fig. 4.11. Same patient as in Fig 4.10. Source localization methods identify a right frontal onset (epileptogenic zone) in a cortical area surrounding a large tuber.

of ictal EEG data in a patient with TSC and intractable complex partial seizures. The identification of a dialeptic episode on scalp video-EEG recording points to a right hemisphere onset. Source localization identifies the right frontal lobe as the possible epileptogenic zone. When mapped on to the MRI (surface rendering), there is a striking congruence between the site of a major cortical tuber and that of the seizure onset (Fig. 4.11).

Magnetoencephalography

An improvement in functional localization can be obtained by combining EEG and magnetoencephalography (MEG) signals. Whereas scalp EEG detects both tangential and radial sources (i.e. activity in the sulci and in the gyri) MEG selectively measures tangential sources (i.e. activity in the sulci). Furthermore, MEG measures magnetic fields that are primarily associated with intracranial currents. The intracranial currents that pass into the skull and scalp contribute only partially (about 5%) to extracranial measured magnetic fields. By contrast, EEG signal is more affected by the volume currents and the interposed tissues. The small volume of intracranial currents in the MEG means that it may be possible not to include the skull and scalp within the source of localization. For this reason, spatial resolution of MEG is about one-third better than that of EEG, because the magnetic field is not distorted by resistive properties of tissues (Fig. 4.12).

The difficulty of localizing the source of epileptic spikes produced by a relatively concentrated neural volume, as in the case of focal epilepsy, favours a magnetic approach. In TSC, which is often characterized by many brain lesions, it is difficult to identify the epileptogenic areas only on the basis of scalp EEGs. We have suggested that MEG, combined with EEG, may be a suitable technique to perform this task (Peresson et al. 1998, Curatolo and Peresson 1999). At the present time we consider that findings gathered with EEG and MEG are not mutually exclusive, but rather complementary. These techniques are the only non-invasive methods (with a time resolution of less than one millisecond) available for studying the physiology and pathology of the central nervous system.

The field distribution obtained by MEG can be used for three-dimensional source localization. Combining MEG data on brain function with MRI data on brain structure, it is possible to localize equivalent current dipole (ECD) in a zone corresponding to involved cortical areas. A head-based three-dimensional co-ordinated system allows computer merging of MEG signal ECD localizations with MRI multiplanar images, a process called magnetic source imaging (MSI). An example of MSI localization is given in Figs 4.13 and 4.14.

MSI can provide both functional and structural information with a good time and space resolution, and, in particular, additional spatial data in TSC patients with convexity foci, allowing more accurate localization of the zone of the cortical focal abnormalities. It remains unclear to what extent MSI could be of assistance in avoiding invasive studies in surgery candidates, and in helping the surgeon to perform individualized and conservative resection in children with intractable localization-related seizures associated with TSC (Figs 4.15, 4.16).

Other functional imaging data

Early 18-FDG PET study findings supported the idea that functional brain abnormalities were a potential source of critical information in patients with early-onset

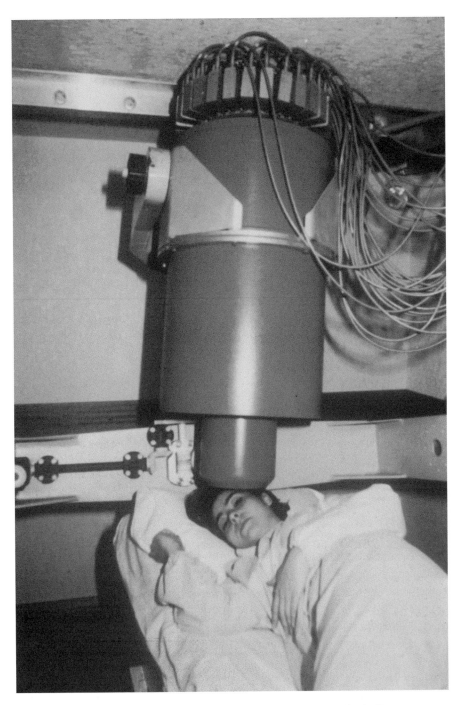

Fig. 4.12. Photograph of the neuromagnetometer system operating in Rome.

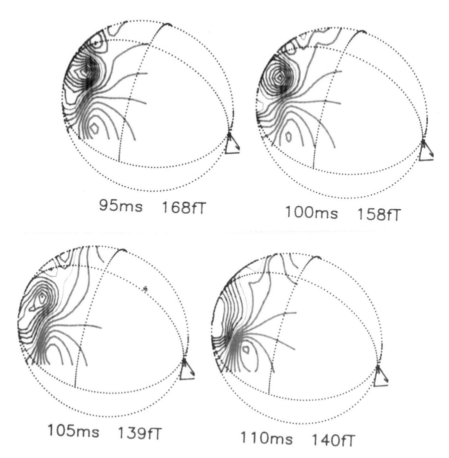

95ms   168fT   100ms   158fT

105ms   139fT   110ms   140fT

Fig. 4.13. Sequence of field mapping in a 14-year-old girl with intractable temporal lobe seizures.

refractory epilepsy (Chugani 1994). This study suggested that some, if not all, of the early seizures in children with infantile spasms are partial in nature. The surgical relevance of these functional data lies in the identification of what they call the area of cortical abnormality (Chugani et al. 1993). This might or might not correlate with the EEG focus of seizure onset and/or an underlying structural abnormality. This concept, although introduced in the broader context of the surgical treatment of infantile spasms, irrespective of the aetiology, carries important implications for patients with TSC and multiple MRI abnormalities. More recently, the use of new radioactive tracers has been advocated as more specific in identifying epileptogenic tubers in patients with TSC (Chugani et al. 1998), suggesting that the serotonin pathway might play an important role in the selective epileptogenicity of some cortical lesions.

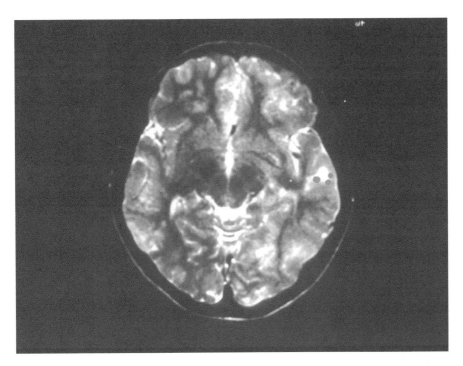

Fig. 4.14. Same patient as in Fig. 4.13. Magnetic source imaging (MSI) localizes the epileptogenic zone in the left temporal region.

TREATMENT

Resective surgery

Surgical treatment in TSC patients in the past has largely been restricted to resection of subependymal nodules or giant cell astrocytomas, and/or treatment of obstructive hydrocephalus secondary to blockage of cerebrospinal fluid pathways. In the last decade, surgical series have been published and have shown encouraging results (Avellino et al. 1997, Baumgartner et al. 1997, Guerreiro et al. 1998). Small series have shown an improvement in seizure control after surgery, with a variable follow-up (Achslogh 1964, Perot et al. 1966, Bye et al. 1989, Erba and Duchowny 1990).

Palmini and colleagues (1991) reported a series of 10 patients treated by craniotomy and seizure foci resection, in which one was seizure-free, one had a greater than 90% reduction of major seizures and at least 75% reduction of minor seizures, three had a greater than 50% reduction of major and minor seizures, three had a less than 50% reduction of major seizures irrespective of minor seizures, and two were lost to follow-up.

Bebin et al. (1993) presented the Mayo Clinic experience of surgical treatment of epilepsy in TSC. Nine patients underwent cortical resection or stereotaxic

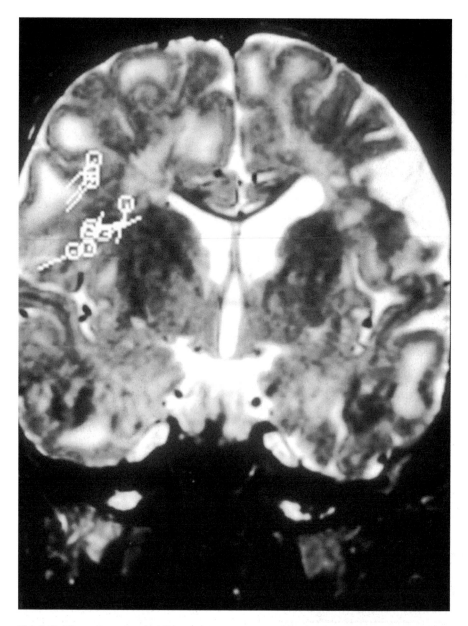

Fig. 4.15. Three-dimensional MSI localization in a 3-year-old girl with intractable partial seizures, who had previous resective surgery. Coronal section showing an epileptogenic zone in the right parietal region.

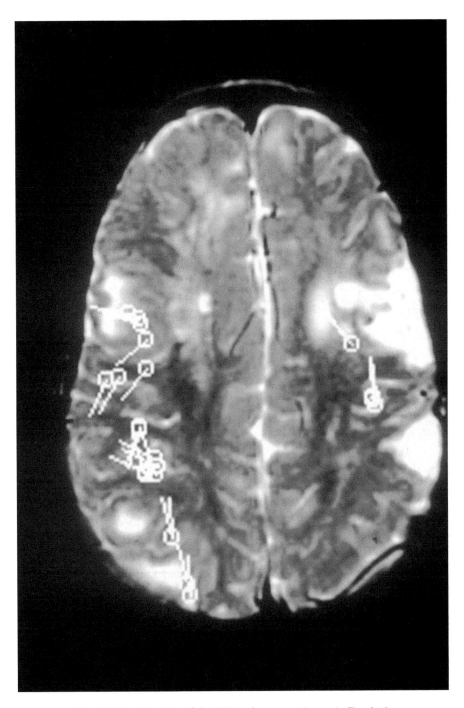

Fig. 4.16. Axial section of the MSI in the same patient as in Fig. 4.15.

lesionectomy, and had excellent or good outcome: six patients were seizure-free after a mean follow-up of 35 months.

Avellino et al. (1997) reported that 6 out of 11 patients were free of seizures after extratemporal resection.

Guerreiro et al. (1998) described 18 patients (9 male) with TSC who underwent surgical treatment of medically refractory epilepsy. Twelve patients had a well-localized epileptogenic lesion and were treated by lesionectomy or focal resection. Of the resections, seven were frontal, four temporal, one fronto-temporal, one occipital, and one fronto-parietal. Four patients underwent more than one operation. Six patients had corpus callosotomy. Among the 12 patients who underwent lesion-ectomy or cortical resection, seven had excellent outcome: five are seizure-free and two have only auras. Another four patients had good or fair outcome. According to Guerreiro these data provide evidence that focal resection can be considered as a treatment option in patients with TSC.

Multiple brain lesions are frequently seen in patients with TSC, but resective surgery can be considered if the main epileptogenic abnormality is correlated with only one lesion. The best outcome in this study was in patients who had focal seizures and good imaging and EEG correlation, despite having multiple seizure types, other imaging abnormalities, or multifocal or generalized EEG findings. In these series, all patients who had excellent outcome had a single obvious tuber on neuroimaging examination.

Neville et al. (2000) described eight children with TSC who had surgery for epilepsy. There were resections in six children and two anterior callosotomies. Of the six children receiving focal resections (frontal, temporal and parietal), four had normal early development, and three of these showed mild/moderate delay at surgery. Two were severely cognitively impaired. After surgery, four were seizure-free, one with marked recovery of cognitive function; two had temporary or no relief of seizures; both had severe cognitive impairment and autism, but one had some relief of autistic features and the other temporary improvement in communication. Invasive monitoring was used in three of these patients. Two children with severe cognitive and autistic impairment had anterior two-thirds callosotomies, one with removal of giant cell astrocytomas, for severe drop attacks. One had total relief of drop attacks and the other had useful reduction and slowing of the attacks and marked improvement in communication.

Jayant et al. retrospectively analysed nine patients with TSC who underwent focal resective surgery for frequent, medically intractable seizures. Age of seizure onset ranged from 3 months to 11 years. Non-invasive (all patients) and invasive (five patients) video-EEG monitoring showed seizures arising from one temporal region in seven patients, left parieto-occipital region in one, and left frontal region in one. Neuroimaging revealed a single temporal lesion in two patients, correspond-ing to the EEG focus, and multiple temporal and extratemporal lesions in seven. In addition, one patient had hippocampal atrophy on the same side as the EEG focus. Temporal resection was performed in seven patients (right 4, left 3), left superior occipital resection in one, and left frontal resection in one. Of the seven patients with temporal resection, six were seizure-free at 5 months to 14 years follow-up, and one patient, with dual pathology, had marked reduction of seizures. The patient with frontal resection had no seizures at one-month follow-up. The patient with occipital resection did not improve. An additional four case reports, including one from Miami Children's Hospital, documented favourable outcome after resection.

The experience of Koh et al. (2000), in which 9 out of 13 patients (69%) were seizure-free, is thus fully consistent with the results from other centres and confirms the feasibility and efficacy of excisional procedures in patients with TSC.

Recently, Romanelli et al. (2001) reported the case of a child with TSC and severe and intractable epilepsy with onset in the first month of life. Video-EEG monitoring at the age of 1 year revealed a left temporal seizure focus. Repeat video-EEG at age 2 years revealed a right posterior quadrant epileptic focus. Although bilateral subdural electrodes confirmed independent right parietal (principal) and left temporal seizure foci, a two-stage procedure was undertaken. The right parietal epileptogenic area was resected first, while the left temporal area continued to show epileptic activity on subdural electrode recordings and was resected two days later. During the more than 24-month follow-up period, there have been no tonic-clonic or complex partial seizures. Simple partial motor seizures involving the right foot were reduced by more than 80% and other simple partial seizures were eliminated. Cognitive and motor development were significantly improved after surgery.

Thiele et al. (2001) reported on the surgical outcome of 21 children, ranging in age from 5 weeks to 22 years. Four children later underwent repeat resective surgery in the same region for continued seizure activity. Eleven of these children underwent resection of a frontal tuber, seven a resection of a temporal tuber, two a resection of an occipital tuber, and four underwent a corpus callosotomy. Subsequent to surgery, the children have been followed up for 1 month to 11 years. All experienced some significant reduction in seizure frequency. Seven of the children have experienced a more than 98% reduction in seizures, six a 70–97% reduction, six a 50–69% reduction, and two a 25–40% reduction. Following surgery, several patients have shown an improvement in cognitive and/or social functioning.

As expected, the best outcome has been reported in patients with focal seizures and good imaging and EEG correlation. A more striking finding was that the coexistence of multiple seizure types, other imaging abnormalities, and/or multifocal or generalized EEG findings was not necessarily associated with a poor response. In the absence of such correlation, palliative procedures such as corpus callosotomy were found to provide at least some improvement, particularly when drop attacks were present.

Since the majority of drug-resistant patients with TSC are not good candidates for surgical intervention, other options should be considered.

Vagus nerve stimulation

The vagal nerve stimulator is a major non-medical alternative treatment for epilepsy management and should be considered when a patient with TSC and intractable epilepsy fails the criteria for resective surgery. Vagus nerve stimulation (VNS) is a novel approach to treating epilepsy. It is approved as add-on therapy in adults and adolescents over 12 years of age with partial-onset seizures which are refractory to antiepileptic medications.

VNS uses an implantable medical device programmed to provide baseline intermittent stimulation of the left vagus nerve. For VNS, a computer-controlled and battery-powered pacemaker generator is used, connected to a nerve stimulation lead. Unlike other types of epilepsy surgery, surgical implantation of this system does not involve a craniotomy. The pacemaker generator is implanted in the chest under the skin, and the lead is implanted in the neck. Despite extensive experimental studies and some human data, the mode of action of VNS is unknown.

No specific seizure type or syndrome has been clearly identified as being the greatest beneficiary of this technique. However, children with partial seizures preceded by aura may have a good chance of obtaining excellent results because of the stimulator ability to arrest the seizures if used during an aura.

Murphy et al. described an open-label, retrospective, multicentre study to determine the outcome of intermittent stimulation of the left vagal nerve in 10 children with TSC and medically refractory epilepsy. Nine experienced at least a 50% reduction in seizure frequency, and five had a 90% or greater reduction. No adverse events were encountered. Comparison with published and registry patients revealed improved seizure control in the TSC patients.

Several studies have reported that the efficacy of VNS improves significantly with time. According to the physicians, one-third of patients treated with VNS as part of their long-term treatment regimen experienced a significant improvement in overall quality of life, one-third experienced a good improvement, and one-third experienced little or no improvement. Currently, there is no way to determine which individuals will respond to VNS or how quickly an individual may respond to therapy (Whittemore 2000).

Other options: the ketogenic diet

The ketogenic diet was developed in the early 1900s as a treatment for drug-resistant seizures. The diet contains a very large proportion of saturated fat (animal fats and some vegetable oils), and a drastically reduced proportion of protein and carbohydrate, so that about 90% of the body's daily energy requirements come from fat. This produces a rise in blood acetone level and a decrease in blood sugar concentration. The mechanisms of action by which the ketogenic diet work are still not clear. Ketosis, acidosis, changes in fluid and electrolyte balance, and hyperlipidemia have all been proposed as factors responsible for the antiepileptic effect. The antiepileptic effect induced by ketosis takes place over 7 to 10 days, despite rapid initiation of the ketotic state, suggesting that ketosis may alter brain metabolism in such a way as to induce an anticonvulsant effect. The real problem with the diet is that it is both extraordinarily nasty and very difficult to prepare. Children who are intractable to currently available antiepileptic therapy may improve on the diet; those under 10 years of age demonstrate a more favourable response than older children and adults. Patients with myoclonic/atonic seizures tend to achieve better seizure control than those with other seizure types.

REFERENCES

Achanya JN, Kotagal P, Dinner DS, Wyllie E, Bingaman W (2000) Surgical treatment of epilepsy in patients with tuberous sclerosis. TSC Millennium Symposium "From gene to treatment". Edinburgh, 13–15 September – Abstracts Book.

Achslogh J (1964) La chirurgie de l'épilepsie dans les phakomatoses. *Neurochirurgie* 10: 523–49.

Aicardi J and Peer Review Groups, Mumford JP, Dumas C, Wood S (1996) Vigabatrin as initial therapy for infantile spasms; a European retrospective survey. *Epilepsia* 37: 638–42.

Arndt CF, Derambure P, Defoort S, Hache JC (1999) Is visual impairment related to vigabatrin reversible? *Epilepsia* 40(2): 256.

Avellino AM, Berger, MS, Rostomily, RC, Shaw CM, Ojemann GA (1997) Surgical management and seizure outcome in patients with tuberous sclerosis. *J Neurosurg* 87: 391–6.

Baumgartner JE, Wheless JW, Kulkarni S, Northrup H, Au KS, Smith A, Brookshire B (1997) On the surgical treatment of refractory epilepsy in tuberous sclerosis complex. *Pediatr Neurosurg* 27(6): 311–18.

Bebin EM, Kelly PJ, Gomez MR (1993) Surgical treatment for epilepsy in cerebral tuberous sclerosis. *Epilepsia* 34: 651–7.

Blanke O, Lantz G, Seeck M, Spinelli L, Grave de Peralta R, Thut G, Landis T, Michel CM (2000) Temporal and spatial determination of EEG-seizure onset in the frequency domain. *Clin. Neurophysiol* 11: 763–72.

Bruni O, Cortesi F, Giannotti F, Curatolo P (1995) Sleep disorders in tuberous sclerosis: a polysomnographic study. *Brain Dev* 17: 52–6.

Bye AM, Matheson JM, Tobias VH, et al. (1989) Selective epilepsy surgery in tuberous sclerosis. *Aust Paediatr J* 25: 243–5.

Chen LS, Mitchell WJ, Horton EJ, Snead OC III (1995) Clinical utility of video-EEG monitoring. *Pediatr Neurol* 12: 220–4.

Chiron C, Dulac O, Beaumont D, Palacios L, Pajot N, Mumford J (1991) Therapeutic trial of Vigabatrin in refractory infantile spasms. *J Child Neurol* 6(2): 2552–9.

Chugani HT (1994) The role of PET in childhood epilepsy. *J Child Neurol* 9 (suppl 1): S82–S88.

Chugani HT, Shields DA, Shewnon DD, Sankar R, Comayr Y, Winter HV, Peacock WJ (1993) Surgery for intractable infantile spasms: neuroimaging perspectives. *Epilepsia* 34(4): 764–71.

Chugani DC, Chugani HT, Muzik O, et al. (1998) Imaging epileptogenic tubers in children with tuberous sclerosis complex using alpha-11C-methyl-L-tryptophan positron emission tomography. *Ann Neurol* 44: 858–66.

Concas A, Follesa P, Barbaccia ML, Purdy RH, Biggio G (1999) Physiological modulation of GABA(A)receptor plasticity by progesterone metabolites. *Eur J Pharmacol* 375: 225–35.

Crino PB, Henske EP (1999) New developments in the neurobiology of the tuberous sclerosis complex. *Neurology* 53: 1384–90.

Curatolo P (1994) Vigabatrin for refractory partial seizures in children with tuberous sclerosis. *Neuropediatrics* 25: 55–6.

Curatolo P, Cusmai R (1988) MRI in Bourneville disease: relationship with EEG findings. *Neurophysiol Clin* 18: 49–157.

Curatolo P, Peresson M (1999) Magnetoencephalography. In: Gomez MR (ed) *Tuberous Sclerosis Complex*. New York: Raven Press, pp 75–84.

Curatolo P, Cusmai R, Cortesi F, Jambaqué I, Chiron C, Dulac O (1991) Neurologic and psychiatric aspects of tuberous sclerosis. *Ann NY Acad Sci* 615: 8–16.

Curatolo P, Seri S, Verdecchia M, Bombardieri R (2001a) Infantile spasms in tuberous sclerosis complex. *Brain Dev* 173: 502–7.

Curatolo P, Verdecchia M, Bombardieri R (2001b) Vigabatrin for tuberous sclerosis. *Brain Dev* 23: 649–53.

Curatolo P, Verdecchia M, Bombardieri R (2002) Tuberous sclerosis complex: a review of neurological aspects. *EJPN* 6: 15–23.

Cusmai R, Chiron C, Curatolo P, Dulac O, Tran Dinh S (1990) Topographic comparative study of magnetic resonance imaging and electroencephalography in 34 children with tuberous sclerosis. *Epilepsia* 31: 747–55.

Dulac O, Lemaitre A, Plouin P (1984) The Bourneville syndrome: clinical and EEG features of epilepsy in the first year of life. *Boll Lega It Epil* 45/46: 39–42.

Eke T, Talbot JF, Lawden MC (1997) Severe persistent visual field constriction associated with vigabatrin. *BMJ* 314: 180–1.

Erba G, Duchowny MS (1990) Partial epilepsy and tuberous sclerosis: indication for surgery in disseminated disease. *J Epilepsy* 3 (suppl): 315–19.

Franz DN, Tudor C, Leonard J (2000) Topiramate as therapy for tuberous sclerosis complex-associated seizures. *Epilepsia* 41(7): 87.

Franz DN, Tudor C, Leonard J, Egelhoff JC, Byars A, Valerius K, Sethuraman G (2001a) Lamotrigine therapy of epilepsy in tuberous sclerosis. *Epilepsia* 42(7): 935–40.

Franz DN, Leonard J, Tudor C, Chuck G, Egelhoff J (2001b) Levetiracetam therapy of epilepsy in tuberous sclerosis. *J Child Neurol* 16: 679.

Franz DN, Leonard J, Tudor C, Chuck G, Egelhoff J (2001c) Oxcarbazepine therapy of epilepsy in tuberous sclerosis. *J Child Neurol* 16: 680.

Genton P (2000) When antiepileptic drugs aggravate epilepsy. *Brain Dev* 22: 75–80.

Giordano L, Valseriati D, Vignoli A, Morescalchi F, Gandolfo E (2000) Another case of reversibility of visual-field defect induced by vigabatrin monotherapy: is young age a favorable factor? *Neurol Sci* 21: 185–6.

Guerreiro MM, Andermann F, Andermann E, et al. (1998) Surgical treatment of epilepsy in tuberous sclerosis: strategies and results in 18 patients. *Neurology* 51: 1263–9.

Guerrini R, Dravet C, Genton P, et al. (1998) Lamotrigine and seizure aggravation in severe myoclonic epilepsy. *Epilepsia* 39: 508–12.

Hancock E, Osborne JP (1999) Vigabatrin in the treatment of infantile spasm in tuberous sclerosis: literature review. *J Child Neurol* 14: 71–4.

Jambaqué I, Chiron C, Dumas C, Mumford J, Dulac O (2000) Mental and behavioural outcome of infantile epilepsy treated by vigabatrin in tuberous sclerosis patients. *Epilepsy Res* 38: 151–60.

Koh S, Jayakar P, Dunoyer C, Whiting SE, Resnick TJ, Alvarez LA, Morrison G, Ragheb J, Prats A, Dean P, Gilman J, Duchowny MS (2000) Epilepsy surgery in children with tuberous sclerosis complex: presurgical evaluation and outcome. *Epilepsia* 41(9): 1206–13.

Maitra R, Reynolds JN (1998) Modulation of GABA(A) receptor function by neuroactive steroids: evidence for heterogeneity of steroid sensitivity of recombinant GABA(A) receptor isoforms. *Can J Physiol Pharmacol* 76: 909–20.

Mauri-Llerda JA, Iniguez C, Tejero-Juste C, Santos-Lasaosa S, Escalza-Cortina I, Ascaso-Puyuelo J, Abad-Alegria F, Morales-Asin F (2000) Visual field changes secondary to Vigabatrin treatment. *Rev Neurol* 31: 1104–8.

Meldrum BS (1996) Update on the mechanism of action of antiepileptic drugs. *Epilepsia* 37 (suppl 6): 4–11.

Michel CM, Grave de Peralta R, Lantz G, Gonzalez S, Spinelli L, Blanke O, Landis T, Seeck M (1999) Spatiotemporal EEG analysis and distributed source estimation in presurgical epilepsy evaluation. *J Clin Neurophysiol* 16: 239–66.

Miller SP, Tasch T, Sylvain M, Farmer JP, O'Gorman AM, Shevell MI (1998) Tuberous sclerosis complex and neonatal seizures. *J Child Neurol* 13: 619–23.

Mitchell WG, Shah NS (2000) Vigabatrin (VGB) for infantile spasms: non-dose dependent response. *Epilepsia* 41(7): 187.

Murphy JV (1999) Left vagal nerve stimulation in children with medically refractory epilepsy. *J Pediatr* 134(5): 563–6.

Neville BGR, Cross HC, Boyd SG, Heyman L, Gupta S, Harkness W (2000) Surgery for epilepsy in children with tuberous sclerosis. TSC Millennium Symposium "From gene to treatment", Edinburgh, 13–15 September – Abstracts Book.

Olsen RW, Avoli M (1997) GABA and epileptogenesis. *Epilepsia* 38: 399–407.

Palmini A, Andermann F, Olivier A, Tampieri D, Robitaille Y (1991) Focal neuronal migration disorders and intractable partial epilepsy: results of surgical treatment. *Ann Neurol* 30: 750–7.

Peresson M, Lopez L, Narici L, Curatolo P (1998) Magnetic source imaging and reactivity to rhythmical stimulation in tuberous sclerosis. *Brain Dev* 20: 512–18.

Perot P, Weir B, Rasmussen T (1966) Tuberous sclerosis: surgical therapy for seizures. *Arch Neurol* 15: 498–506.

Plouin P, Dulac O, Jalin C, Chiron C (1993) Twenty-four-hour ambulatory EEG monitoring in infantile spasms. *Epilepsia* 34: 686–91.

Romanelli P, Weiner HL, Devinsky O, et al. (2001) Multiple subpial transections and bilateral resective epilepsy surgery in a child with tuberous sclerosis. International School of Neurological Sciences – XI Annual Symposium of the Child Neurology Section, p 35.

Schmidt D and Bourgeois B (2000) A risk-benefit assessment of therapies for Lennox–Gastaut syndrome. *Drug Saf* 22(6): 467–77.

Seri S, Cerquiglini A, Cusmai R, Curatolo P (1991) Tuberous sclerosis: relationships between topographic mapping EEG, VEPs and MRI findings. *Neurophysiol Clin* 21: 161–72.

Seri S, Cerquiglini A, Pascual Marqui M, Michel C, Pisani F, Curatolo P (1998) Frontal lobe epilepsy: EEG-MRI fusioning. *J Child Neurol* 13: 34–8.

Smith SS, Gong QH, Hsu F, Markowitz RS, French-Mullen JMH, Li X (1998) GABA(A) receptor alpha4 subunit suppression prevents withdrawal properties of an endogenous steroid. *Nature* 392: 926–9.

Spiegel EA, Wycis HT, Baird HW III (1958) Pallidotomy and pallidoamygdalotomy in certain types of convulsive disorders. *Arch Neurol Psychiatry* 80: 714–28.

Stephenson JPB (1988) A study of TS seizures using visual recording techniques. Tuberous Sclerosis Symposium. Nottingham, 15–16 Sept. Abstract

Thiele EA (2000) Epilepsy surgery for tuberous sclerosis patients with seizures that do not respond to medications. *Tuberous Sclerosis Alliance – Perspective* 91: 4–5.

Thiele EA, Duffy FH, Poussaint TY, Prather PA, Riviello JJ, Bourgeois BFD, Holmes GL, Black PM (2001) Intractable epilepsy and tuberous sclerosis complex: role of epilepsy surgery in the pediatric population. *J Child Neurol* 16: 681. Abstract.

Uldall P, Bucholt JM (1999) Clinical experiences with topiramate in children with intractable epilepsy. *Europ J Paediatr Neurol* 3(3): 105–11.

van Veelen CWM, Hardus P, Verduin WM, Berendschot TJM, van Rijen PC, Postma G, Stilma JS (2000) Concentric contraction of the visual field in patients with temporal lobe epilepsy using vigabatrin, long term results. *Epilepsia* 41(7): 136.

Verdecchia M, Temin P, Dorofeeva M, Di Michele F, Porfirio MC, Furnari C, Curatolo P (1998) Relationship between neurosteroid gamma-aminobutyric-acid A modulators and seizure frequency in epileptic children. *Ann Neurol* 44: 565.

Versino M, Veggiotti P (1999) Reversibility of vigabatrin-induced visual-field defect. *Lancet* 354: 486.

White R, Hua Yue, Scheithauer B, Lynch DR, Henske EP, Crino PB (2001) Selective alterations in glutamate and GABA receptor subunit mRNA expression in dysplastic neurons and giant cells of cortical tubers. *Ann Neurol* 49: 67–78.

Whittemore V (2000) Vagus nerve stimulation is it right for you? *NTSA Perspective 2000* 88: 3.

Wolf HK, Birkholz T, Wellmer J, Blumcke I, Pietsch T, Wiestler OD (1995) Neurochemical profile of glioneuronal lesions from patients with pharmacoresistant focal epilepsies. *J Neuropathol Exp Neurol* 54: 689–97.

5
INTELLECTUAL AND COGNITIVE IMPAIRMENTS

Patrick F Bolton

INTRODUCTION

Following the first descriptions of tuberous sclerosis (TSC) by Bourneville (1880), clinicians for a long time considered that learning disability was a core characteristic of the syndrome. Indeed, diagnosis was based on the presence of three features: facial angiofibroma (in those days referred to as adenoma sebaceum), epilepsy and learning disability (Vogt 1908). However, as the features of the syndrome have become better delineated and the genetic basis better understood, it has become apparent that learning disability is not an inevitable consequence of the disease, but an associated feature found in a subset of individuals. Early estimates of the prevalence of learning disability in individuals with tuberous sclerosis were primarily based on clinic populations, and so were potentially biased towards overestimating the frequency of associated intellectual impairments, simply because individuals with TSC and intellectual impairments were more likely to be referred to clinics. The results of population-based prevalence studies of learning disability in TSC are summarized in Table 5.1.

The majority of studies only attempted a crude estimation of the frequency of learning disability, relying on clinical details such as attendance at special schools, and the ability to speak, read, write and hold down a job, as the means for assessing intellectual ability. Nevertheless, these studies all confirmed that learning disability

TABLE 5.1
Recent prevalence studies of learning disability

Study	N	Learning disability (N)	Learning disability (%)
Nevin and Pearce 1968	18	12	61
Hunt and Lindenbaum 1984	69	44	69
Webb et al. 1991a	26	10	38
Shepherd and Stephenson 1992	104	58	56
Gillberg et al. 1994	28	18	64
Webb et al. 1996	131	82	63
Joinson et al., submitted-b	108	52	40

only occurs in a proportion of individuals with tuberous sclerosis and that a substantial number of people with the disease function in the normal range of ability. Several of these studies seemed to suggest that when individuals with tuberous sclerosis suffered from learning disability, it tended to be of a severe or profound form (Harrison and Bolton 1997). However, the relatively crude estimates of ability level prevented any systematic investigation of the nature of the distribution of intellectual ability in individuals with tuberous sclerosis. As a result it has been unclear, until recently, whether intellectual level was generally decreased in individuals with tuberous sclerosis, or whether there was a bimodal distribution, with a group of individuals functioning in the normal or near normal range, and another separate group functioning in the intellectually impaired range (Fig. 5.1). Clarification of this issue was important because it would potentially throw light on the mechanisms underlying the association between tuberous sclerosis and learning disability (Harrison and Bolton 1997).

Another shortcoming of the research conducted in the twentieth century concerned the absence of any comparison or control group in any of the studies reported in the literature. As a consequence, it was not possible to determine whether individuals with tuberous sclerosis, of normal ability, performed at the same or a lower level than expected on tests of intelligence, given their background and circumstances (Harrison and Bolton 1997). In addition to these uncertainties, there were some inconsistencies in reports concerning the pattern of intellectual impairments in individuals with tuberous sclerosis (Harrison and Bolton 1997). For

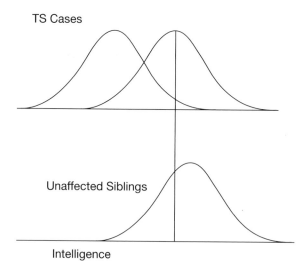

Fig. 5.1. Hypothetical bimodal distribution in intelligence in TSC cases versus unaffected sibling controls.

example, Webb et al. conducted one of the largest recent population studies of learning disability in tuberous sclerosis. They found that males were more likely to suffer from learning disability than females, and speculated that the sex differences in the risk of learning disability may derive from protective effects of factors determining female sex (Webb et al. 1996). A major limitation of this study was the reliance on a history of educational and occupational attainments and the person's level of literacy to determine whether or not a learning disability was present. Clearly, this limitation may have led to some inaccuracies in the estimation of the rates of learning disability, so a more systematic evaluation of this question was obviously necessary.

The first population-based study of tuberous sclerosis to measure intellectual level using standardized tests of intelligence was conducted by Gillberg and colleagues on a sample of 28 children with TSC from the western region of Sweden (Gillberg et al. 1994). Ten individuals (36%) had IQ scores in the normal range, seven (25%) had mild learning disability, and 11 (39%) had severe/profound learning disability. Unfortunately, the degree of disability was estimated using just the Wechsler intelligence scales, so conclusions about the form of IQ distribution in this population were limited. This is because the Wechsler scales do not estimate IQ scores below 50 (i.e. moderate, severe and profound degrees of learning disability cannot be differentiated). Moreover, the sample size was small and there was no comparison group. Nevertheless, the findings suggested that although individuals with TSC do suffer from mild forms of intellectual impairment, they tend either to be normally intelligent or to suffer from moderate to profound learning disability. Moreover, the study found no evidence for a sex difference in the rates of learning disability (Gillberg et al. 1994).

To address the inconsistencies and uncertainties in the published reports, Joinson and colleagues (Joinson et al. 2003) recently undertook detailed psychometric evaluation of all available TSC cases in the Wessex region. This sample has been serially ascertained over the last 10 to 15 years (Webb et al. 1996, O'Callaghan et al. 1998). There were 179 identified individuals with tuberous sclerosis, and it was possible to test 108 of these using standardized tests of intellectual and cognitive function and adaptive behaviour. Whenever possible, individuals were assessed using the Wechsler scales, but in the younger and more intellectually impaired individuals, IQ was estimated using the Ravens Coloured Matrices, the British Picture Vocabulary Scales, and/or the Vineland Adaptive Behaviour Scales. The assessed sub-group was no different in age, sex, rates of epilepsy and learning disability (estimated from available clinical details) from the group that it was not possible to test. As an additional element to the study design, intellectual and cognitive assessments were completed in all available unaffected siblings.

The results were striking in demonstrating a clear bimodal distribution in intellectual abilities. Around 40% of the sample had learning disability, with most of the individuals having severe or profound learning disability. The remaining 60% of cases, although functioning in the normal range, nevertheless showed a significantly lower mean IQ when compared with the unaffected siblings. Also of importance, the study found no sex differences in the rates of learning disability or in the mean level of intellectual ability. The results clearly suggested that a specific set of factors may underlie severe and profound learning disability in people with tuberous sclerosis. Consistent with this view, the rate of epilepsy, especially infantile spasms, was significantly higher in the group with severe/profound learning disability than in the normally intelligent individuals with TSC (Joinson et al. 2003).

The slightly reduced overall level of ability in the individuals with normal intelligence with TSC, when compared with their unaffected siblings, could have arisen in three main ways. First, it could reflect a general decrement in IQ arising from the effects of TSC on intellectual function (including tuber number and epilepsy). A similar downward shift in IQ has been reported, for example, in individuals with hemiplegic cerebral palsy (Goodman and Yude 1996). Second, it could have arisen from population admixture. That is, amongst those with IQ > 69 there are cases of normal ability who are no different from their siblings, and mildly affected cases (IQ 70–85, for example) who have some of the risk factors for severe/profound learning disability but who have been comparatively unscathed. Third, it might have arisen due to truncated ascertainment – that is, the tendency for more mildly affected cases to go unidentified. The possibility of truncated ascertainment has been highlighted by a study of so-called secondarily ascertained cases of tuberous sclerosis (Webb et al. 1991a). This study was conducted to overcome problems of ascertainment bias, by selecting individuals whose parents were known to have TSC before the child was born. The individuals were themselves therefore secondarily ascertained. This sample selection strategy meant that cases would be most representative of the full range of manifestations of TSC. It was noteworthy that although the overall rate of learning disability in this study was lower (38%) than in any other study, it was close to the estimated rate in the Joinson et al. study, suggesting that truncation in ascertainment may not be a factor leading to the reduced IQ in the normally intelligent individuals in the Joinson et al. study (2003). Again, however, the evaluation of the presence of learning disability was very crude and the overall sample size very small, so there remains a good deal of uncertainty about the accuracy of the estimates.

The very marked bimodal distribution in intellectual abilities in the Wessex study is consistent with findings from other reports (Shepherd and Stephenson 1992, Gillberg et al. 1994), and suggests that there may be a distinct set of factors that lead to learning disability in tuberous sclerosis. What might these factors be? One possibility concerns the nature of the genetic mutations giving rise to tuberous sclerosis. Recent reports have suggested that individuals with *TSC2* mutations may have a more severe form of tuberous sclerosis than individuals with *TSC1* mutations

(Jones et al. 1997, Dabora et al. 2001). The exact reasons why the severity of the tuberous sclerosis should be more marked in individuals with *TSC2* compared with *TSC1* remain unknown. It may be that second-hit somatic mutations occur more frequently in the *TSC2* gene or that *TSC2* mutations have a dominant negative effect. Whatever the explanation, one of the consequences would be more extensive brain involvement, which in turn is likely to lead to more severe intellectual impairments.

Although differences in the kind of genetic mutation may partly explain the bimodal distribution, it seems unlikely that these would account for the very marked bimodality observed in the Joinson et al. study. Indeed, we already know that individuals with *TSC1* mutations can have marked intellectual impairments, so what other factors might therefore serve to determine whether individuals with tuberous sclerosis develop severe/profound learning disability? Two possibilities warrant consideration. The first is that the cortical tubers and subependymal nodules, which are known to vary in number and location (Shepherd et al. 1995a), give rise to severe or profound learning disability if they are especially numerous or if they involve certain key brain regions or structures (Harrison and Bolton 1997). The second possibility is that the epilepsy which derives from the cortical and subcortical brain abnormalities may have an adverse effect on intellectual development, with the seizures leading to brain dysfunction and marked intellectual impairment, if they are very severe, frequent or of a specific kind (Harrison and Bolton 1997). Of course, the two explanations are not mutually exclusive, and some combination of the two might account for the findings. What evidence is there, however, to support either of these two principal explanations?

Improvements in brain imaging techniques, using MRI, have emerged over the last 10 to 15 years and, as a result, it has become possible to examine the relationship between the brain abnormalities and intellectual impairments in tuberous sclerosis in much greater depth than ever before. Several reports (Roach et al. 1987, Inoue et al. 1988, Jambaqué et al. 1991, Menor et al. 1992, Shepherd et al. 1995b, Bolton and Griffiths 1997) and a meta-analysis (Goodman et al. 1997) of selected studies have shown that the degree of cognitive impairment is associated with the overall number of cortical tubers. However, as the degree of intellectual impairment in these studies was usually only crudely classified, indicating whether learning disability was present or absent, it is unclear whether or not the relationship between tuber number and intellectual ability was monotonically linear. Moreover, to date, there has been very little systematic investigation of the relationship between the number of tubers in specific locations and the degree of intellectual impairment (Harrison and Bolton 1997). Recent research into the neural basis of intelligence suggests that the frontal lobes play a central role (Duncan et al. 2000). This raises the possibility that the extent of frontal involvement in tuberous sclerosis would be most closely correlated with the degree of intellectual impairment.

Advocates of the view that seizures may be important in shaping intellectual development in tuberous sclerosis point to the finding that almost all individuals with learning disability and tuberous sclerosis have a history of seizures and often present with infantile spasms (Gomez et al. 1982). They also point to cases where there was an apparently normal period of early development prior to the onset of seizures, and then an apparent regression or loss of skills. A recent examination of the role of tuber count and a history of infantile spasms in predicting intellectual level in tuberous sclerosis has been undertaken in a subset of cases who had MRI scans in the Wessex study sample. The analyses indicated that both tuber number and a history of infantile spasms independently predicted intellectual impairments (O'Callaghan et al., submitted).

At present, therefore, the roles of structural abnormalities and seizures in determining intellectual outcome remain unclear: on the basis of the current research it remains possible that either or both are relevant. Further clarification of the issue will be difficult to achieve, as the questions are best addressed by intervention studies. However, as yet there is no obviously superior treatment for infantile spasms in tuberous sclerosis, although recent studies suggest that Vigabatrin holds promise (Chiron et al. 1997, Hancock and Osborne 1999). Indeed, a recent report by Jambaqué and colleagues suggested that individuals who responded to Vigabatrin treatment for their seizures had improved developmental outcome. This lends some support to the notion that the seizures may be important in influencing intellectual development (Jambaqué et al. 2000). It must be noted, however, that treatment responsiveness in itself does not prove that the seizures were causing intellectual impairments. It might instead be that those individuals with less severe brain involvement, and hence better developmental prognoses, are more likely to respond to drug treatment for their seizures.

The findings reported to date, and especially those from the recent Wessex study (Joinson et al. 2003), provide important information for the purposes of genetic counselling and advising families about prognosis. Thus, it is clear from these investigations that the rate of learning disability is far lower than originally believed, and is roughly 40%. Importantly, it seems that individuals are most likely either to be functioning in the normal range or to have moderate to profound learning disability: the likelihood of the latter being related to genetic status, the number of cortical tubers on MRI, and a history of early-onset seizures, particularly infantile spasms (Joinson et al. 2003).

SPECIFIC COGNITIVE DEFICITS

Given the nature of the brain involvement in tuberous sclerosis, it could be predicted that normally intelligent individuals with the disease might be prone to developing specific cognitive impairments (Harrison and Bolton 1997). Jambaqué et al. conducted the first small-scale, uncontrolled, study of IQ and cognitive performance in 23 individuals with tuberous sclerosis (Jambaqué et al. 1991). Amongst the seven normally intelligent children in the clinic series, five individuals were reported to have specific developmental problems (dyspraxia; speech delay; visuo-spatial disturbance; memory impairment; dyscalculia). In addition, although not discussed, three of the five children had verbal and performance IQ estimates that showed a discrepancy of 15 or more points (Jambaqué et al. 1991). The findings provided some support for the notion that specific developmental disorders may be associated with tuberous sclerosis. However, the absence of a control group and the fact that the cases were all referred to a clinic preclude any firm conclusions.

Harrison and colleagues speculated that the heterogeneity in the nature of the brain abnormalities characterizing tuberous sclerosis would likely give rise to a range of specific cognitive impairments, rather than neuropsychological impairments of any particular kind (Harrison et al. 1999). In order to investigate this question, and to circumvent the possible biases associated with the study of clinic samples, they conducted a controlled study of the normally intelligent children, aged 5 and above, residing in the Bath district of the UK (Harrison et al. 1999). These cases had previously been identified as part of the Wessex epidemiological studies of tuberous sclerosis (Webb et al. 1991b). Unaffected siblings and spouses of individuals with tuberous sclerosis were recruited and assessed to control for non-TSC familial factors that predispose to specific cognitive disorders. The neuropsychological test battery employed was chosen to test a broad range of cognitive skills, but with a specific emphasis on tests of frontal lobe functions, as frontal lobe tubers are so commonly found in tuberous sclerosis. The principal neuropsychological tests used in the study are described in Table 5.2, and further details can be found in the original report (Harrison et al. 1999).

Sample size was small so conclusions were limited, but, nevertheless, the results showed that, as a group, individuals with tuberous sclerosis were prone to neuropsychological impairments of one form or another, when compared with their unaffected siblings or spouses (Harrison et al. 1999). On the basis of these findings, and again in recognition of the propensity of the brain abnormalities in tuberous sclerosis to involve the frontal lobes, further investigations of normally intelligent adults with tuberous sclerosis were undertaken (Bolton et al., submitted). The test battery used for this larger study was based on the tests employed in the study by Harrison et al., and included tests from the Cambridge Automated Neuropsychological Test Battery (CANTAB) (Sahakian and Owen 1992). In this larger sample of 19 cases, impairments on two subtests of the CANTAB battery were identified in the group of individuals with tuberous sclerosis compared with controls. In particular, poor performance on the spatial span subtest as well as the intra-dimensional/extra-dimensional (ID/ED) set shifting task was identified (Bolton et al., submitted). Performance on spatial span tasks is thought to depend on right temporal and ventromedial frontal structures. Previous research using the ID/ED shift task has

TABLE 5.2
Neuropsychological test battery

Controlled Word Association
This test measures verbal fluency (VF), e.g. for the letter 'B' (phonological VF), and for the category 'animals' (semantic VF). The subject is instructed to say as many words as they can think of beginning with B or that are examples of animals. Phonological VF is impaired in people with certain types of frontal brain damage, whereas semantic VF is impaired in people with temporal lobe damage (Benton 1968, Miller 1984, Hodges et al. 1992).

Hayling Sentence Completion Test
This test measures latency of completion of everyday sentences with a word missing at the end. Subjects are then tested for the ability to inhibit an automatic response and generate nonsense words to complete similar sentences (measured as an error score) (Burgess and Shallice 1996).

Mini Mental State Examination (Folstein et al. 1975)
This is a quick and broad assessment of cognitive dysfunction whose utility lies in suggesting areas of dysfunction that might then be further explored. It also functions as a test of both language reception and production, so can be used as a quick test of the subject's ability to both receive and produce linguistic information.

Raven's Advanced Progressive Matrices (Raven 1958)
This is a non-verbal test of intellect. Recent research has suggested that it is sensitive to impairments of fluid intelligence and frontal lobe damage.

The National Adult Reading Test (Nelson 1982)
This test has been shown to be a relatively robust indicator of premorbid intelligence, relying upon a correlation between vocabulary size and general intelligence.

CANTAB TESTS (Sahakian and Owen 1992)
Spatial span
This is a test analogous to the Corsi block-tapping test (Milner 1971) in that it requires subjects to monitor and recall a sequence of blocks that change colour.

Spatial working memory
This task tests a subject's ability to retain information regarding memory for locations previously visited. Errors are scored according to the number of occasions on which the subject returned to a box in which a blue token had already been found. An efficient means of completing the test is to follow a predetermined search sequence, starting with a particular box and then returning to that same box once a token has been found. This yields a 'strategy' measure, obtained by counting the number of occasions on which the subject does not begin with the previously chosen starting box. Thus a high score implies low use of strategy and a low score an effective use of strategy.

Stockings of Cambridge
This is a modified version of the Tower of London spatial planning task which allows for the measurement of both speed and accuracy of thinking.

TABLE 5.2 (*continued*)

Pattern recognition
In this task subjects are presented with two series of 12 abstract patterns and are instructed to remember them. After a five-second delay, each pattern, paired with a novel pattern, is presented in reverse order and subjects are instructed to touch the pattern they have previously seen.

Spatial recognition
In this task five squares are presented sequentially in different locations around the screen. Subsequently, in the recognition phase, each square is presented with a novel location and subjects are asked to touch the location they have previously seen a square appear in. This procedure is repeated a further three times.

ID/ED set shift
This task requires subjects to learn a series of nine two-alternative, forced-choice discriminations using feedback provided automatically by computer. Two critical stages occur within the test, one at the sixth rule change where subjects must shift to new exemplars of the most recent dimension, and a second at the eighth rule change where subjects must shift to a second dimension. This protocol provides two popularly used outcome measures, "Stages completed" and "Total errors".

suggested that patients with basal ganglia (Downes et al. 1989) or prefrontal lobe dysfunction (Owen et al. 1991) perform poorly on this task, though probably for different reasons (Owen et al. 1993). These findings are notable considering that patients with neurological disorders that do not involve fronto-striatal networks do not exhibit impaired ID/ED shift performance. So, for example, the performance of patients with temporal lobe lesions, or mild dementia of the Alzheimer type, and that of neurosurgical patients with amygdalo-hippocampectomy is comparable to the performance of neurologically normal controls. ID/ED set shifting deficits are found more consistently in patients with Huntington's than in patients with Parkinson's disease. Accordingly, Lawrence and colleagues have proposed that damage to the caudate nuclei is the likely cause of dysfunction (Lawrence et al. 1996). Both bilateral and unilateral lesions to the caudate nucleus are extremely rare, so there has been very limited opportunity to test exactly how critical this structure is for successful ID/ED shift completion. However, amongst the small number of caudate lesion studies reported, a number have suggested dysfunction on tests analogous to the ID/ED shift, specifically the Wisconsin Card Sorting Test (WCST). One study using the WCST with caudate-lesioned patients found evidence of marked impairment (Mendez et al. 1989); and, more recently, Petty and colleagues have reported a case of bilateral caudate damage where the patient's WCST deficit was so pronounced that he failed to achieve even one category and made 48 errors (Petty et al. 1996).

Taken together, the findings raise the possibility that the ID/ED set shifting impairments stem from lesions to the caudate, but why should this be so in tuberous sclerosis? Subependymal nodules are found in a large proportion of patients with TSC and these nodules are often found in the striathalamic groove, between the head of caudate and thalamus. It seems possible therefore that the ID/ED shift deficits may stem from subependymal nodules encroaching into the caudate nucleus. Clearly, such a possibility must remain speculative until the issue is studied in detail.

Another obvious line of enquiry for neuropsychology studies in tuberous sclerosis concerns the high rates of hyperactivity in children with TSC (Gillberg et al. 1994). It is well recognized that children with marked hyperactivity are prone to attentional difficulties, so the reports of frequent hyperactive behaviours in normally intelligent children with tuberous sclerosis raised the likelihood of attention impairments. De Vries and Bolton studied this in a population-based sample of individuals with tuberous sclerosis from the eastern region of the UK (de Vries and Bolton 1999). They identified 20 children with normal or near-normal intelligence, and 20 unaffected siblings. They assessed them for the presence of hyperactivity and evaluated them using the Test of Everyday Attention for Children. Results indicated that the TSC children were prone to hyperkinesis, with around 50% of the sample meeting ICD-10 criteria for a diagnosis of hyperkinetic syndrome (de Vries and Bolton 1999). All the children with hyperkinesis were impaired on the Test of Everyday Attention for Children, but, in addition, the TSC children who did not meet criteria for a diagnosis of hyperkinesis performed poorly on the attentional measures, compared with their unaffected siblings (de Vries and Bolton 1999). They seemed to have particular difficulties in the domain of sustained attention. It is not yet clear what the brain basis for these impairments might be, or indeed whether the seizure disorder or its treatment might in part underlie the attentional deficits found in these children. So, here again, further work, looking at the relationship between the brain abnormalities, seizure disorders and attentional impairments, will be required.

LANGUAGE IMPAIRMENTS

It has often been questioned whether children of normal intelligence with tuberous sclerosis may be prone to language disorders. However, the issue has not been investigated in any systematic fashion until recently. Joinson and colleagues examined the question amongst the normally intelligent individuals in the Wessex epidemiological sample (Joinson et al. submitted). There were 60 individuals with TSC and normal intelligence and 28 unaffected sibling controls, who were assessed using an interview schedule that has been devised and validated for obtaining histories of developmental abnormalities (Bolton et al. 1994, Fombonne et al. 1997). Using this schedule, 17% of the individuals with TSC were reported to have significant delays in language acquisition (no words by age 2 or phrase speech by age 3), compared with 0% in the unaffected siblings comparison group. In the subset of children in the sample, it was possible to formally test speech and language skills using the Clinical Evaluation of Language Fundamentals (revised). These assessments confirmed that the TSC children were significantly more likely to have language problems than their unaffected sibling controls (Joinson et al. submitted). The language difficulties principally involved receptive language skills, and they were sometimes accompanied by problems in social communication. Although these social communication difficulties were similar in kind to those seen in children with autism spectrum disorders, this diagnosis was given to only one of the children with language impairments.

Social communication problems have also been reported in children with idiopathic forms of receptive language disorder, where it has been questioned whether this represents a subtle partial form of autism spectrum disorder (Howlin et al. 2000, Mawhood et al. 2000). The results reported by Joinson and colleagues (Joinson et al. submitted), when considered in conjunction with the known association with TSC and autism spectrum disorders, raise similar questions that will need to be investigated in larger series and prospectively. It was also of interest that the receptive language disorders in the study by Joinson and colleagues were equally likely to occur in girls and boys. Although the numbers were too small to draw any firm conclusions, the findings do suggest that the pathophysiological mechanisms supersede any protective effects associated with being female.

EDUCATIONAL ATTAINMENTS

The association between specific cognitive impairments and TSC amongst normally intelligent individuals raises the question as to whether there are identifiable difficulties in scholastic attainment in this group. Again, this issue has not been studied to any great extent, but the question has been subject to preliminary analysis in the Wessex study (Joinson et al., in preparation). Normally intelligent individuals with TSC and their unaffected siblings were evaluated using the Wechsler Wide Scale Achievement Test, which evaluates reading, spelling and mathematical skills. The rates of disorder in the TSC individuals and their unaffected siblings were no different, suggesting that TSC does not confer a risk for specific disorders of educational attainment. Some caution in accepting this conclusion is warranted, as the number of cases was small and the rate of problems in the unaffected siblings was quite high, suggesting that perhaps siblings with educational difficulties may have been more likely to participate in the study.

CONCLUSIONS AND CLINICAL IMPLICATIONS

It is evident that early conceptualizations of the intellectual and cognitive impairments associated with TSC have had to be revised substantially in recent times. The initial view that TSC inevitably led to learning disability has now been shown to be very misleading. Current estimates suggest that learning disability occurs much less frequently than originally believed, affecting around 40% of individuals (Joinson et al. 2003). The likelihood of learning disability developing appears to be associated with the nature of the genetic mutation, the extent of brain abnormality, and the age of onset and type of seizure disorder (Goodman et al. 1997, Jones et al. 1997, Dabora et al. 2001, Joinson et al. 2003, O'Callaghan et al., submitted). The degree to which these factors jointly or independently contribute to shaping developmental outcome will have to be the subject of future research. In order to investigate these questions, prospective and longitudinal studies of a large representative population will be required. Similar considerations apply to clarifications of the range and extent of specific cognitive disorders and the delineation of the mechanisms that underlie their emergence. However, the mechanisms involved are likely to be different according to the nature of the cognitive impairment, with perhaps structural and functional disruptions to the development of different neural networks resulting in distinct, partly overlapping cognitive impairments.

It is already clear that tuberous sclerosis is proving to be a particularly informative model system for studying contemporary issues in developmental, cognitive and behavioural neuroscience. It is to be hoped that the advances made in understanding the manner in which cognitive and behavioural development may go awry in tuberous sclerosis will pave the way for the development of better, more effective treatments. The findings reviewed here provide the outline for counselling families about the risks of adverse development outcomes. They also provide some details that can be used in advising about prognosis. However, although the bare basics are now better delineated, over the next 10 years the picture, and our concepts, will have to undergo further revision as the results of ongoing and new research are assimilated.

REFERENCES

Benton AL (1968) Differential behavioural effects of frontal lobe disease. *Neuropsychologia* 6: 53.

Bolton PF, Griffiths, PD (1997) Association of tuberous sclerosis of temporal lobes with autism and atypical autism [see comments]. *Lancet* 349 (9049): 392–5.

Bolton P, Macdonald H, Pickles A, et al. (1994) A case-control family history study of autism. *Journal of Child Psychology and Psychiatry* 35: 877–900.

Bolton PF, de Vries P, Harrison J, Sahakian B, et al. (submitted) Specific cognitive deficits in tuberous sclerosis.

Bourneville DM (1880) Sclérose tubéreuse des circonvolutions cérébrales: idiotie et épilepsie hémiplégique. *Arch Neurol (Paris)* 1: 81–91.

Burgess PW, Shallice T (1996) Response suppression, initiation and strategy use following frontal lobe lesions. *Neuropsychologia* 34(4): 263–73.

Chiron C, Dumas C, Jambaqué I, et al. (1997) Randomized trial comparing vigabatrin and hydrocortisone in infantile spasms due to tuberous sclerosis. *Epilepsy Res*, 26(2): 389–95.

Dabora SL, Jóźwiak S, Franz DN, et al. (2001) Mutational analysis in a cohort of 224 tuberous sclerosis patients indicates increased severity of TSC2, compared with TSC1, disease in multiple organs. *Am J Hum Genet* 68(1): 64–80.

de Vries P, Bolton P (1999) Hyperactivitiy in tuberous sclerosis. Paper presented at the World Congress on Psychiatric Genetics, Monterey, California.

Downes JJ, Roberts AC, Sahakian BJ, et al. (1989) Impaired extra-dimensional shift performance in medicated and unmedicated Parkinson's disease: evidence for a specific attentional dysfunction. *Neuropsychologia* 27(11): 1329–43.

Duncan J, Seitz RJ, Kolodny J, et al. (2000) A neural basis for general intelligence. *Science* 289(5478): 457–60.

Folstein MF, Folstein SE, McHugh PR (1975) 'Mini Mental State' a practical method for grading the cognitive state of patients for the clinician. *J Psychiatric Res* 12: 189–98.

Fombonne E, Bolton P, Prior J, et al. (1997) A family study of autism: cognitive patterns and levels in parents and siblings. *J Child Psychol Psychiatry* 38(6): 667–83.

Gillberg IC, Gillberg C, Ahlsen G (1994) Autistic behaviour and attention deficits in tuberous sclerosis: a population-based study. *Dev Med Child Neurol* 36(1): 50–6.

Gomez MR, Kuntz NL, Westmoreland BF (1982) Tuberous sclerosis, early onset of seizures, and mental subnormality: study of discordant homozygous twins. *Neurology* 32(6): 604–11.

Goodman R, Yude C (1996) IQ and its predictors in childhood hemiplegia. *Dev Med Child Neurol* 38: 881–90.

Goodman M, Lamm SH, Engel A, et al. (1997) Cortical tuber count: a biomarker indicating neurologic severity of tuberous sclerosis complex [see comments]. *J Child Neurol* 12(2): 85–90.

Hancock E, Osborne JP (1999) Vigabatrin in the treatment of infantile spasms in tuberous sclerosis: literature review. *J Child Neurol* 14(2): 71–4.

Harrison JE, Bolton PF (1997) Annotation: tuberous sclerosis. *J Child Psychol Psychiatry*, 38(6): 603–14.

Harrison JE, O'Callaghan FJ, Hancock E, et al. (1999) Cognitive deficits in normally intelligent patients with tuberous sclerosis. *Am J Med Genet* 88(6): 642–6.

Hodges JR, Patterson K, Oxbury S, et al. (1992) Semantic dementia: progressive fluent aphasia with temporal lobe atrophy. *Brain* 115: 1783–1806.

Howlin P, Mawhood L, Rutter M (2000) Autism and developmental receptive language disorder – a follow-up comparison in early adult life. II: Social, behavioural, and psychiatric outcomes. *J Child Psychol Psychiatry* 41(5): 561–78.

Hunt A, Lindenbaum RH (1984) Tuberous sclerosis – a new estimate of prevalence within the Oxford region. *J Med Genet* 21(4): 272–7.

Inoue Y, Nakajima S, Fukuda T, et al. (1988) Magnetic resonance images of tuberous sclerosis. Further observations and clinical correlations. *Neuroradiology* 30(5): 379–84.

Jambaqué I, Cusmai R, Curatolo P, et al. (1991) Neuropsychological aspects of tuberous sclerosis in relation to epilepsy and MRI findings. *Dev Med Child Neurol* 33(8): 698–705.

Jambaqué I, Chiron C, Dumas C, et al. (2000) Mental and behavioural outcome of infantile epilepsy treated by vigabatrin in tuberous sclerosis patients. *Epilepsy Res* 38(2–3): 151–60.

Joinson C, O'Callaghan F, Osborne J, et al. (2003) Learning disability and epilepsy in an epidemiological sample of individuals with tuberous sclerosis complex. *Psychol Medicine* 33: 335–44.

Joinson C, O'Callaghan F, Osborne J, et al. (in preparation) Specific cognitive deficits in an epidemiological sample of individuals with tuberous sclerosis complex and normal intelligence.

Joinson C, O'Callaghan F, Osborne J, et al. (submitted) Language impairments in an epidemiological sample of individuals with tuberous sclerosis complex and normal intelligence.

Jones AC, Daniells CE, Snell RG, et al. (1997) Molecular genetic and phenotypic analysis reveals differences between TSC1 and TSC2 associated familial and sporadic tuberous sclerosis. *Hum Mol Genet* 6(12): 2155–61.

Lawrence AD, Sahakian BJ, Hodges JR, et al. (1996) Executive and mnemonic functions in early Huntington's disease. *Brain* 119 (pt 5): 1633–45.

Mawhood L, Howlin P, Rutter M (2000) Autism and developmental receptive language disorder – a comparative follow-up in early adult life. I: Cognitive and language outcomes. *J Child Psychol Psychiatry* 41(5): 547–59.

Mendez MF, Adams NL, Lewandowski KS (1989) Neurobehavioral changes associated with caudate lesions. *Neurology* 39(3): 349–54.

Menor F, Marti-Bonmati L, Mulas F, et al. (1992) Neuroimaging in tuberous sclerosis: a clinicoradiological evaluation in pediatric patients. *Pediatr Radiol* 22(7): 485–9.

Miller E (1984) Verbal fluency as a function of a measure of verbal intelligence and in relation to different types of cerebral pathology. *Br J Clin Psychol* 23: 53–7.

Milner B (1971) Interhemispheric differences in the localisation of psychological processes in man. *Br Med Bull* 27: 272–7.

Nelson H (1982) *National Adult Reading Test*. Windsor: NFER-Nelson.

Nevin NC, Pearce WG (1968) Diagnostic and genetical aspects of tuberous sclerosis. *J Med Genet* 5(4): 273–80.

O'Callaghan FJ, Shiell AW, Osborne JP, et al. (1998) Prevalence of tuberous sclerosis estimated by capture-recapture analysis [letter] [see comments]. *Lancet* 351(9114): 1490.

O'Callaghan F, Joinson C, Bolton P, et al. (submitted) Evidence that in tuberous sclerosis infantile spasms are associated with learning disability independently of the effect of cortical tuber count.

Owen AM, Roberts AC, Polkey CE, et al. (1991) Extra-dimensional versus intra-dimensional set shifting performance following frontal lobe excisions, temporal lobe excisions or amygdalo-hippocampectomy in man. *Neuropsychologia* 29(10): 993–1006.

Owen AM, Roberts AC, Hodges JR, et al. (1993) Contrasting mechanisms of impaired attentional set-shifting in patients with frontal lobe damage or Parkinson's disease. *Brain* 116 (pt 5): 1159–75.

Petty RG, Bonner D, Mouratoglou V, et al. (1996) Acute frontal lobe syndrome and dyscontrol associated with bilateral caudate nucleus infarctions. *Br J Psychiatry* 168(2): 237–40.

Raven JC (1958) *Advanced Progressive Matrices*. London: HK Lewis & Co.

Roach ES, Williams DP, Laster DW (1987) Magnetic resonance imaging in tuberous sclerosis. *Arch Neurol* 44(3): 301–3.

Sahakian BJ, Owen AM (1992) Computerized assessment in neuropsychiatry using CANTAB: discussion paper. *J Royal Soc Med* 85: 399–401.

Shepherd CW, Stephenson JBP (1992) Seizures and intellectual disability associated with tuberous sclerosis complex in the west of Scotland. *Dev Med Child Neurol* 34(9): 766–74.

Shepherd CW, Houser OW, Gomez MR (1995a) Magnetic-resonance-imaging in tuberous sclerosis complex. *Epilepsia* 36 (suppl 3): S245–S245.

Shepherd CW, Houser OW, Gomez MR (1995b) MR findings in tuberous sclerosis complex and correlation with seizure development and mental impairment. *Am J Neuroradiol* 16: 149–55.

Vogt H (1908) Zur diagnostik der tuberosen Sklerose. *Z. Erforsh, Behandl, jugendl, Schwachsinns* 2: 1–12.

Webb DW, Fryer AE, Osborne JP (1991a) On the incidence of fits and mental retardation in tuberous sclerosis. *J Med Genet* 28: 395–7.

Webb DW, Thomson JL, Osborne JP (1991b) Cranial magnetic resonance imaging in patients with tuberous sclerosis and normal intellect. *Arch Dis Child* 66(12): 1375–7.

Webb DW, Fryer AE, Osborne JP (1996) Morbidity associated with tuberous sclerosis: a population study. *Dev Med Child Neurol* 38: 146–55.

6
AUTISM

Michael Dowling and Paolo Curatolo

Autism is one of the most devastating of the behavioural disorders, characterized by a trio of repetitive stereotyped behaviours, impairment in social interaction and impairment in communication. There is recent evidence for a strong genetic component to autism, with a high concordance in monozygotic twins, a low concordance in dizygotic twins and a 3–7% recurrence risk in families with primary autism. This recurrence risk, which is lower than the 25 to 50% risk expected for simple Mendelian inheritance, in conjunction with the twin data, suggests that autism is a genetically heterogeneous multigenic disorder, due to the additive and epistatic effect of many different genes and a modest environmental component. Prevalence estimates range from 0.4 to 2 per 1000 children, with a strong and as yet unexplained male preponderance (2.5 to 4:1).

In 1932, Critchley and Earl described autistic behaviours in tuberous sclerosis patients 11 years before Kanner's classic paper describing early infantile autism. They observed that "the essential feature of the psychology of epyloia is a combination of intellectual defect with a primitive form of psychosis. The intellectual defect is always pronounced . . . the psychosis always resembles a primitive form of catatonic schizophrenia . . . the depth of psychosis is independent of the degree of intellectual defects, although the two processes are so inextricably intertwined as to render impossible any accurate estimation of the part played by either in any given case" (Critchley and Earl 1932: 320). "All manner of bizarre attitudes and stereotyped movements occur and these are most striking in the hands and fingers. . . . These movements appear to have some significance for the patients; they occur when the appearance of dissociation is most marked and the eyes usually fixate the moving hand. The patients grow solitary, silent and apathetic and liable to sudden brief outburst of motiveless excitement" (ibid.: 321). But it was not until nearly a century after Bourneville's original description of tuberous sclerosis complex (TSC) (1880) that it became apparent that there was a high frequency of autistic behaviour in patients with TSC (Riikonen and Amnell 1981, Hunt and Shepherd 1993).

EPIDEMIOLOGICAL STUDIES
Simple calculation of the expected frequency of autism in TSC, if the two are independently occurring conditions, given the individual prevalence rates of 2/1000 and 1/6000 respectively, makes it unlikely that there would be many patients

identified with both disorders. The percentage of autistic children who also have
TSC is not known. However, in a study of over 300,000 French schoolchildren,
Fombonne et al. (1997) identified 174 children with autism and found that 1.1% of
these autistic children were also afflicted with TSC.

This percentage is probably an underestimation because not all autistic children
are usually examined in order to detect signs for diagnosing TSC. Different studies
have shown that 3 to 4% of autistic subjects may have TSC. Conversely, studies of
TSC patients have identified much higher rates of autism, ranging from 17% to as
high as 61%. These studies are summarized in Table 6.1.

After early identification of the coincidence of the disorders noted in
numerous case studies, Hunt and Dennis (1987) published a systematic study of
psychological problems in children with TSC. Their analysis was based on a 321-
item interview including a specific 13-item questionnaire focusing on autistic
behaviours such as object attachment, social interactions, etc., with a score of 7/13
assigned as a cut-off score defining autism. In this study, half of the 90 TSC patients

TABLE 6.1
Frequency and demographic characteristics of autism in tuberous sclerosis

Authors	N of TSC patients	N of patients with autism	% with autism	M:F	Assessment
Hunt and Dennis 1987	90	45	50%	24:22	Hunt and Dennis questionnaire
Riikonen and Simell 1990	24	4	17%		
Curatolo et al. 1991	23	6	26%		Hunt and Dennis questionnaire
Smalley et al. 1992	13	7	54%	5:2	ADI
Hunt and Shepherd 1993	21	5	24%	3:2	Hunt and Dennis questionnaire
Gillberg et al. 1994	28	17	61%	7:10	CARS, DSM-IIIR
Calderon et al. 1994	27	7	26%	2:5	DSM-IIIR criteria
Webb et al. 1996	131	6	5%		Hunt and Dennis questionnaire
Bolton and Griffiths 1997	18	9	50%		ICD-10 criteria
Baker et al. 1998	20	4	20%	3:1	ABC, ADI Direct exam
Gutierrez et al. 1998	28	8	29%	1:1	ADI, ADI-R, ADOS for conf.

met their criteria for autism. All of the TSC patients identified as autistic were also identified as having learning disability, and 40/45 had a history of infantile spasms. Subsequent authors, including Curatolo and co-workers (1991), who identified autism in 6 out of 23 patients (26%) with TSC, used the same diagnostic questionnaire. All six had severe learning disability, with IQ < 40. Curatolo et al. extended the epidemiological study to include analysis of imaging results, which will be discussed further below. A similar incidence (24%) was noted by Hunt and Shepherd (1993), using the same questionnaire in a careful study specifically designed to determine the prevalence of autism in children aged 3 to 11 years born in the west of Scotland.

A standardized interview, the Autism Diagnostic Interview (ADI) or the Autism Behavior Checklist, with direct examination, was used in more recent studies (Le Couteur et al. 1989). Using the ADI, 7 out of 13 TSC patients (54%) were found to be autistic by Smalley and co-workers (1992). In a subsequent study by the same group, with an expansion on their original TSC population of 13 to 28 patients, only 8 patients (29%) were identified with autism by revised ADI criteria with the addition of a confirmatory direct observation interview (Gutierrez et al. 1998). It is unclear whether the difference between these two studies (54% vs. 29%) is due to the more stringent criteria for autism, or simply due to the small number of patients or the possible identification and enrolment of less severely affected patients over time.

An incidence in the same range (20%) was also identified using the ABC and ADI (Baker et al. 1998), while investigations applying DSM-IIIR or ICD-10 criteria found incidences of autism in TSC of 26%, 50%, or as high as 61% (Calderon et al. 1994, Gillberg et al. 1994, Bolton and Griffiths 1997). The highest incidence of 61% noted by Gillberg and co-workers may be due to a lower threshold for the diagnosis of autism in their population. In their report they note that, in addition to the 17 patients identified with autism, an additional six cases exhibited autistic-like conditions and one patient was identified with Asperger syndrome, giving a total of 24 cases of autistic spectrum disorders out of 28 patients. The lowest frequency (5%) may also be misleading. Webb and his co-workers (1996) studied a population of 131 TSC patients, but the original Hunt and Dennis autism questionnaire was only applied to the 26 children with learning disorders and behaviour problems, identifying six patients with autism.

A review of the sex ratios for autistic patients is revealing, with the smaller studies demonstrating a male or female predominance, but the larger studies showing an approximately 1:1 ratio. When pooling the data from all seven studies where a sex ratio is reported, the pooled numbers are very close to 1:1, clearly different from the male preponderance (2.5 to 4:1) well known from general studies of autism. No sex-related differences have been reported for the neurologic, dermatologic, or other manifestations of TSC.

Despite the differences in TSC populations and diagnostic criteria for autism, these studies, as a whole, reveal that a significant proportion of TSC patients exhibit distinct symptomatology of autism. The pathogenesis of autism in TSC is still largely unknown and many different hypotheses can be raised. In patients with tuberous sclerosis, autism or autistic behaviour could be a consequence of: (1) the location of the cortical or subcortical tubers; (2) a generalized defect in brain development; (3) a spectrum of behaviours associated with learning disability; (4) the effects of seizures and/or EEG abnormalities (see also Chapter 8). An alternative explanation is that this typical pattern of autistic behaviour seen in TSC reflects more direct effects of an abnormal genetic program. This could open a path for the study and treatment of biological bases of behaviour, a current focus of neurosciences.

LOCALIZATION OF CORTICAL TUBERS IN ASSOCIATIVE AREAS
Neuroimaging studies in autistic patients have failed to identify any underlying abnormalities, with the exception of an association with larger brain volumes in autistic children, corresponding to the observed larger head circumference (without frank macrocephaly). Other studies have attempted the classical neurologic localization of function by studying patients with acquired autistic behaviours after stroke or localized brain injury, with limited success. Other neuropathologic studies have implicated the temporal lobes, limbic system, or the cerebellum (reviewed in Bauman and Kemper 1985, Bachevalier 1994, Courchesne et al. 1994, Rapin and Katzman 1998). Because of the presence of easily identifiable cortical lesions in TSC, several studies of autism in TSC have attempted to correlate the behavioural disorder with the location of cortical tubers.

Curatolo and co-workers (1991) found evidence suggesting that two subpopulations existed. Patients with TSC and autism with early onset (before age 2) presented prevalent parietotemporal cortical lesions, while those with later onset (3 to 5 years) had both frontal and posterior tubers. In their study of 23 patients the greatest correlation was with tuber number, rather than localization: 5 of the 6 autistic patients had more than 8 tubers while only 6 of the 17 nonautistic patients had more than 8 tubers.

Bolton and Griffiths (1997) found a very strong association between temporal lobe tubers and autism. In their study of 18 TSC patients, temporal lobe tubers were found in 8 out of 9 autistic patients, but were not found in any of the 9 nonautistic patients. In the autistic patients, the lateralization of the temporal tubers was on the left for three patients, on the right for four, with bilateral temporal tubers for the remaining two. Overall, the autistic patients had more tubers (mean of six tubers for autistic vs. two for nonautistic subjects). In tuberous sclerosis patients overall, the number of cortical tubers is greatest in the frontal lobes, followed by the parietal, temporal, cerebellar and occipital lobes. Bolton and Griffiths noted that, as a group, their patients demonstrated the same distribution of tubers. This accentuates the

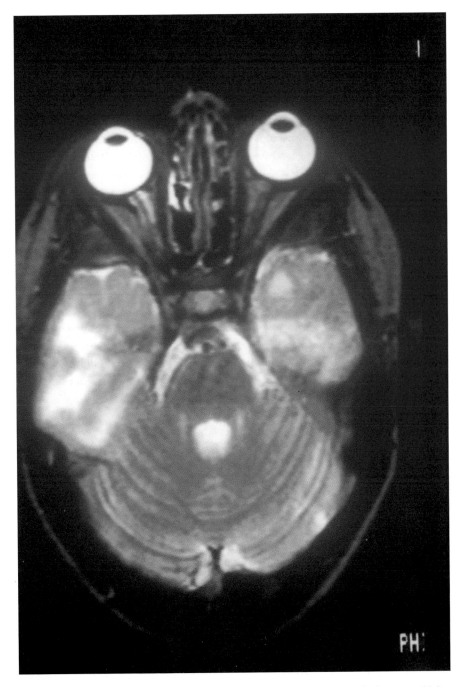

Fig. 6.1. Axial magnetic resonance imaging showing large cortical tubers in both temporal lobes in a 4-year-old boy with autism.

significance of their findings of a correlation of the less common temporal lobe tubers with autism. One limitation of their study was the mixed use of CT and MRI, which may have underestimated tubers in patients investigated with CT imaging only.

In another recent study of 14 children with TSC, all studied by MRI and brain-stem auditory evoked potentials, Seri and co-workers (1999) found that all seven of the autistic patients had temporal lobe lesions (Fig. 6.1), while none of the seven nonautistic patients had temporal lobe lesions. Further, they identified abnormalities in auditory evoked potentials, which were present only in the autistic patients. The total lesion burden was 39 for the autistic and 38 for the nonautistic patients, indicating a comparable severity of CNS involvement between the two groups.

In contrast to these studies implicating the temporal lobe lesions with autism in TSC, Baker and co-workers (1998) found no temporal lesions in the four autistic patients identified in their study of 20 TSC patients. However, both CT and MRI were used and, again, temporal lobe lesions may have been overlooked on CT.

Another recent study of 29 TSC patients examined by MRI and a battery of neuropsychological tests, including the CARS (Childhood Autism Rating Scale), found no relation between CARS scores and the total number of lesions or the localization of tubers in the cerebrum. However, they found that patients with more cerebellar tubers had higher (more autistic) CARS scores (Weber et al. 2000). In this study, IQ was negatively correlated with tuber number. Interestingly, despite the increased incidence of autistic features in patients with learning disability, comparison of autistic patients to others revealed no differences in total tuber number, IQ, or location of other tubers. CARS scores in the autistic range were dependent only on the presence or absence of cerebellar tubers.

The discrepancies in the above studies, favouring temporal versus cerebellar lesions, are difficult to explain. However, many of the earlier studies of tuber local-ization were at least partly CT-based, with the possibility of underestimation of cerebellar lesions due to limitations of CT in imaging the posterior fossa. For example, Bolton and Griffiths' (1997) study included 18 patients, with six imaged with CT only. They did analyse for cerebellar as well as temporal tubers. In this study, cerebellar tubers were identified in 3 out of 9 TSC patients with autism vs. only 1 out of 9 TSC patients without autism. On the other hand, the analysis in Baker's group did not include an evaluation of cerebellar lesions at all. What is clear is that the analysis of tuber localization by number or simply by lobe or hemisphere is too crude and ignores the fact that there are widespread reciprocal connections between the cerebellum and cortical and subcortical structures. These tuber-specific structure/function studies may overlook the underlying nature of TSC as a more global disorder of cellular proliferation, migration and differentiation in the developing brain.

Recent molecular studies suggest that hamartin and tuberin are involved even earlier in neural development. *TSC2* expression is observed in nine-day mouse embryos and in neuroblastoma cell lines; tuberin expression is upregulated by induction of neuronal differentiation. Antisense inhibition of tuberin expression may inhibit this neuronal differentiation (Soucek et al. 1998). Perhaps the autistic features seen in TSC could be due to a more subtle disordered early neuronal differentiation and proliferation, more akin to that suggested by multiple studies of "primary" autism (Rapin and Katzman 1998).

Co-immunoprecipitation and studies using the yeast two-hybrid system suggest that hamartin and tuberin interact (van Slegtenhorst et al. 1998). It is likely that they form a complex which functions to control cell growth and differentiation, perhaps though the GTPase activating properties demonstrated for tuberin, which may explain their apparent tumor suppressor properties (Wienecke et al. 1995). Pathological studies suggest that during the proliferative phase of development in TSC, an abnormal population is formed at the germinal matrix which fails to show normal differentiation, forming the so-called "neuroastrocytes" which give rise to subependymal nodules and giant cell astrocytomas. Some of these cells show abnormal migration, forming heterotopias in the subcortical white matter, while others migrate to the cortical plate where they form aggregates of dysplastic cortex, the cortical tubers.

Both the severity of the underlying genetic mutation and the timing of loss of heterozygosity at the wild type allele are thus likely to be critical in determining the severity and extent of the structural abnormality. Often, several of the pathologic abnormalities in TSC are found in a contiguous abnormal wedge of tissue extending from the subependymal zone to the cerebral cortex, including subependymal nodules, white matter heterotopias and cortical tubers. Thus, in autistic TSC patients, attempts to localize functional deficits based on the distribution of cortical tubers may be complicated by the variable extent of the underlying, more subtle and more widespread subcortical lesion.

COMORBIDITY

The variable cerebral pathology of TSC results in a similarly variable neurologic phenotype. Learning disability is a common feature of TSC, with approximately 50% of patients with moderate to profound impairment (Jóźwiak et al. 1998). Patients with fewer than five tubers had considerable variation in cognitive function, while those with 10 or more lesions were severely impaired (Roach et al. 1987). Goodman et al. (1997), in a meta-analysis, demonstrated a positive linear relationship between total tuber number and degree of intellectual impairment.

The high incidence of learning disability in patients with TSC may cloud studies of autism. Several of the epidemiologic studies of autism in TSC have suggested associations between learning disability and autism. Hunt and Dennis (1987) found that all of their autistic patients had learning disability. Other studies have also identified learning disability as a significant risk factor for autism in TSC patients. However, learning disability, by itself, is not sufficient to account for all cases; patients with intellectual impairment from other causes, such as cerebral palsy or Down syndrome, do not have a similarly increased risk of autism (Wing and Gould 1979). Despite the increased risk in TSC, autism has been identified in TSC patients without significant intellectual impairment. In 17 patients identified as autistic, 14 had learning disability – 7 severe (IQ < 50), 7 mild (IQ 51–70) – and 3 had near normal intelligence (IQ 71–84) (Gillberg et al. 1994). This group also included a patient with Asperger syndrome with normal intelligence. Similarly, Bolton and Griffiths (1997) found that 2 out of 9 of their autistic patients had normal intelligence.

The complexity of these issues is well demonstrated by the results of a study of cognitive deficits in TSC patients with normal intelligence (Harrison et al. 1999). A group of seven TSC patients with IQs in the normal range (mean 99) underwent an extensive battery of neuropsychological tests. Using the 5th percentile as a cut-off for all these tests, only two of the seven patients were within the normal range in all subtests. Interestingly one of these "normal" patients had four tubers and had recently undergone surgical removal of a subependymal giant cell astrocytoma. The second had four tubers of more than 1.5 cm. A third patient scored below the 5th percentile in only one of the 15 subtests and she had nine tubers and several subependymal nodules. These three patients all also had a history of epilepsy, unlike the other four patients evaluated. Thus, while tuber number may correlate with learning disability, normal cognitive function is compatible with extensive cerebral involvement and seizures as well.

EPILEPTIC PATHWAYS TO AUTISM IN TSC

In population studies of autism, seizures occur at an increased frequency, with recurrent seizures in up to one-third of all autistic patients (Olsson et al. 1988). Wong (1993) undertook a prospective study of the prevalence of epilepsy in 246 children with autistic spectrum disorders, comparing them to children with developmental dysphasia and Down syndrome. She found a 6.5% prevalence for epilepsy in the autistic children, with no seizures observed in the other groups, with onset of the seizures predating diagnosis of autism in all but one patient.

Other studies have noted that children with autistic spectrum disorders without seizures have an increased incidence of abnormal EEGs. Epileptiform EEGs were noted in 15–20% of autistic children without history of clinical seizures (Tuchman and Rapin 1997). Prolonged video-EEG studies of children with autism and regression reveal epileptiform EEGs in 46% (Tuchman and Rapin 1997), and a recent magnetoelectroencephalography study of children with autism and regression identified epileptiform activity in 82% (Lewine et al. 1999). What remains unclear is whether seizures or epileptiform discharges have an effect on cognitive function that results in autistic behaviour, or whether those discharges or seizures are the result of the same underlying pathology that gives rise to autism (Tuchman 2000).

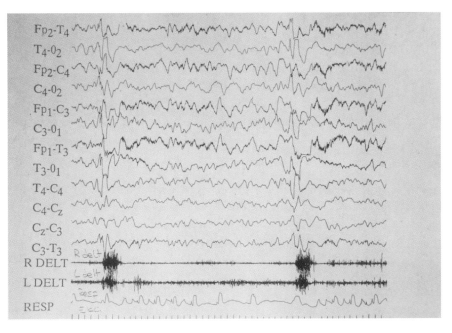

Fig. 6.2. Ictal EEG showing epileptic spasms in a child with subsequent autism.

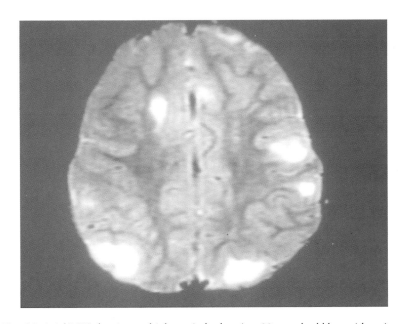

Fig. 6.3. Axial MRI showing multiple cortical tubers in a 20-month-old boy with autism.

Epilepsy is a common sequel of TSC, affecting up to 92% of patients (Gomez 1998). Like learning disability, epilepsy has been identified as a risk factor for autism in TSC. Several of the epidemiological studies reviewed earlier suggest an increased incidence of autism in TSC patients with epilepsy, with infantile spasms apparently presenting a greater risk (Curatolo and Cusmai 1987) (Figs 6.2, 6.3). Hunt and Dennis (1987) found that 40 out of 69 patients (58%) with infantile spasms had autism, while 5 out of 21 patients without infantile spasms had autism. Overall, among autistic patients, 40 out of 45 had a history of infantile spasms. Similar increased rates of infantile spasms (IS) among autistic TSC patients are seen in other studies: IS in 5 out of 6 autistic patients but also in 9 out of 17 nonautistic patients (Curatolo et al. 1991); IS in 3 out of 5 autistic patients but also in 4 out of 16 nonautistic patients (Hunt and Shepherd 1993); and IS in 11 out of 17 autistic patients but also in 5 out of 11 nonautistic patients (Gillberg et al. 1994).

Gutierrez et al. (1998) also concluded that infantile spasms were a risk factor for autism in TSC patients, but that the presence of other types of seizures, and their severity or control, were not important contributing factors to autism. The high incidence of infantile spasms in nonautistic patients and the large number of autistic TSC patients without infantile spasms suggest that there is not a causative link between infantile spasms and autism. Rather, as with learning disability, discussed above, it is the nature and severity of the underlying pathology which predisposes patients independently to both infantile spasms and autism.

In a study of tuberous sclerosis and infantile spasms, Riikonen and Simell (1990) noted that of 241 children presenting with infantile spasms, 24 had TSC. Of these 24 TSC patients, only four had autism. A fifth patient was reported as having other behaviour problems (poor contact with other children and extreme shyness). All of these 24 children had below normal intelligence (IQ < 85), and only one was seizure-free at follow-up 2.5–19 years later). In this study focusing only on TSC patients with infantile spasms, the incidence of autism (maximum of 5 out of 24) is no greater, and actually lower, than that noted in most of the studies of autism in TSC reviewed earlier. Thus this study does not support a causal role for infantile spasms in autism in TSC patients.

Another study focusing on psychiatric disorders in children with earlier infantile spasms found 24 cases of autism among 192 patients with infantile spasms (Riikonen and Amnell 1981). In this population, aetiological factors for infantile spasms were identified as brain malformations, birth injuries, early infections, familial disorders, and, for eight patients, tuberous sclerosis. Two of these eight TSC patients were identified as autistic. The incidence of autism in the non-TSC group, 22 out of 184 with infantile spasms, is lower than in most studies of the incidence of autism in TSC, suggesting again that, while infantile spasms may be a risk factor, there may be some other aspect of TSC, other than infantile spasms alone, predisposing to autism or autistic behaviour.

OUTCOME OF EPILEPSY INTERVENTION ON COGNITIVE/ BEHAVIOURAL DEVELOPMENT

If seizures or even epileptiform discharges contribute to or are causal for autism, then, presumably, treatment with antiepileptic medications or surgery may improve outcomes. There have been no controlled clinical trials addressing these issues. Tuchman (2000) reviewed the data on children with autistic spectrum disorders with abnormal EEGs both with and without clinical seizures. He emphasized that only anecdotal evidence supports the use of antiepileptic medications in patients without clinical seizures, and cautioned that there was no current justification for epilepsy surgery in children with autism or autistic regression with EEG abnormalities, in the absence of intractable epilepsy.

Deonna and colleagues (1993) reported two cases of "autistic regression" in patients with tuberous sclerosis with either seizures or EEG abnormalities. In one patient, early development was normal, with autistic behaviour coincident with seizures beginning at 13 months. His behaviour steadily improved after his seizures were controlled with medication. The second patient suffered a severe regression of cognitive function and showed autistic behaviour at 22 months. He was treated with antiepileptic medications without clear evidence of seizures and with a normal EEG, but did not improve. At 3.5 years his EEGs revealed a very active frontal spike focus during sleep, but despite further treatment with antiepileptic medications he made minimal cognitive progress.

The remarkably high response rate (80–100%) to Vigabatrin in TSC patients with infantile spasms presented an opportunity to determine whether controlling IS could affect cognitive and behavioural outcomes and prevent the development of autistic behaviour (Chiron et al. 1990). In seven TSC patients with IS, all responded to Vigabatrin with cessation of spasms, but five continued to have rare partial seizures. Six of the seven patients had dramatic increases in developmental quotients from 10 to 45 points, and autistic behaviours were noted to disappear in five of the six IS patients who had autism (Jambaqué et al. 2000). In contrast, six other TSC patients without IS who had partial seizures were also treated with Vigabatrin. In this partial seizure group, five of the six continued to have rare seizures but their developmental quotients were unchanged. Only one patient in the partial seizure group was noted to be autistic at Vigabatrin initiation. His behaviour and development quotient (< 30) were unchanged by Vigabatrin. This study suggests that early effective control of IS may lead to improved cognitive and behavioural outcomes.

Vigabatrin is believed to act via increased GABA concentrations due to its irreversible inhibition of GABA transaminase. The authors of the above study note that any specific effect of the drug on cognition could be ruled out since patients in both the IS and partial seizure group received the same medication and the patients in the partial seizure group had no significant change in cognitive status. However, the patients in the IS group were younger than those in the partial seizure

group. Infantile spasms occur in younger patients, at a time of active CNS development when the differential effects of increased GABA levels, on both seizure control
and development, are unclear. It is also possible that there is a more direct relationship between GABA and autistic behaviour in TSC, as hypothesized by Gutierrez
et al. (1998).

In a recent study on behavioural and cognitive outcome in TSC infants treated
by Vigabatrin for early seizures, Jambaqué et al. (2000) hypothesized that the significant improvement of cognition and behaviour observed after Vigabatrin treatment
may be due to the control of the secondary generalization induced by infantile
spasms. This control seems to be a key factor for both cognitive and behavioural
outcome.

Unfortunately in recent years there have been reports of the appearance of visual
field defects following Vigabatrin treatment (see also Chapter 4).

IS AUTISM A DIRECT EFFECT OF THE ABNORMAL GENETIC PROGRAM?

The *TSC2* gene was originally identified in linkage studies because of a fortuitous
contiguous gene syndrome. A family was identified with both TSC and polycystic
kidney disease. The mother and her daughter both suffered from polycystic kidney
disease and carried a balanced chromosomal translocation involving 16p13.3. They
both had no evidence of TSC, but the other child, a boy, had severe learning
disability, with seizures, and repetitive autistic behaviours. On examination, he had
facial angiofibromatosis, hypopigmented macules, with subependymal calcifications
noted by head CT, and multiple cysts detected by renal ultrasound. He carried the
unbalanced karyotype with a deletion of the distal end of chromosome 16p, implying
a close linkage of the two genes. Further analysis revealed that the genes for tuberous
sclerosis (*TSC2*) and the gene for polycystic kidney disease (*PKD1*) are only 60 base
pairs apart. Interestingly, this patient, with a large deletion, is also described as being
autistic. Perhaps the deletion in the gene-rich region of chromosome 16p13.3 also
includes another gene important for the development of autism.

Smalley et al. (1994) investigated psychiatric and behavioural disorders,
including autism and pervasive developmental disorder, in a single kindred with
a known *TSC2* mutation. They found that, within this family, individuals with TSC
had a significantly higher incidence of anxiety disorders than family members
without TSC, and suggested that anxiety disorders may be a manifestation of *TSC2*
mutations. They also point out that anxiety disorders have been shown to be
clustered in relatives of autistic patients as well, suggesting that a gene predisposing
to autism may be linked to the *TSC2* gene.

In a later study, Gutierrez et al. (1998) compared the rates of anxiety disorders
among first-degree relatives of 10 TSC patients with autism or pervasive developmental disorder (PDD) vs. 12 TSC patients without behavioural abnormalities.

They found increased rates of social phobia in family members of the autistic/PDD TSC patients, again suggesting a possible linked genetic locus involving behavioural anomalies, independent of TSC itself. In this latter study the genotype – i.e. whether the 22 probands studied carried a mutation at the *TSC1* or *TSC2* locus – was not determined. Reanalysis of these groups once their genotype is determined may provide further evidence linking behavioural abnormalities to the *TSC2* locus.

In a comprehensive genotype/phenotype analysis of 150 families, mutations were characterized in 120 families (Jones et al. 1997). In addition to finding that *TSC1* mutations were significantly under-represented in sporadic cases, compared with *TSC2* mutations, intellectual disability was found to be significantly more frequent among sporadic cases with *TSC2* mutations than among those with *TSC1* mutations. In this study, intellectual disability was very broadly defined as a developmental quotient of <70, or on the basis of the impossibility of mainstream schooling, or, for adults, institutionalization or requirement for supervision in the community. Intellectual disability was reported in 59 out of 88 *TSC2* mutations (67%) vs. 4 out of 13 *TSC1* mutations (31%). The observed increased severity of mutations at the *TSC2* locus may, as Jones et al. suggested, be due to some role of tuberin (the *TSC2* gene product). However, the number and location of tubers, the presence of seizures, or specific behaviour phenotypes, such as autism, were not defined in the study, making impossible the genotype/phenotype analysis of autistic behaviours in TSC.

At present, other than these intriguing studies, there are no data linking autistic behaviour in TSC with the *TSC2* locus. Analysis of a large number of familial and sporadic cases of TSC revealed that *TSC2* mutations are both more frequent and more likely to involve large rearrangements, including deletions, than the *TSC1* locus (Jones et al. 1997, Sampson et al. 1997). Mosaicism for deletions of the *TSC2/ PKD1* locus has also been detected frequently, indicating that this may be a recombination hot-spot. There are no reports of autism occurring in the setting of polycystic kidney disease without TSC (Sampson et al. 1997).

Recently the terminal 2 megabases of the short arm of human 16 have been sequenced (Daniels et al. 2001). This region contains the *TSC2* locus and there is linkage evidence for bipolar affective disorder and epilepsy, as well as for autism, in this same area. A locus of susceptibility to autism has been identified in the 16p13.3 chromosomal region (Philippe et al. 1999). Meanwhile, the mutations in *TSC1* and *TSC2* have been identified for several hundred TSC patients. What is now needed is the behavioural assessment of these patients, to determine if there is an association between one of the two TSC loci and autism, or, more specifically, between large deletions at these loci and autism. Thus, the answers to some of these questions are at hand.

TREATMENT

Treatment for both autism and tuberous sclerosis requires a multidisciplinary, comprehensive and individualized approach. In addition to the routine screening of the TSC population for cardiac, renal and other organ system involvement, the high incidence of autism and other behavioural problems necessitates neuropsychiatric evaluation (Curatolo et al. 2002). A full discussion of the treatment of autism is beyond the scope of this review, but early and intensive intervention with a highly structured environment supplemented with appropriate psychotropic medications can be very beneficial (Rapin 1997).

Treatment in children with TSC and pervasive developmental disorders is difficult and time-consuming. Home-based approaches to autism and TSC may be beneficial to both the child and his/her family. Parents should be regarded as co-therapists. All parents need to receive as much education as possible about autism and TSC. Parents and professionals should try their best to encourage social interaction between TSC children and peers. Both speech therapy and social skills training could be beneficial, and the first step should be to improve the clinical setting and to assist the child to optimize communication skills and adaptive behaviours.

In children with specific behaviour problems, psychopharmacology has a clear role. Unfortunately we do not at the moment have a specific drug treatment to improve communication and learning. However, the major goals of drug therapy could be to act on target symptoms, such as aggressiveness, obsessions, compulsive behaviour and hyperactivity.

Children with persistent seizures should be closely monitored in order to evaluate possible drug interaction and the risk of an increase of seizure frequency. It is well known that clomipramine, bupropion, chlorpromazine and clozapine may lower the seizures threshold. The child with prominent compulsive and ritualistic behaviour may largely benefit from serotonin-reuptake-inhibitors, such as Fluoxetine and Sertraline. Haloperidol may cause a reduction of the aggressiveness, hyperactivity and repetitive behaviours. However, lethargy and extrapyramidal movement disorders are the main drawbacks. Risperidone is a new antipsychotic agent with high affinity for the serotonin type 2 and dopamine type 2 receptors. Somnolence is a commonly reported adverse event associated with Risperidone treatment.

Antiepileptic drugs can also provide indirect benefits in relation to the behavioural problems associated with TSC. It is well known that sodium valproate can improve aggressiveness, motor hyperactivity and irritable mood. It is clear from the above discussion of the beneficial effects of Vigabatrin on developmental outcome that early control of infantile spasms is important. Certainly, evaluation of TSC patients with autism for seizures is warranted; however, the role of seizure control in treating autistic behaviour remains unclear. More data on behavioural outcomes with different antiepileptic agents and different seizure types or localizations are needed.

The role of surgery in treating autistic behaviours in TSC patients is unclear. PET scanning techniques in TSC patients with autism may provide new insight into the aetiological questions discussed above. Earlier studies of patients with infantile spasms, with PET scanning, found a high correlation of bitemporal hypometabolism on 2-Deoxy-2 [18F] fluoro-D-glucose PET scans with poor developmental outcomes (Chugani et al. 1996). Of 110 children with infantile spasms evaluated for potential surgical intervention, Chugani et al. identified a subset of 18 children with bitemporal hypometabolism. In long-term follow-up, all 18 had severe developmental delay, with minimal language development, and 10 out of 14 who were further evaluated met DSM-IV criteria for autistic disorder. Such functional imaging techniques may contribute to our understanding of the role of epileptogenic tuber localization in autistic patients.

One caveat specific to the care of patients affected with TSC and learning disability or behavioural problems is to maintain a high index of suspicion for the development of a subependymal giant cell astrocytoma. This is illustrated by the case of a 27-year-old woman with TSC and a severe learning disorder with no language. She developed tantrums, with clumsiness, ataxia and further cognitive deterioration for six months before diagnosis with a giant cell astrocytoma (Webb et al. 1996). These tumours occur in 5 to 14% of TSC patients and can present with seizures, or change in seizure control, behavioural changes, focal neurological deficits, or through obstruction of CSF outflow, with headache, nausea and vomiting (Weiner et al. 1998).

Behaviour changes in this population can result in increased use of medications, with subsequent neurologic signs and symptoms then erroneously attributed to medication side effects. Subependymal giant cell astrocytoma should be considered for all behavourial or neurological changes in patients with TSC.

CONCLUSIONS

Despite the great deal of progress in the last few years, the neural basis of autism in TSC is still largely unknown and represents a major challenge for child neurologists.

The epidemiological studies of autism, despite differing tuberous sclerosis populations and varying diagnostic criteria, all arrive at a surprisingly high incidence of autism, of from 17 to 61%. Thus, the importance of evaluating children with TSC for autism cannot be overstressed. The incidence of autism may be significantly higher than the rates of cardiac and renal abnormalities, for which screening is routinely conducted in this population. It is to be hoped that early diagnosis of autism will allow for earlier treatment and the potential for better outcome.

Clearly, the underlying pathology of TSC predisposes to multiple overlapping morbidities, including learning disability, seizures, and a spectrum of behavioural abnormalities, with a high incidence of autism or autistic spectrum disorders. From the current evidence, no one factor (learning disability, tuber localization, occurrence of infantile spasms, focal EEG abnormalities, or seizures) can be causally linked with the abnormal behaviour. Rather, it may be that all of the aetiological categories detailed above may be causal for autism in TSC. Some patients may exhibit autistic behaviour secondary to specifically located cortical tubers, others may be affected by specific epileptic phenomena, with others perhaps harbouring a deletion in an adjacent but otherwise independent gene which is critical in the genesis of autism.

The better identification of patients, especially the identification of less severely affected patients, presumably with a lower cortical lesion burden, combined with improved imaging with MRI or functional imaging techniques, may aid in studies of the localization of behaviour in the developing brain. Similarly, the improved treatments for epilepsy in TSC patients, including the remarkable response of infantile spasms to Vigabatrin, as well as the continuing success of epilepsy surgery, may allow for the elimination or reduction of epilepsy as a variable in attempts to distinguish between the various possible aetiologies of autism in TSC. Improved seizure control may allow for a more independent analysis of the effects of lesion localization, learning disability, or genotype on behaviour. Finally, as the underlying genetic mutations in more and more patients with tuberous sclerosis are characterized, genotype/phenotype correlations with autistic behaviour can be made.

REFERENCES

Bachevalier J (1994) Medial temporal lobe structures and autism: a review of clinical and experimental findings. *Neuropsychologia* 32(6): 627–48.

Baker P, Piven J, Sato Y (1998) Autism and tuberous sclerosis complex: prevalence and clinical features. *J Autism Dev Disord* 28(4): 279–85.

Baron-Cohen S (2000) The cognitive neuroscience of autism: evolutionary approaches. In: Gazzaniga MS (ed) *The New Cognitive Neurosciences*. Cambridge, MA: MIT Press, pp 1249–57.

Bauman M, Kemper TL (1985) Histoanatomic observations of the brain in early infantile autism. *Neurology* 35: 866–74.

Bolton PF, Griffiths PD (1997) Association of tuberous sclerosis of temporal lobes with autism and atypical autism. *Lancet* 349: 392–5.

Bourneville DM (1880) Sclérose tubéreuse des circonvolutions cérébrales: idiotie et épilepsie hémiplégique. *Arch Neurol (Paris)* 1: 81–91.

Calderon Gonzalez R, Trevino Welsh J, Calderon Sepulveda A (1994) Autism in tuberous sclerosis. *Gac Med Mex* 130(5): 374–9.

Chiron C, Dulac O, Luna D (1990) Vigabatrin in infantile spasms. *Lancet* 335: 363–4.

Chugani HT, Da Silva, Chugani DC (1996) Infantile spasms: III. Prognostic implications of bitemporal hypometabolism on positron emission tomography. *Ann Neurol* 39(5): 643–9.

Courchesne E, Townsend J, Saitoh O (1994) The brain in infantile autism: posterior fossa structures are abnormal. *Neurology* 44: 214–23.

Critchley M, Earl CJC (1932) Tuberose sclerosis and allied conditions. *Brain* 55: 311–46.

Curatolo P, Cusmai R (1987) Autism and infantile spasms in children with tuberous sclerosis. *Dev Med Child Neurol* 29: 550–1.

Curatolo P, Cusmai R, Cortesi F, Chiron C, Jambaqué I, Dulac O (1991) Neuropsychiatric aspects of tuberous sclerosis. *Ann NY Acad Sci* 615: 8–16.

Curatolo P, Verdecchia M, Bombardieri R (2002) Tuberous sclerosis complex: a review of neurological aspects. *Eur J Ped Neurol* 6: 15–23.

Daniels RJ, Peden JF, Lloyd C, Horsley SW, Clark K, Tufarelli C, Kearney L, Buckle VJ, Doggett NA, Flint J, Higgs DR (2001) Sequence, structure and pathology of the fully annotated terminal 2 Mb of the short arm of human chromosome 16. *Hum Mol Genet* 10(4): 339–52.

Deonna T, Zeigler A, Moura-Sera J, Innocenti G (1993) Autistic regression in relation to limbic pathology and epilepsy: report of two cases. *Dev Med Child Neurol* 35: 158–76.

Fombonne E, Du Mazaubrun C, Cans C, Grandjean H (1997) Autism and associated medical disorders in a French epidemiological survey. *J Am Acad Child Adolesc Psychiatry* 36(11): 1561–9.

Gillberg IC, Gillberg C, Ahlsen G (1994) Autistic behavior and attention deficits in tuberous sclerosis: a population based study. *Dev Med Child Neurol* 36: 50–6.

Gomez MR (1998) Neurologic and psychiatric features. In: Gomez MR (ed) *Tuberous Sclerosis*. New York: Raven Press, pp 21–36.

Goodman M, Lamm SH, Engel A, Shepherd CW, Houser OW, Gomez MR (1997) Cortical tuber count: a biomarker indicating neurologic severity of tuberous sclerosis complex. *J Child Neurol* 12: 85–90.

Gutierrez GC, Smalley SL, Tanguay PE (1998) Autism in tuberous sclerosis complex. *J Autism Dev Disord* 28(2): 97–103.

Harrison JE, O'Callaghan FJ, Hancock E, Osborne JP, Bolton PF (1999) Cognitive deficits in normally intelligent patients with tuberous sclerosis. *Am J Med Genet* 88(6): 642–6.

Hunt A, Dennis J (1987) Psychiatric disorder among children with tuberous sclerosis. *Dev Med Child Neurol* 29: 190–8.

Hunt A, Shepherd C (1993) A prevalence study of autism in tuberous sclerosis. *J Autism Dev Disord* 23(2): 323–39.

Jambaqué I, Cusmai R, Curatolo P, Cortesi F, Perrot C, Dulac O (1991) Neuropsychological aspects of tuberous sclerosis in relation to epilepsy and MRI findings. *Dev Med Child Neurol* 33: 689–705.

Jambaqué I, Chiron C, Dumas D, Mumford J, Dulac C (2000) Mental and behavioral outcome of infantile epilepsy treated by vigabatrin in tuberous sclerosis patients. *Epilepsy Research* 38: 151–60.

Jones AC, Daniells CE, Snell RG, Tachataki M, Idziaszczyk SA, Krawczak M, Sampson JR, Cheadle JP (1997) Molecular genetic and phenotypic analysis reveals differences between TSC1 and TSC2 associated familial and sporadic tuberous sclerosis. *Hum Mol Genet* 6(12): 2155–61.

Józwiak S, Goodman M, Lamm SH (1998) Poor mental development in patients with tuberous sclerosis complex. *Arch Neurol* 55: 379–84.

Le Couteur A, Rutter M, Lord C, Rios P, Robertson S, Holdgrafer M, McLennan J (1989) Autism diagnostic interview: a standardized investigator-based instrument. *Autism Dev Disord* 19(3): 363–87.

Lewine JD, Andrews R, Chez M, Patil AA, Devinsky O, Smith M, Kanner A, Davis JT, Funke M, Jones G, Chong B, Provencal S, Weisend M, Lee RR, Orrison WW Jr (1999) Magneto-encephalographic patterns of epileptiform activity in children with regressive autism spectrum disorders. *Pediatrics* 104(3): 405–18.

Olsson I, Steffenburg S, Gillberg C (1988) Epilepsy in autism and autisticlike conditions. A population-based study. *Arch Neurol* 45(6): 666–8.

Philippe A, Martinez M, Guilloud-Bataille, Gillberg C, Rastam M, Sponheim E, Coleman M,

Zappella M, Aschauer H, van Malldergerme L, Penet C, Feingold J, Brice A, Leboyer M, et al. (1999) Genome-wide scan for autism susceptibility genes. *Hum Mol Genet* 8: 805–12.

Rapin I (1997) Autism. *New England J Med* 337(2): 97–104.

Rapin I, Katzman R (1998) Neurobiology of autism. *Ann Neurol* 43: 7–14.

Riikonen R, Amnell G (1981) Psychiatric disorders in children with earlier infantile spasms. *Dev Med Child Neurol* 23: 747–60.

Riikonen R, Simell O (1990) Tuberous sclerosis and infantile spasms. *Dev Med Child Neurol* 32: 203–9.

Roach ES (1997) Tuberous sclerosis: function follows form. *J Child Neurol* 12(2): 75–6.

Roach ES, Williams DP, Laster DW (1987) Magnetic resonance imaging in tuberous sclerosis. *Arch Neurol* 44: 301–3.

Sampson J, Maheshwar M, Aspinwall R, et al. (1997) PKD1 gene involvement and renal cystic disease in tuberous sclerosis. *Am J Hum Genet* 61: 843–51.

Seri S, Cerquiglini A, Pisani F, Curatolo P (1999) Autism in tuberous sclerosis: evoked potential evidence for a deficit in auditory sensory processing. *Clin Neurophysiol* 110: 1825–30.

Smalley SL (1998) Autism and tuberous sclerosis. *J Autism Dev Disord* 28(5): 407–14.

Smalley SL, Tanguay PE, Smith M, Guitierrez G (1992) Autism and tuberous sclerosis. *J Autism Dev Disord* 22(3): 339–55.

Smalley SL, Burger F, Smith M (1994) Phenotypic variation of tuberous sclerosis in a single extended kindred. *J Med Genet* 31(10): 761–5.

Soucek T, Holzl G, Bernaschek G, Hengstschlager M (1998) A role of the tuberous sclerosis gene-2 product during neuronal differentiation. *Oncogene* 16: 2197–204.

Tuchman RF (1994) Epilepsy, language, and behavior: clinical models in childhood. *J Child Neurol* 9: 95–102.

Tuchman R (2000) Treatment of seizure disorders and EEG abnormalities in children with autism spectrum disorders. *J Autism Dev Disord* 30(5): 485–9.

Tuchman RF, Rapin I (1997) Regression in pervasive developmental disorders: seizures and epileptiform electroencephalogram correlates. *Pediatrics* 99(4): 560–6.

van Slegtenhorst M, Nellist M, Nagelkerken B, Cheadle J, Snell R, van den Ouweland A, Reuser A, Sampson J, Halley D, van der Sluijs P (1998) Interaction between hamartin and tuberin, the TSC1 and TSC2 gene products. *Hum Mol Genet* 7(6): 1053–7.

Webb DW, Fryer AE, Osborne JP (1996) Morbidity associated with tuberous sclerosis: a population study. *Dev Med Child Neurol* 38: 146–55.

Weber AM, Egelhoff JC, McKellop JM, Franz DN (2000) Autism and the cerebellum: evidence from tuberous sclerosis. *J Autism Dev Disord* 30(6): 511–17.

Weiner DM, Ewalt DH, Roach ES, Hensle TW (1998) The tuberous sclerosis complex: a comprehensive review. *J Am Coll Surg* 187: 548–60.

Wienecke R, Konig A, DeClue JE (1995) Identification of tuberin, the tuberous sclerosis-2 product – tuberin possesses specific rap1GAP activity. *J Biol Chem* 270: 16409–14.

Wing L, Gould J (1979) Severe impairments of social interaction and associated abnormalities in children: epidemiology and classifications. *J Autism Dev Disord* 9: 11–29.

Wong V (1993) Epilepsy in children with autistic spectrum disorder. *J Child Neurol* 8: 316–22.

7

NEUROIMAGING

Alessandro Bozzao, Guglielmo Manenti and Paolo Curatolo

Basic CNS pathologic findings in TSC include subependymal nodules (SENs), cortical/subcortical tubers, subependymal giant cell astrocytoma (SEGA), heterotopic dysplastic neurons in white matter, and ventricular enlargement. According to the "second hit" hypothesis, each of these lesions is thought to arise from a single cell carrying a *TSC1* or *TSC2* mutation. In individuals with TSC, one copy of the responsible genes has a germline mutation of *TSC1* and *TSC2*. Lesions would arise from a single cell, only if a further event (or "second hit") causes a somatic mutation rendering both copies of the gene non-functional in that cell and its progeny, as it does with retinoblastoma and neurofibromatosis (Gutmann 1998). The result of this dysfunction seems to be a change in the cell genetic program affecting differentiation and/or proliferation. Therefore, most TSC lesions could be described as hamartias, hamartomas or hamartoblastomas, according to the state of maturation of the precursor cell at the time of the "second hit". This hypothesis is also consistent with the pathological similarities in the four major brain manifestations in TSC (cortical tuber, white matter abnormalities, subependymal nodule and subependymal giant cell astrocytoma) consisting of highly cellular dysplastic masses, composed of abnormal giant or balloon cells. Some of these abnormal cells show characteristics of astrocytes, while others exhibit neuronal differentiation or an intermediate form between the two with abnormal neuro-glial interaction (Trombley and Mirra 1981).

The formation and maturation of the cerebral neocortex involve complex processes (Barkovich et al. 1992, Barkovich 2000). Giant pluripotential cells generated in the subependymal and periventricular regions of the developing brain differentiate into glial and neuronal precursors. Whereas a proportion of these precursors undergo programmed cell death, most of the neurons that will form the cerebral cortex migrate to their destination along radial glial fibres originating from glial cell precursors. These fibres have specific chemotactic properties and serve as guides for neuron migration from the subependymal region to the cortical surface. Radial migration is most active during the third to fifth month of gestation but it continues after birth until approximately 5 months of age. Neurons destined for layer I, which is eventually the more superficial layer of the cortex, are the first to migrate. The other pools of neurons subsequently migrate inside-out, successively forming layers VI to II. After their arrival in the predetermined place in the cortex, neurons establish synaptic contacts to complete the cortical organization. Abnormalities in these processes result in malformations due to abnormal neuronal and glial prolif-eration in the germinal matrix, abnormal neuronal migration, and abnormal cortical organization (Barkovich et al. 1996).

The first abnormal step in TSC is abnormal neuronal and glial differentiation and proliferation. Two populations of primitive pluripotential giant cells are gener-ated in the germinal matrix: the first one consists of normal primitive cells which become normal astroglia and neurons forming the normal cerebral cortex; the second one consists of abnormal primitive cells which fail to clearly differentiate into neurons and glial cells (Braffman et al. 1992).

The second step is abnormal migration. Some of the abnormal giant primitive cells remain in the germinal matrix where they constitute subependymal tubers and giant cell astrocytomas. Other abnormal giant cells may undergo incomplete migra-tion, forming heterotopic clusters and bands of abnormal cells in the white matter, extending from the subependymal zones to the subcortical white matter. Other undifferentiated giant balloon cells may reach the cortex, forming cortical tubers.

Finally, abnormal cortical organization may account for some focal cortical dysplasias. Most of these pathologic findings are readily imaged with current tech-nology.

In the past, CT was widely used as the first-choice imaging technique to evaluate TSC lesions. CT allows an optimal visualization of calcified SENs and cortical tubers, while small and non-calcified lesions are not well detected. CT features of tubers generally demonstrate low attenuation as compared to adjacent parenchyma, may calcify, and rarely enhance with iodinated contrast.

CT has detected tubers during the first decade of life which have disappeared or resolved by the third decade. The resolution could be due to gliosis, but delayed myelination is a more logical explanation, although no pathologic proof is reported. These findings are similar to those reported in the other hamartomatoses (Sevick et al. 1992). On CT, SEGAs appear as heterogeneous, partially calcified, large lesions at the foramina of Monro. Traditionally any lesion showing enhancement on CT after administration of iodinated contrast medium, or progressively growing in serial imaging studies, is considered a SEGA. A surveillance program involving annual computed cranial tomography was reported to reduce surgical morbidity and the risk of tumour recurrence (Torres et al. 1998).

During the last two decades MRI has become the imaging method of choice in the evaluation of TSC, and it is now considered the most sensitive imaging technique to make a presumptive diagnosis of the disease. Using spin-echo imaging sequences, MRI has been less fruitful than CT in demonstrating calcifications; however, these sequences allow the detection of tubers to such an extent that MRI has definitively become the examination of choice for the evaluation of TSC.

Recent advances in MRI include fluid-attenuated inversion recovery (FLAIR) (Rydberg et al. 1994) and magnetization transfer (MT) imaging sequences (Grossman et al. 1994). FLAIR sequences demonstrate a greater sensibility than conventional ones in disclosing cortical tubers in the myelinated brain (Figs 7.1–7.3) (Maeda et al. 1995). Their sensitivity for the detection of TSC in the developing and still unmyelinated brain has yet to be determined. However, T1-weighted imaging is still superior for delineation of subependymal nodules. MT technique allows a better visualization of enhancement when used in combination with short TR sequences; enhancement is thus visualized at the burden of cortical tubers. However, on short TR images with MT, cortical tubers and subependymal nodules show higher signal than normally myelinated white matter, revealing more tubers than conventional sequences (Figs 7.4 and 7.5) (Girard et al. 1997).

There are no reports concerning the use of diffusion weighted images in TSC. Diffusion imaging is capable of showing those areas with reduced free water content and it is typically employed to discover cytotoxic edema in acute ischemia. In our experience, which involved 12 patients, most cortical tubers produced high signal on apparent diffusion coefficient maps (ADC), thus suggesting increased free water or reduced myelination (Figs 7.6 and 7.7).

SUBEPENDYMAL NODULES (SENs)
SENs are hamartomatous lesions that are typically located along the walls of the lateral ventricles, often adjacent to the caudate nucleus (Figs 7.8 and 7.9); they have

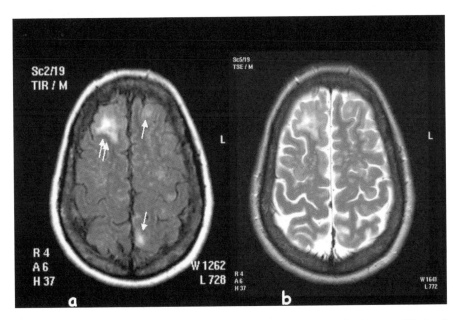

Fig. 7.1. Subcortical tubers (arrows) shown on FLAIR (a) and T2-weighted images (b). Small tubers are much more evident on FLAIR images.

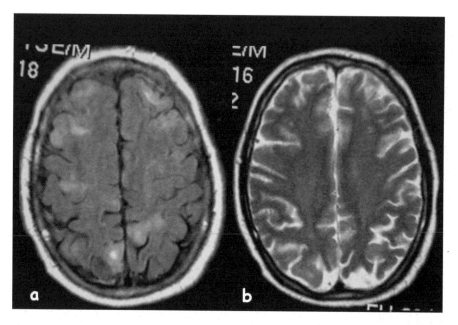

Fig. 7.2. Subcortical tubers shown on FLAIR (a) and T2-weighted images (b). Most of the tubers are appreciable only on FLAIR images.

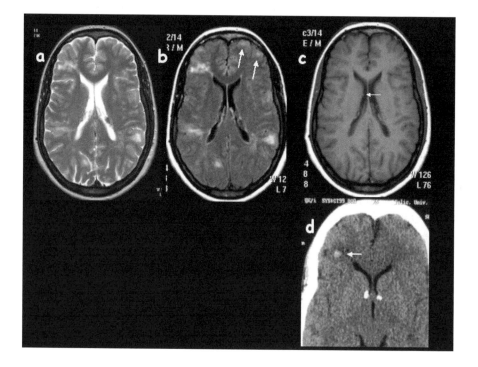

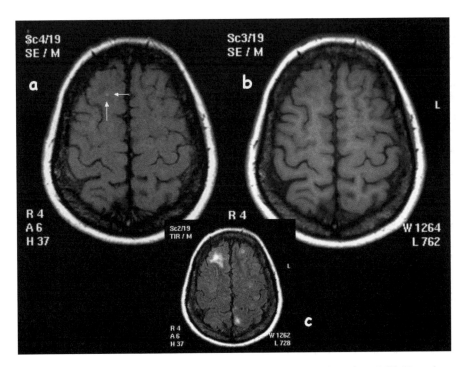

Fig. 7.4. Cortical tubers shown on T1-weighted images with MT (a), without MT (b), and on FLAIR images. Mild hyper-intense signal is evident in the core of the tuber on MT-T1 image (arrows), probably due to unmyelinated white matter.

never been observed in the third ventricle. SENs, found in the vast majority of patients, are often multiple and generally small (1 cm or less). SENs develop during fetal life and grow in proportion to the remainder of the brain. Growth tends to stop after the first decade (Hosoya et al. 1999).

MRI of SENs shows these lesions to have a signal iso-intense to white matter on T1-weighted sequences (Fig. 7.8), and iso- or hypo-intense on T2-weighted sequences. Large calcifications are seen with T2-weighted MRI as a signal void, whereas smaller SENs are more readily imaged with CT, especially if calcified. Dell et al. (1988) have reported that the MRI signal intensity of SENs varies depending on whether calcium carbonate or phosphate is present (Fig. 7.9). When phosphate was present the T1-weighted signal was increased. By contrast, in the presence of the

---

Fig. 7.3. Cortical tubers and subependymal nodules (SENs). Tubers are more evident on FLAIR images (b) than on T2 (a) and T1 (c). SENs are shown as hypo-intense nodules in the ependymal layer on T2 sequences (a), due to calcifications, and protrude inside the ventricle on T1-weighted images (c). Calcifications are shown by CT both in the tubers and in the SENs in the same patient.

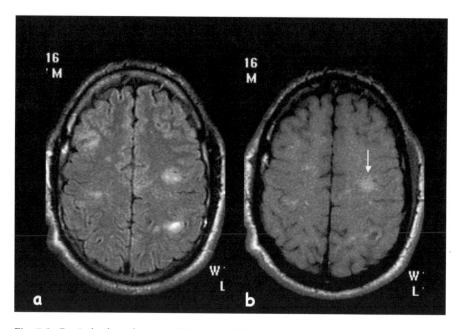

Fig. 7.5. Cortical tubers shown on T1-weighted images with MT and FLAIR images. Hyperintense signal is evident inside some cortical tubers (arrow).

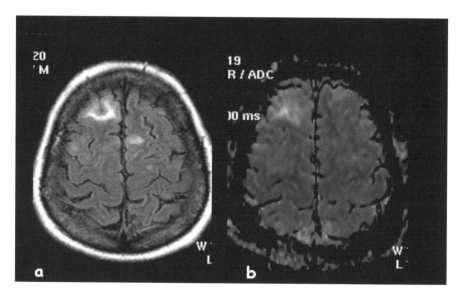

Fig. 7.6. Cortical tuber in the frontal region producing high signal on apparent diffusion coefficient maps (ADC) (b) compared to FLAIR image (a).

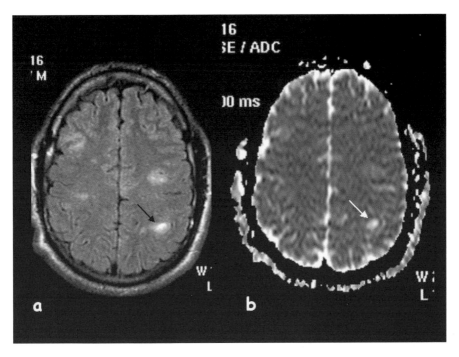

Fig. 7.7. Cortical tuber in the parietal region (arrow) producing high signal on apparent diffusion coefficient maps (ADC) (b) compared to FLAIR image (a). Small tubers are not appreciable on ADC map.

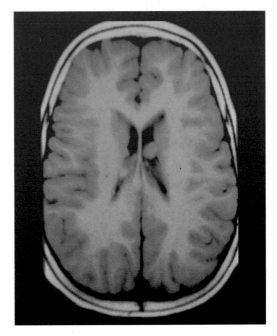

Fig. 7.8. SENs typically located along the outer walls of the lateral ventricles adjacent to the caudate nucleus are shown on T1-weighted images.

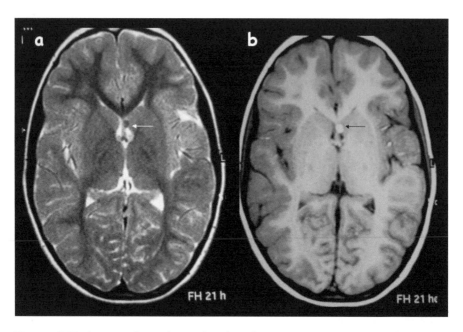

Fig. 7.9. SEN adjacent to the caudate nucleus shows hypo-intense signal on T2-weighted images (a) and iso-intense signal to the white matter on T1 (b) (arrows).

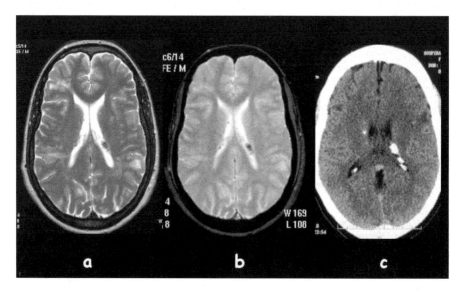

Fig. 7.10. Calcified SENs are shown on T2 TSE (a), -gradient echo (b) -weighted images and on CT. Gradient echo better depicts the calcifications.

carbonate radical, the T1-weighted signal was hypo-intense. MR gradient echo pulse sequences with short flip angle are particularly useful because of the magnetic susceptibility of calcified lesions, leading to a hypo-intense signal (Fig. 7.10). Some SENs enhance following intravenous gadolinium administration. Any SENs located near the foramen of Monro that enhance must be carefully evaluated by serial imaging studies.

SUBEPENDYMAL GIANT CELL ASTROCYTOMAS (SEGAs)
MRI of SEGAs often shows a heterogeneous mass with lower signal than normal white matter on T1, and higher than the adjacent white and grey matter on T2 (Fig. 7.11). Hypo-intense areas within these tumours may be secondary to calcifications, tumour vessels, or intra-tumoral haemorrhage. All SEGAs enhance following gadolinium administration. The nodules over 5 mm in diameter that are incompletely calcified and enhanced by gadolinium are at higher risk of growing, particularly in children with a familial history of tuberous sclerosis (Nabbout et al. 1999). It is advisable to systematically perform an MRI examination before 2 years of age and to repeat it every one to three years, depending on the level of clinical suspicion in each child.

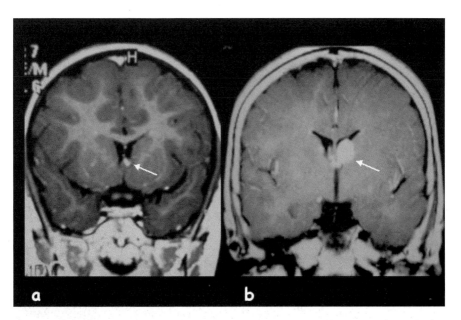

Fig. 7.11. Progressive growth of an enhancing lesion at the foramen of Monro in a TSC patient. Coronal T1-weighted image with gadolinium (a) shows a small enhancing lesion's marked growth in the three-year follow-up (b).

CORTICAL TUBERS

Cortical and subcortical tubers are hypomyelinated hamartias involving mainly the cerebral cortex and underlying white matter. The cranial MRI findings of tubers are now well characterized as increased signal lesions of the cerebral cortex or subcortical white matter, often evident with T2-weighted MRI. Nixon demonstrated similar abnormalities with MRI of postmortem brain specimens from patients with TSC (Nixon et al. 1989). Cerebellar lesions demonstrated by MRI are apparently more common than once believed and are always associated with supratentorial ones (Fig. 7.12). Patients with cerebellar tubers are significantly older and have more global cortical lesions than those with isolated cerebral tubers. Furthermore, they are often associated with focal cerebellar volume loss (Marti-Bonmati et al. 2000).

Tubers are usually multiple, variable in size and cortical location, and may tend to calcify (Sener et al. 1992, Wilms et al. 1992). Tubers may be associated with underlying white matter abnormalities, including occasional migration lines, curvilinear bands or wedges extending from the periventricular region to the cerebral cortex (Iwasaki et al. 1990). These white matter abnormalities may represent hypomyelinated lesions and are pathologically similar to the subcortical part of tubers (Sheithauer 1992). Spin-echo MRI sequences show that tubers generally enlarge the gyri and appear as regions of low T1 and high T2 signal (Figs 7.1–7.3, 7.5). These signal abnormalities are related to defective myelination of neuronal fibres and

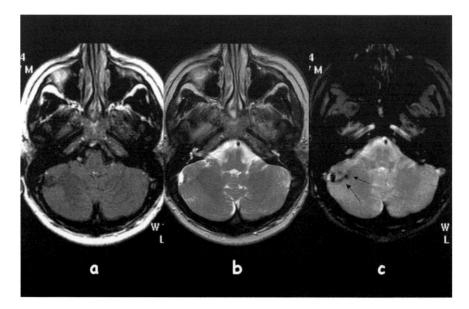

Fig. 7.12. Cerebellar tuber shown on FLAIR, T2-TSE and T2-gradient echo images. As expected, the calcified tuber is more evident on gradient echo image (arrows).

gliosis. Cyst formation may occur as a consequence of lysis of dysplastic cells. FLAIR imaging sequences have been reported as more sensitive than spin-echo sequences in detecting smaller tubers. (Figs 7.1–7.3) (Maeda et al. 1995).

In very young patients with immature white matter, the MRI appearance of tubers varies. In early infancy, many tubers are not detectable. When detected, the tubers do not show the characteristic findings noted in the myelinated brain. Instead the tuber may appear relatively hypo-intense compared to the adjacent unmyelinated white matter on T2-weighted sequences.

Baron and Barkovich described the MRI findings in seven neonates and infants less than 3 months of age (Baron and Barkovich 1999). In these young patients the nodular subependymal and parenchimal lesions tend to be hyper-intense on T1-weighted images and hypo-intense on T2-weighted images, just the opposite of what is seen in older children (Baron and Barkovich 1999). The reason for the increased T1 signal in tubers during early infancy is unknown. Presumably this paradox reflects either the texture of the tuber or a peculiar protein concentration that creates increased T1 signal (Altman et al. 1988).

Several imaging descriptions have been used in literature to define tubers, including sulcal islands, gyral cores, spindles and wedges (Houser et al. 1991, Shepherd et al. 1995). Presumably, all these different definitions reflect the dynamic profile of myelination, and are related to the question of whether a tuber is located in an unmyelinated, myelinating or myelinated brain.

Magnetic resonance spectroscopy (MRS) may play a role in the estimation of histological changes in tubers. MRS has shown a decrease of N-acetyl-aspartate (NAA)/creatinine ratios in the tubers, which is considered to reflect a reduction of neurons. Conversely, the increase of myoinositol/creatinine ratios in the tubers is thought to reflect an increase of glial cells (Mizuno et al. 2000). The reduced NAA/creatinine ratio is probably due to a reduced level of NA.

WHITE MATTER LESIONS

White matter lesions appear as radial bands, wedge-shaped and nodular foci mostly affecting the supratentorial white matter. White matter abnormalities have been reported in 95% of patients with TSC (Griffiths et al. 1998). Radial white matter lesions run from the ventricles through the cerebral mantle to the normal cortex or to the cortical tuber (Fig. 7.13). From an histological point of view these anomalies are almost identical to those observed in the cortical tubers. Radial bands are composed of clusters of heterotopic cells and are indicative of a disorder of migration associated with abnormal cell differentiation. Therefore, on MRI, white matter lesions are similarly hyper-intense on long TR and hypo-intense on short TR images (Braffman et al. 1992).

Wedge-shaped lesions are triangular in configuration and have their apex near the ventricle and their base at the cortex. This pattern is usually evident in the

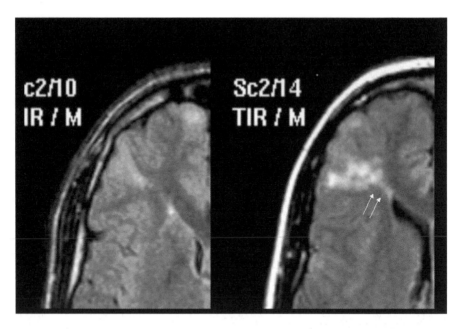

Fig. 7.13. White matter lesions involving the white matter from the cortex to the underlying ventricle (arrows), associated with a cortical tuber in the frontal region.

T2-weighted imaging. The site, shape and histopathological findings of white matter lesions confirm that TSC is a disorder of both histogenesis and cell migration. In particular, the different location between the lateral ventricles and the cerebral cortex could be the result of different timing of neuronal and glial migration arrest (Houser et al. 1991).

Focal or multiple lesions located in the deep or periventricular white matter have been described (Martin et al. 1987, Canapicchi et al. 1996). Since these lesions have been reported in older patients they could result from cystic degenerative phenomena (Canapicchi et al. 1996).

OTHER CNS FINDINGS IN TSC

Other rare findings associated with TSC include cerebro-vascular occlusive disease and vascular ectasias or aneurysm. Magnetic resonance angiography is a reasonable screening tool for these vascular problems if involvement of large vessels is suspected (Fig. 7.14). According to some authors, vascular dysplasias in general, and aneurysms (mainly intracranial) in particular, could be added to the other non-primary diagnostic features for the clinical diagnosis of tuberous sclerosis (Beltramello et al. 1999).

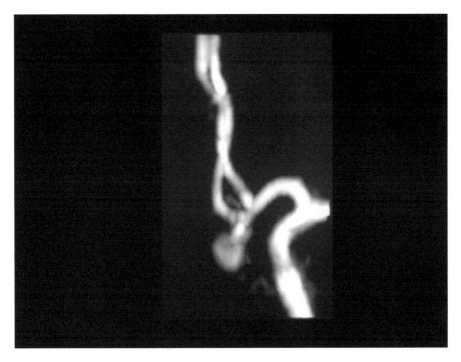

Fig. 7.14. MR angiography in a patient affected by TSC showing an aneurysm of the anterior communicating artery.

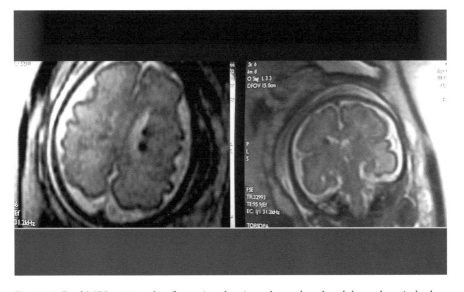

Fig. 7.15. Fetal MRI at 27 weeks of gestation showing subependymal nodules and cortical tuber.

FETAL MRI

MRI has a prominent role in the evaluation of pregnancies at risk for TSC (Curatolo and Brinchi 1993). The disease has been detected as early as 22 weeks gestation, by ultrasonographic detection of cardiac tumours. In these cases, fetal MRI can detect brain lesions in the locations typical for TSC as early as 26 weeks. The concomitant presence of both subependymal nodules and cortical tubers, two major features, allows a definitive diagnosis to be made (Fig. 7.15).

REFERENCES

Altman NR, Purser RK, Post MJD (1988) Tuberous sclerosis: characteristics at CT and MR imaging. *Radiology* 167:527–32.

Barkovich AJ (2000) Congenital malformations of the brain and skull. *Pediatric Neuroimaging, 3rd edn.* Philadelphia: Lippincott Williams and Wilkins.

Barkovich AJ, Gressens P, Evrard P (1992) Formation, maturation, and disorders of brain neocortex. *Am J Neuroradiol* 13: 423–46.

Barkovich AJ, Kuzniecky RI, Dobyns WB, Jackson GD, Becker LE, Evrard P (1996) A classification scheme for malformations of cortical development. *Neuropediatrics* 27: 59–63.

Baron Y, Barkovich AJ (1999) MR imaging of tuberous sclerosis in neonates and young infants. *Am J Neuroradiol* 20(5): 907–16.

Beltramello A, Puppini G, Bricolo A, Andreis IA, et al. (1999) Does the tuberous sclerosis complex include intracranial aneurysms? A case report with a review of the literature. *Pediatr Radiol* 29(3): 206–11.

Braffman BH, Bilaniuk LT, Naidich TP, Altman NR, Post MJ, et al. (1992) MR imaging of tuberous sclerosis: pathogenesis of this phakomatosis, use of gadopentate dimeglumine, and literature review. *Radiology* 183: 227–38.

Canapicchi R, Abbruzzese A, Guerrini R, Bianchi MC, Montanaro D, Cioni G (1996) Neuroimaging of tuberous sclerosis. In: Guerrini R, Andermann F, Canapicchi R, Roger J, Zifkin BG, Pfanner P (eds) *Dysplasias of Cerebral Cortex.* Philadelphia: Lippincott Raven, pp. 151–62.

Curatolo P, Brinchi V (1993) Antenatal diagnosis of tuberous sclerosis. *Lancet* 341: 176–7.

Dell LA, Brown MS, Orrison WW, et al. (1988) Physiologic intracranial calcification with hyperintensity on MR imaging: case report and experimental model. *Am J Neuroradiol* 9: 1141–5.

Girard N, Zimmerman RA, Schnur RE, Haselgrove J, Christensen K (1997) Magnetization transfer in the investigation of patients with tuberous sclerosis. *Neuroradiology* 39(7): 523–8.

Griffiths PD, Bolton P, Verity C (1998) White matter abnormalities in tuberous sclerosis complex. *Acta Radiol* 39(5): 482–6.

Grossman RI, Gomori JM, Ramer KN, Lexa FJ, Schnall MD (1994) Magnetization transfer: theory and clinical applications in neuroradiology. *Radiographics* 14: 279–90.

Gutmann DH (1998) Parallels between tuberous sclerosis complex and neurofibromatosis I: common threads in the same tapestry. *Semin Pediatr Neurol* 276–86.

Hosoya M, Naito H, Nihei K (1999) Neurological prognosis correlated with variations over time in the number of subependymal nodules in tuberous sclerosis. *Brain Dev* 21(8): 544–7.

Houser WO, Shepherd CW, Gomez MR (1991) Imaging of intracranial tuberous sclerosis. *Ann NY Acad Sci* 615: 81–93.

Iwasaki S, Nakagawa H, Kichikawa K, et al. (1990) MR and CT of tuberous sclerosis: linear abnormalities in the cerebral white matter. *Am J Neuroradiol* 11: 1029–34.

Maeda M, Tartaro A, Matsuda T, Ishii Y (1995) Cortical and subcortical tubers in tuberous sclerosis and FLAIR sequence. *JCAT* 19: 660–7.

Marti-Bonmati L, Menor F, Dosda R (2000) Tuberous sclerosis: differences between cerebral and cerebellar cortical tubers in a pediatric population. *Am J Neuroradiol* 21(3): 557–60.

Martin N, De Broucker T, Cambier J, Marsault C, Nahum H (1987) MRI evaluation of tuberous sclerosis. *Neuroradiology* 29: 437–43.

Mizuno S, Takahashi Y, Kato Z, Goto H, Kondo N, Hoshi H (2000) Magnetic resonance spectroscopy of tubers in patients with tuberous sclerosis. *Acta Neurol Scand* 102(3): 175–8.

Nabbout R, Santos M, Rolland Y, Delalande O, Dulac O, Chiron C (1999) Early diagnosis of subependymal giant cell astrocytoma in children with tuberous sclerosis. *J Neurol Neurosurg Psychiatry* 66(3): 370–5.

Nixon JR, Miller GM, Okazari H, Gomez MR (1989) Cerebral tuberous sclerosis: postmortem magnetic resonance imaging and pathologic anatomy. *Mayo Clin Proc* 64: 305–11.

Rydberg JN, Hammond CA, Grimm RC, et al. (1994) Initial clinical experience in MR imaging of the brain with fast fluid attenuated inversion-recovery pulse sequence. *Radiology* 193: 173–80.

Sener RN, Meral A, Farmaka H, Kalender N (1992) CT of gyriform calcification in tuberous sclerosis. *Pediatr Radiol* 22: 525–6.

Sevick RJ, Barkovich AJ, Edwards MSB, Koch T, Berg B, Lempert T (1992) Evolution of white matter lesions in neurofibromatosis type 1: MR findings. *AJR* 159: 171–5.

Sheithauer BW (1992) The neuropathology of tuberous sclerosis. *J Dermatol* 19: 897–903.

Shepherd CW, Houser OW, Gomez MR (1995) MR findings in tuberous sclerosis complex and correlation with seizure development and mental impairment. *Am J Neuroradiol* 16: 149–55.

Torres OA, Roach ES, Dlgado MR, Sparagana SP, Sheffield E, Swift D, Bruce D (1998) Early diagnosis of subependymal giant cell astrocytoma in patients with tuberous sclerosis. *J Child Neurol* 13(4): 173–7.

Trombley IK, Mirra SS (1981) Ultrastructure of tuberous sclerosis: cortical tuber and subependymal tumor. *Ann Neurol* 9: 174–81.

Wilms G, van Hijcks E, Demarael P, Smet MH, Plets C, Brucher JM (1992) Gyriform calcifications in tuberous sclerosis simulating the appearance of Sturge-Weber disease. *Am J Neuroradiol* 13: 295–8.

8

POSITRON EMISSION TOMOGRAPHY

Eishi Asano, Diane C Chugani and Harry T Chugani

Positron emission tomography (PET) is a non-invasive functional imaging tool which measures regional uptake and affinity of metabolic substrates in the brain and other organs. For the brain, PET has been utilized clinically to localize epileptogenic zones for epilepsy surgery, and also to study cognitive aspects of various disease conditions, including tuberous sclerosis complex (TSC). The purpose of this chapter is to review the usefulness of PET in the localization of epileptic foci and assessment of cognitive dysfunction in patients with TSC.

EPILEPSY IN TSC

Epilepsy occurs in 70–90% of all those affected with TSC, and for many of these children, seizures cannot be adequately controlled by medication (Gomez 1988, Webb et al. 1996). Several investigations have reported good seizure outcome in TSC patients who underwent surgical resection of epileptogenic zones (Bebin et al. 1993, Avellino et al. 1997, Guerreiro et al. 1998, Koh et al. 2000). Cortical tubers and malformed cortices have been found to be epileptogenic and were surgically removed in patients with TSC (Bebin et al. 1993, Koh et al. 2000). Good outcome was likely to be obtained in patients who showed concordance in localization from seizure semiology, electroencephalography (EEG), and a prominent cortical lesion defined by neuroimaging modalities (Bebin et al. 1993).

In chronological terms, X-ray (Bata and Kopcsanyi 1967), computed tomography (CT) (Harwood-Nash et al. 1975), PET (Szelies et al. 1983), magnetic resonance imaging (MRI) (Kandt et al. 1985, Takanashi et al. 1995) and single photon emission computed tomography (SPECT) (Sieg et al. 1991) have all been utilized to localize the cortical lesions in TSC. In CT, cortical tubers are often radiologically isodense to normal cortex and can be seen only in the few cases in which they are calcified (Harwood-Nash et al. 1975, Curatolo et al. 1991). PET has been used to detect cortical tubers in TSC since 1983 (Szelies et al. 1983), and subsequent newer PET methods are beginning to play an important role in the presurgical evaluation of TSC patients with refractory epilepsy.

ROLE OF 2-DEOXY-2-[^{18}F]FLUORO-D-GLUCOSE (FDG) PET IN EPILEPSY SURGERY FOR TSC

Using interictal PET scanning with 2-deoxy-2-[^{18}F]fluoro-D-glucose (FDG), Szelies et al. (1983) clearly demonstrated cortical tubers as nodular hypometabolic regions with 30–60% lower glucose metabolic rate than in the homologous contralateral region. It was suggested that hypometabolism in cortical tubers is due to decreased numbers of neurons and abnormal dendritic pattern in the tubers (Huttenlocher and Heydemann 1984, Machado-Salas 1984). Rintahaka and Chugani (1997) confirmed that hypometabolic regions on FDG images corresponded to cortical tubers on MRI. In addition, we have recently reported that FDG images often detected small cortical tubers not observed on T2-weighted MR images, but which were observed on fluid-attenuated inversion recovery (FLAIR) MR images (Asano et al. 2000a). We also found that glucose hypometabolic regions were usually larger than lesions on MRI, and that cortical tubers on MRI showed severely hypometabolic regions, whereas relatively mild hypometabolism was seen over the surrounding cortex, with dysplastic features on pathology but often normal on MRI (Fig. 8.1) (Asano et al. 2000a, 2000b). Our preliminary data, using chronic subdural EEG recording, suggested that ictal activity often originated from mildly hypometabolic regions adjacent to cortical tubers in patients with TSC (Asano et al. 2000b).

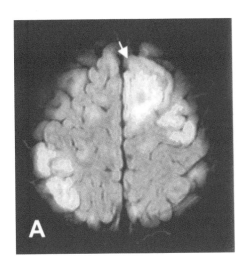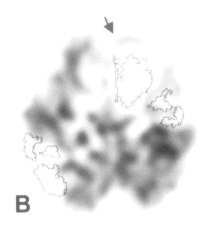

Fig. 8.1. Coregistered MRI and PET images in a 12-year-old boy with TSC and intractable epilepsy.
(A) The FLAIR MR-image shows multiple cortical tubers (encircled areas) in the left frontal and the right parietal lobes. (B) The FDG image shows a region of cortical hypometabolism corresponding to the cortical tubers. Relatively mild hypometabolism is seen over the cortex adjacent to the largest tuber in the left frontal lobe (arrow).

From a developmental perspective, previous FDG PET studies in non-TSC patients have shown that epileptic patients with glucose hypometabolism in the bilateral homotopic regions did not achieve normal development post-operatively, even if surgical resection of the epileptogenic zone on one side resulted in seizure-free outcome (Chugani et al. 1996, Blum et al. 1998). Therefore, we suggest that FDG PET has two major roles in epilepsy surgery for TSC: (1) to detect cortical tubers as well as surrounding dysplastic cortices with high sensitivity; (2) to assess the full extent of functional abnormality in the contralateral hemisphere, thereby predicting the post-operative cognitive function.

ROLE OF α-[¹¹C]METHYL-L-TRYPTOPHAN (AMT) PET IN EPILEPSY SURGERY FOR TSC

Both FDG PET and MRI are limited in presurgical evaluation for epilepsy surgery in patients with TSC due to their inability to differentiate between epileptogenic and non-epileptogenic lesions, in cases of multiple cortical tubers and multifocal EEG abnormalities (Rintahaka and Chugani 1997, Fukushima et al. 1998). This problem was addressed by implementation of the PET tracer, α-[¹¹C]methyl-L-tryptophan (AMT) (Chugani et al. 1998a, Asano et al. 2000a). AMT showed 20–188% higher uptake in epileptogenic compared to non-epileptogenic tubers in two-thirds of patients with medically intractable epilepsy (Fig. 8.2) (Chugani et al. 1998a). Thus, AMT PET can be used to identify specifically epileptogenic tubers in over half of TSC patients.

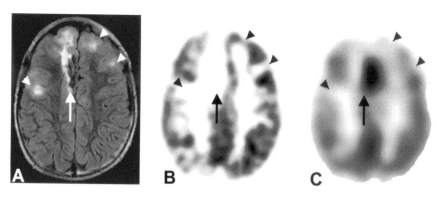

Fig. 8.2. Coregistered MRI and PET images in a 7-year-old boy with TSC and intractable epilepsy.
(A) The FLAIR MR-image shows multiple cortical tubers in the right and left frontal lobes (arrow and arrowheads). The largest tuber (arrow) in the right medial frontal region shows heterogeneous intensity due to calcification. (B) The FDG image shows regions of cortical hypometabolism corresponding to the cortical tubers. (C) The AMT image shows increased tracer uptake in the right medial frontal region (arrow) and decreased tracer uptake in the remaining tubers (arrowheads). Note that AMT uptake in the scalp was manually removed.

Subsequently, we undertook an analysis of all tubers visible on MRI and FDG PET, to examine further the relationship between AMT uptake and epileptic activity on EEG (Asano et al. 2000a). AMT uptake values for the tubers in the epileptic lobes were significantly higher than for those in the non-epileptic lobes (Asano et al. 2000a). Cortical tubers with AMT uptake equal to or greater than normal cortex were specifically related to epileptiform activity (specificity greater than 90%) (Asano et al. 2000a). In addition, we have encountered patients with TSC, in whom dysplastic cortex adjacent to a tuber showed mild glucose hypometabolism and prominently increased AMT uptake, where subdural EEG recording demonstrated origin of ictal discharges (Fig. 8.3) (Asano et al. 2000b). Therefore, we suggest that AMT PET (which provides specificity) combined with FDG PET (which provides sensitivity) will improve the detection of epileptogenic zones in TSC patients being evaluated for epilepsy surgery.

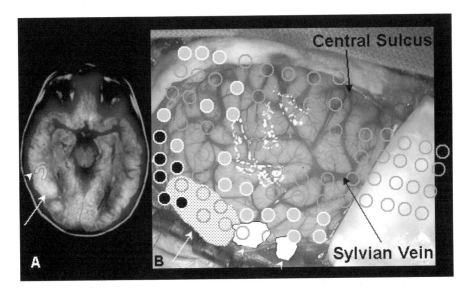

Fig. 8.3. An MRI/PET fusion image and a photograph of the brain surface in a 6-year-old boy with TSC and intractable epilepsy.
(A) The FLAIR MRI and AMT PET fusion image shows a cortical tuber (encircled area) in the right posterior temporal region and increased AMT uptake in the posterior edge of the tuber (arrow). (B) The intraoperative photograph shows the exposed temporal, parietal and frontal lobes in the right hemisphere, where 8 by 8 and 4 by 5 grid electrode arrays (electrode locations are denoted by circles) were placed for chronic intracranial EEG monitoring. Electrodes are colour-coded: black = seizure onset, grey = seizure spread, and grey circle = no early ictal involvement. The dotted area represents the region with increased AMT uptake (arrow). Encircled white areas represent the contour of cortical tubers (arrowheads). The patient underwent resection of the right temporal and parietal cortices, including the cortical tubers, the regions with increased AMT uptake and regions showing seizure onset and early ictal involvement. The patient has been seizure-free since the resective surgery (28-month follow-up period).

AMT was initially developed as a PET tracer for the measurement of brain serotonin synthesis in humans (Diksic et al. 1990, Muzik et al. 1997, Chugani et al. 1998b). However, tryptophan is also metabolized by indoleamine 2,3-dioxygenase in the brain under some pathologic conditions such as ischemia, immune activation and epilepsy, resulting in increased concentration of kynurenine pathway metabolites including quinolinic acid (Yamazaki et al. 1985, Chugani et al. 1998c). We have recently demonstrated that resected epileptogenic tissues with increased AMT uptake did not have increased serotonin synthesis, but had five times higher quinolinic acid than non-epileptogenic tissues (Chugani et al. 1998c). Several metabolites of the kynurenine pathway, including quinolinic acid, kynurenine and 3-hydroxykynurenine, are convulsants through their action as agonists at N-methyl-D-aspartate receptors (Lapin 1982, Perkins and Stone 1982). Local application of these metabolites to the brain in experimental animals results in epileptiform discharges and seizures (Schwarcz et al. 1984). Therefore, it has been postulated that metabolites of the kynurenine pathway might play a role in the initiation and maintenance of seizures in human seizure disorders (Feldblum et al. 1988). Further biochemical research with surgically resected epileptogenic tissues will answer the question of whether high AMT uptake is a persistent feature of epileptogenic tubers, or whether seizures induce biochemical changes which are detected as increased AMT uptake within a certain time-frame after a seizure.

AUTISM IN TSC

Autism is a developmental disorder which is diagnosed based upon behavioural criteria in three domains: stereotypical behaviours, social interactions, and verbal and non-verbal communication (Lord et al. 1994). It is estimated that autism occurs in 17 to 61% of individuals with TSC (Hunt and Dennis 1987, Jambaqué et al. 1991, Hunt and Shepherd 1992, Bolton and Griffiths 1997), establishing autism as a major neuropsychological concern in TSC. The incidence of autism in girls with TSC is equal to that in boys with this condition (Smalley et al. 1992, Gillberg et al. 1994), an observation which is in strong contrast to a fourfold higher incidence of autism in males for the entire population of autistic individuals (Bryson 1996).

The pathogenic mechanisms of autism in TSC are poorly understood, although previous studies have shown clinical risk factors for autism. Infantile spasms are common in autistic children with TSC, and one study reported that 57% of children with TSC who had infantile spasms were autistic (Hunt and Dennis 1987). In contrast to this finding, a Finnish series study showed that 13% of children with infantile spasms from other causes were autistic (Riikonen and Amnell 1981). These data suggest that there is a considerable difference in the prevalence of autism between TSC and non-TSC children with infantile spasms, and the relationship between infantile spasms and autism remains unclear. Our recent study in TSC demonstrated that 15 subjects with a history of infantile spasms had more severe communication disturbances than 11 subjects without, but that there was no significant difference in severity of stereotypical behaviours or social interaction between subjects with or without a history of infantile spasms (Asano et al. 2001). Therefore, we speculate that infantile spasms in early life have major effects with regard to communication and intellectual decline, but relatively minor effects with regard to the development of stereotypical behaviours and lack of social interaction, in children with TSC.

Radiographic studies using MRI and CT have indicated that tubers in the temporal lobes are associated with autism. Three previous studies have shown that 43–100% of autistic TSC patients had cortical tubers in the temporal lobes, whereas all the non-autistic TSC patients were free from temporal tubers (Smalley et al. 1995, Bolton and Griffiths 1997, Seri et al. 1999). However, other studies reported that a considerable percentage of non-autistic TSC patients had temporal tubers and that some of them even had normal intelligence (Bebin et al. 1993, Guerreiro et al. 1998, Asano et al. 2001). Our recent study demonstrated that TSC children with learning disability had more cortical tubers in the dorsal frontal cortex and lateral temporal cortex than those without learning disability, but that there was no significant difference in the topography of cortical tubers between TSC children with or without a diagnosis of autism (Asano et al. 2001).

ROLE OF PET IN THE STUDY OF AUTISM IN TSC

We recently examined the relationship between autism and functional brain abnormalities in 26 children with TSC, using FDG and AMT PET scanning (Asano et al. 2001). Based on the results of the Autism Diagnostic Interview-Revised and the overall adaptive behavioural composite (OABC) from the Vineland Adaptive Behavior Scale, subjects were divided into three groups: autistic (OABC < 70; N = 9), non-autistic with learning disability (OABC < 70; N = 9), and normal intelligence (OABC ≥ 70; N = 8). The results showed that the autistic group had decreased glucose metabolism in non-lesional lateral temporal cortex bilaterally (Fig. 8.4), increased glucose metabolism in the deep cerebellar nuclei (Fig. 8.5), and increased AMT uptake in the caudate nuclei (Fig. 8.4), compared to the non-autistic group with learning disability (Asano et al. 2001). In addition, glucose hypometabolism in the lateral temporal cortices was significantly correlated with severity of communication disturbance ranked by the Gilliam Autism Rating Scale (Asano et al. 2001). Glucose hypermetabolism in the deep cerebellar nuclei and increased AMT uptake in the caudate nuclei were both related to stereotypical behaviours and impaired social interaction, as well as communication disturbance (Asano et al. 2001).

Increased caudate AMT uptake in the autistic group, and a positive correlation between this finding and autistic features, is important in light of the potential role of the caudate nucleus in stereotypical or repetitive behaviours. A role of the caudate

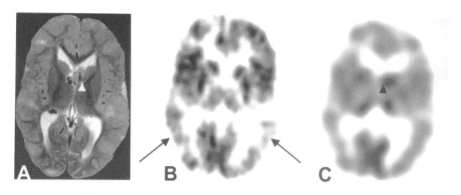

Fig. 8.4. Coregistered MRI and PET images in a 6-year-old boy with TSC and autism.
(A) The FLAIR MR image shows multiple cortical tubers in the left and right temporal, the right frontal and the right occipital lobes, as well as multiple subependymal nodules adjacent to the left and right caudate nuclei and the right thalamus. (B) The FDG PET image shows severe hypometabolism corresponding to the cortical tubers, as well as mild hypometabolism bilaterally in the non-tuberous temporal regions (arrows). (C) The AMT PET image shows prominently increased tracer uptake in the subependymal nodule adjacent to the left caudate nucleus, and appears to influence AMT uptake in the caudate nucleus.

nucleus in autism was previously suggested due to the difference in volume of the caudate in monozygotic twins discordant for autism (Kates et al. 1998). Volumetric MRI measurements showed that the twin with social and language development delays had cortical atrophy of the superior temporal gyrus and frontal lobe, while the twin with strictly defined autism had, in addition, a markedly smaller caudate, amygdala, hippocampus and cerebellar vermis (Kates et al. 1998).

The caudate nuclei are considered to be inhibitory structures organizing a "fronto-striato-thalamo-frontal" circuit (Alexander et al. 1986), disruptions of which can result in stereotypical or repetitive behaviours, as seen in many conditions such as stroke (Kumral et al. 1999), obsessive-compulsive disorder (Trivedi 1996) and Tourette's syndrome (Braun et al. 1993). Our finding of increased uptake of AMT in the caudate nuclei and adjacent subependymal nodules may point toward a mechanism for the disruption of striatal function, resulting in stereotyped behaviour in TSC. Increased metabolism of tryptophan via the kynurenine pathway in subependymal nodules might result in increased quinolinic acid and a disruption in caudate function. Indeed, chronic infusion of quinolinic acid into the caudate nucleus in rats resulted in motor stereotypies (Bazzett et al. 1996). Taken together, these data suggest that increased production of quinolinic acid in the caudate nuclei or adjacent subependymal nodules might be one mechanism underlying stereotyped behaviour in autistic children with TSC.

The FDG PET results (Asano et al. 2001) showed that the autistic TSC children had increased FDG uptake in the deep cerebellar nuclei, compared to the

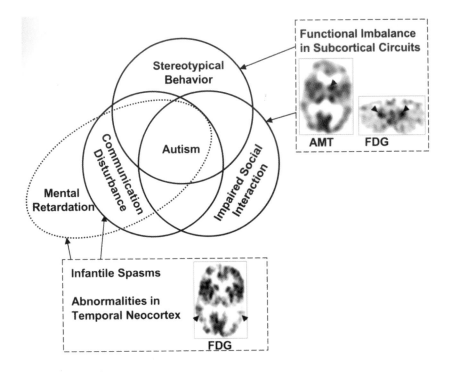

Fig. 8.5. Model of autism in TSC.
Note that the majority of autistic children with TSC have learning disability and that learning disability is especially related to language dysfunction (dotted line). Our recent study showed that the autistic group had decreased glucose metabolism in non-lesional lateral temporal cortex bilaterally (lower), increased glucose metabolism in the deep cerebellar nuclei (upper right), and increased AMT uptake in the caudate nuclei (upper left), compared to the non-autistic group with learning disability.

non-autistic children with learning disability (Fig. 8.5). Moreover, this finding was positively correlated with the severity of autistic features. The dentate nucleus, which is the largest among the four deep cerebellar subnuclei, receives inhibitory afferents from Purkinje cells in the cerebellar cortex and projects to the ventral lateral nucleus of the contralateral thalamus in the dentatorubrothalamic tract (Asanuma et al. 1983). In turn, neurons in the thalamic ventral lateral nucleus project to the frontal cortex (Allen and Tsukahara 1974, Middleton and Strick 1994).

These subcortical circuits involving dentate nucleus have been suggested to play an important role in higher cognitive function (Middleton and Strick 1994), and abnormalities in this circuit have been demonstrated in autistic individuals (Chugani et al. 1997). We showed unilaterally decreased AMT uptake in the frontal cortex and thalamus and elevated AMT uptake in the contralateral deep cerebellar nuclei (Chugani et al. 1997). Purkinje cells in the cerebellum are decreased in number in individuals with idiopathic autism (Bauman and Kemper 1985). On the other hand, hamartin and tuberin are expressed abundantly in neurons and astrocytes in the developing and adult cerebellum (Gutmann et al. 2000). In addition, tuberin localizes predominantly to the Purkinje cells, whereas hamartin is distributed along neuronal or astrocytic processes, where these products can physically interact. Therefore, we suggest that abnormal expression of tuberin in Purkinje cells might disrupt Purkinje-mediated inhibition and result in increased FDG uptake in the deep cerebellar nuclei (Fig. 8.5).

In summary, we propose that infantile spasms and neurodevelopmental abnormalities in temporal neocortex may be risk factors for intellectual and communication delays, while functional imbalance in subcortical circuits may be necessary to cause stereotypical behaviours and impaired social interaction in children with TSC (Fig. 8.5). Further, we suggest that patients with TSC exhibit different behavioural symptoms based upon the combination of brain functional abnormalities present.

SUMMARY AND FUTURE PROSPECTS
The application of functional neuroimaging with FDG and AMT PET has shed new light on mechanisms involved in epileptogenesis, learning disability and autism in TSC. Increasing sensitivity of the new generations of PET scanners allows a reduction in the radioactive dose administered, thus increasing the predilection to apply these imaging modalities in children. Further development of novel radio-labelled tracers, guided by knowledge of the biochemical characteristics underlying this disorder, derived from basic and genetic studies, is the logical next step in the application of PET for the study of pathophysiology in TSC.

ACKNOWLEDGEMENTS
This study was supported by NIH grant NS38324 and a grant from the National Tuberous Sclerosis Association. We are indebted to the staff of the PET Center for their assistance in performing these studies.

REFERENCES
Alexander GE, DeLong MR, Strick PL (1986) Parallel organization of functionally segregated circuits linking basal ganglia and cortex. *Annu Rev Neurosci* 9: 357–81.
Allen GI, Tsukahara N (1974) Cerebrocerebellar communication systems. *Physiol Rev* 54: 957–1006.
Asano E, Chugani DC, Muzik O, et al. (2000a) Multimodality imaging for improved detection of epileptogenic foci in tuberous sclerosis complex. *Neurology* 54: 1976–84.
Asano E, Chugani DC, Juhasz C, et al. (2000b) Epileptogenic zones in tuberous sclerosis complex: subdural EEG versus MRI and FDG PET. *Epilepsia* 41 (suppl l7): 128.
Asano E, Chugani DC, Muzik O, Behen M, Vanisse MA, Rothermel R, Mangner TJ, Chakraborty PK, Chugani HT (2001) Autism in tuberous sclerosis is related to both cortical and subcortical dysfunction. *Neurology* 57: 1269–77.

Asanuma C, Thach WT, Jones EG (1983) Distribution of cerebellar terminations and their relation to other afferent terminations in the ventral lateral thalamic region of the monkey. *Brain Res* 286: 237–65.

Avellino AM, Berger MS, Rostomily RC, Shaw CM, Ojemann GA (1997) Surgical management and seizure outcome in patients with tuberous sclerosis. *J Neurosurg* 87: 391–6.

Bata G, Kopcsanyi I (1967) Intracerebral calcification and familial epilepsy. Diagnosis of tuberous sclerosis in children. *Acta Paediatr Acad Sci Hung* 8: 343–54.

Bauman M, Kemper TL (1985) Histoanatomic observations of the brain in early infantile autism. *Neurology* 35: 866–74.

Bazzett TJ, Falik RC, Becker JB, Albin RL (1996) Chronic intrastriatal administration of quinolinic acid produces transient nocturnal hypermotility in the rat. *Brain Res Bull* 39: 69–73.

Bebin EM, Kelly PJ, Gomez MR (1993) Surgical treatment for epilepsy in cerebral tuberous sclerosis. *Epilepsia* 34: 651–7.

Blum DE, Ehsan T, Dungan D, et al. (1998) Bilateral temporal hypometabolism in epilepsy. *Epilepsia* 39: 651–9.

Bolton PF, Griffiths PD (1997) Association of tuberous sclerosis of temporal lobes with autism and atypical autism. *Lancet* 349: 392–5.

Braun AR, Stoetter B, Randolph C, et al. (1993) The functional neuroanatomy of Tourette's syndrome: an FDG-PET study. I. Regional changes in cerebral glucose metabolism differentiating patients and controls. *Neuropsychopharmacology* 9: 277–91.

Bryson SE (1996) Brief report: epidemiology of autism. *J Autism Dev Disord* 26: 165–7.

Chakraborty PK, Chugani HT (2001) Autism in tuberous sclerosis complex is related to both cortical and subcortical dysfunction. *Neurology* 57: 1269–77.

Chugani HT, Da Silva E, Chugani DC (1996) Infantile spasms: III. Prognostic implications of bitemporal hypometabolism on positron emission tomography. *Ann Neurol* 39: 643–9.

Chugani DC, Muzik O, Rothermel R, et al. (1997) Altered serotonin synthesis in the dentatothalamocortical pathway in autistic boys. *Ann Neurol* 42: 666–9.

Chugani DC, Chugani HT, Muzik O, et al. (1998a) Imaging epileptogenic tubers in children with tuberous sclerosis complex using alpha-[11C]methyl-L-tryptophan positron emission tomography. *Ann Neurol* 44: 858–66.

Chugani DC, Muzik O, Chakraborty P, Mangner T, Chugani HT (1998b) Human brain serotonin synthesis capacity measured in vivo with alpha-[C-11]methyl-L-tryptophan. *Synapse* 28: 33–43.

Chugani DC, Heyes MP, Kuhn DM, Chugani HT (1998c) Evidence ([C-11]methyl-L-tryptophan PET traces tryptophan metabolism via the kynurenine pathway in tuberous sclerosis complex. *Soc Neurosci Abstracts* 24: 1757. Abstract.

Curatolo P, Cusmai R, Cortesi F, et al. (1991) Neuropsychiatric aspects of tuberous sclerosis. *Ann NY Acad Sci* 615: 8–16.

Diksic M, Nagahiro S, Sourkes TL, Yamamoto YL (1990) A new method to measure brain serotonin synthesis in vivo. I. Theory and basic data for a biological model. *J Cereb Blood Flow Metab* 10: 1–12.

Feldblum S, Rougier A, Loiseau H, et al. (1988) Quinolinic-phosphoribosyl transferase activity is decreased in epileptic human brain tissue. *Epilepsia* 29: 523–9.

Fukushima K, Inoue Y, Fujiwara T, Yagi K (1998) Long-term course of West syndrome associated with tuberous sclerosis. *Epilepsia* 39 (suppl 5): 50–4.

Gillberg IC, Gillberg C, Ahlsen G (1994) Autistic behaviour and attention deficits in tuberous sclerosis: a population-based study. *Dev Med Child Neurol* 36: 50–6.

Gomez MR (1988) Neurologic and psychiatric features. In: Gomez MR (ed) *Tuberous Sclerosis, 2nd edn.* New York: Raven Press, pp 21–36.

Guerreiro MM, Andermann F, Andermann E, et al. (1998) Surgical treatment of epilepsy in tuberous sclerosis: strategies and results in 18 patients. *Neurology* 51: 1263–9.

Gutmann DH, Zhang Y, Hasbani MJ, et al. (2000) Expression of the tuberous sclerosis complex gene products, hamartin and tuberin, in central nervous system tissues. *Acta Neuropathol* 99: 223–30.

Harwood-Nash DC, Fitz CR, Reilly BJ (1975) Cranial computed tomography in infants and children. *Can Med Assoc J* 113: 546–9.

Hunt A, Dennis J (1987) Psychiatric disorder among children with tuberous sclerosis. *Dev Med Child Neurol* 29: 190–8.

Hunt A, Shepherd C (1993) A prevalence study of autism in tuberous sclerosis. *J Autism Dev Disord* 23: 323–39.

Huttenlocher PR, Heydemann PT (1984) Fine structure of cortical tubers in tuberous sclerosis: a Golgi study. *Ann Neurol* 16: 595–602.

Jambaqué I, Cusmai R, Curatolo P, et al. (1991) Neuropsychological aspects of tuberous sclerosis in relation to epilepsy and MRI findings. *Dev Med Child Neurol* 33: 698–705.

Kandt RS, Gebarski SS, Goetting MG (1985) Tuberous sclerosis with cardiogenic cerebral embolism: magnetic resonance imaging. *Neurology* 35: 1223–5.

Kates WR, Mostofsky SH, Zimmerman AW, et al. (1998) Neuroanatomical and neurocognitive differences in a pair of monozygous twins discordant for strictly defined autism. *Ann Neurol* 43: 782–91.

Koh S, Jayakar P, Dunoyer C, et al. (2000) Epilepsy surgery in children with tuberous sclerosis complex: presurgical evaluation and outcome. *Epilepsia* 41: 1206–13.

Kumral E, Evyapan D, Balkir K (1999) Acute caudate vascular lesions. *Stroke* 30: 100–8.

Lapin IP (1982) Convulsant action of intracerebroventricularly administered l-kynurenine sulphate, quinolinic acid and other derivatives of succinic acid, and effects of amino acids: structure-activity relationships. *Neuropharmacology* 21: 1227–33.

Lord C, Rutter M, Le Couteur A (1994) Autism Diagnostic Interview-Revised: a revised version of a diagnostic interview for caregivers of individuals with possible pervasive developmental disorders. *J Autism Dev Disord* 24: 659–85.

Machado-Salas JP (1984) Abnormal dendritic patterns and aberrant spine development in Bourneville's disease – a Golgi survey. *Clin Neuropathol* 3: 52–8.

Middleton FA, Strick PL (1994) Anatomical evidence for cerebellar and basal ganglia involvement in higher cognitive function. *Science* 266: 458–61.

Muzik O, Chugani DC, Chakraborty P, Mangner T, Chugani HT (1997) Analysis of [C-11]-alpha-methyl-tryptophan kinetics for the estimation of serotonin synthesis rate in vivo. *J Cereb Blood Flow Metab* 17: 659–69.

Perkins MN, Stone TW (1982) An iontophoretic investigation of the actions of convulsant kynurenines and their interaction with the endogenous excitant quinolinic acid. *Brain Res* 247: 184–7.

Riikonen R, Amnell G (1981) Psychiatric disorders in children with earlier infantile spasms. *Dev Med Child Neurol* 23: 747–60.

Rintahaka PJ, Chugani HT (1997) Clinical role of positron emission tomography in children with tuberous sclerosis complex. *J Child Neurol* 12: 42–52.

Schwarcz R, Brush GS, Foster AC, French ED (1984) Seizure activity and lesions after intrahippocampal quinolinic acid injection. *Exp Neurol* 84: 1–17.

Seri S, Cerquiglini A, Pisani F, Curatolo P (1999) Autism in tuberous sclerosis: evoked potential evidence for a deficit in auditory sensory processing. *Clin Neurophysiol* 110: 1825–30.

Sieg KG, Harty JR, Simmons M, Preston DF, Erickson HM Jr (1991) Tc-99m HMPAO SPECT imaging of the central nervous system in tuberous sclerosis. *Clin Nucl Med* 16: 665–7.

Smalley SL, Tanguay PE, Smith M, Gutierrez G (1992) Autism and tuberous sclerosis. *J Autism Dev Disord* 22: 339–55.

Smalley SL, McCracken J, Tanguay P (1995) Autism, affective disorders, and social phobia. *Am J Med Genet* 60: 19–26.

Szelies B, Herholz K, Heiss WD, et al. (1983) Hypometabolic cortical lesions in tuberous sclerosis with epilepsy: demonstration by positron emission tomography. *J Comput Assist Tomogr* 7: 946–53.

Takanashi J, Sugita K, Fujii K, Niimi H (1995) MR evaluation of tuberous sclerosis: increased sensitivity with fluid-attenuated inversion recovery and relation to severity of seizures and mental retardation. *Am J Neuroradiol* 16: 1923–8.

Trivedi MH (1996) Functional neuroanatomy of obsessive-compulsive disorder. *J Clin Psychiatry* 57: 26–36.

Webb DW, Fryer AE, Osborne JP (1996) Morbidity associated with tuberous sclerosis: a population study. *Dev Med Child Neurol* 38: 146–55.

Yamazaki F, Kuroiwa T, Takikawa O, Kido R (1985) Human indolylamine 2,3-dioxygenase. Its tissue distribution, and characterization of the placental enzyme. *Biochem J* 230: 635–8.

9
DERMATOLOGICAL AND STOMATOLOGICAL MANIFESTATIONS

Sergiusz Jóźwiak and Robert Schwartz

Tuberous sclerosis complex (TSC) is a prominent neurocutaneous syndrome, having neurological symptoms and signs accompanied by dermatological manifestations. Embryological studies have proven that the common origin of the nervous system and skin from ectoderm offers an explanation for this association.

The dermatological features are an important part of TSC, yet the first descriptions made by von Recklinghausen (1862) and Bourneville (1880) of pathologic lesions of the multifaceted disease that was later to be called "tuberous sclerosis" totally ignored the presence of skin manifestations. In spite of the fact that the first picture representing typical facial angiofibromas was published in 1835 by French dermatologist Pierre-Olive François Rayer (1835), it was not until 1905 that Perusini (1905) and Campbell (1905) discovered the association between the cutaneous and cerebral, renal and cardiac lesions in TSC. The diagnostic triad of TSC, including facial angiofibromas (inaccurately called "adenoma sebaceum"), was described first by Campbell (1905), but is better known as "Vogt's triad" (Vogt 1908).

During the next decades we learned of many other skin manifestations of TSC. Some of them are pathognomonic, but some are not and may be seen in healthy persons. The careful examiner may reveal some skin manifestations of TSC even in the neonatal period. As the child grows, additional cutaneous lesions appear and the diagnosis becomes evident. Because about 30% of cases are familial, and skin manifestations are better seen in adults, it should be stressed that in all suspected paediatric cases careful skin examination should be carried out not only in the child, but also in the parents.

According to Gomez (1987), 96% of patients with TSC have one or more of the main skin lesions of the disease (facial angiofibromas, ungual fibromas, shagreen patch, hypomelanotic macules). Therefore, a thorough skin examination of individuals at risk for TSC is the best and the easiest method to make the diagnosis in most of the cases (Gomez 1988a, Jóźwiak 1992). A Wood's lamp may facilitate this examination.

The diagnostic criteria are based on the different specificity of each lesion and serve as a very useful guide in the diagnostic procedure for an individual patient. The usefulness of skin lesions in the diagnosis of TSC in children should also be evaluated according to their incidence and typical age of appearance. It is well known that several findings traditionally regarded as among the most specific – facial papulonodular angiofibromas and periungual fibromas – are usually not present in infants. Contrarily, hypomelanotic macules, regarded as a tertiary feature, are useful as a diagnostic clue (but never alone) for TSC in infants and newborns. Knowledge of the incidence of the lesions, specificity for TSC and typical age of presentation may be crucial for the proper diagnosis of the disease.

SKIN LESIONS RECOGNIZED AS DIAGNOSTIC FEATURES OF TSC

The cutaneous findings diagnostic of TSC are delineated below. These were included in the 1998 revision of TSC diagnostic criteria (Table 9.1) (Roach et al. 1998). Their incidence, clinical description and course, histopathology, diagnostic significance, differential diagnosis and possible treatment are discussed.

FACIAL ANGIOFIBROMA

The earliest illustration of this lesion was displayed in Rayer's colour atlas of skin diseases in 1835 (Rayer 1835) (Fig. 9.1). Rayer described and illustrated a man with facial erythematous papules: "vascular vegetations . . . a rare and little known condition . . . characterized by small red vascular persistent papules, single or in groups . . . occurring most often on the face". In 1880, Bourneville (1880) described similar lesions in his patients with TSC but considered them as coincidental and not related to cerebral and renal pathology. The first more detailed description of facial angiofibromas is ascribed to Balzer and Ménétrier (1885), but the name of the lesions is usually linked with Pringle, as "Pringle's sign", who reported: "indolent, firm, whitish, or yellowish, sago-grain like, solid papules or little tumours embedded in the skin at different depths, or projecting from it . . . intermingled with these lesions and transgressing their limits in every direction, especially over the cheeks, toward the ears, innumerable capillary dilatations and stellate telangiectases" (Pringle

TABLE 9.1
Skin lesions included in the last revision of diagnostic criteria of TSC (Roach et al. 1998)

Major features
1. Facial angiofibromas
2. Forehead fibrous plaque
3. Nontraumatic ungual or periungual fibroma
4. Hypomelanotic macules (three or more)
5. Shagreen patch (connective tissue nevus)

Minor features
1. "Confetti-like" lesions

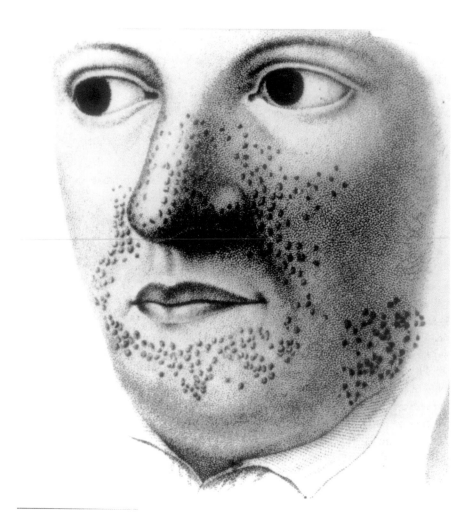

Fig. 9.1. The earliest illustration of tuberous sclerosis, with clusters of facial angiofibromas, displayed in Rayer's colour atlas of skin diseases published in 1835.

1890). Pringle and other authors of the time inaccurately labelled the lesions "adenoma sebaceum". This term is still sometimes used in the current literature.

Incidence

Studies on TSC patients before 1960 described an incidence of facial angiofibromas exceeding 90%. Critchley and Earl found the lesions in 28 out of 29 examined patients (1932). However, this is a biased figure, as the existing diagnostic criteria for TSC at that time required facial angiofibromas as one of the obligatory findings. With the implementation of new diagnostic techniques and an increased number of *formes frustes* of TSC, recent studies have reported lower incidence of the lesions. According to different authors the facial angiofibromas are present in 47 to 88% of patients with TSC (Nevin and Pearce 1968, Rogers 1988, Webb et al. 1996), with higher incidence in individuals over 5 years of age. In our study, facial angiofibromas were found in 74.5% (79 out of 106) of paediatric patients (Jóźwiak et al. 1998b). Webb et al. (1996) found the lesions in 88% of patients aged over 30 years.

Clinical description
The typical facial angiofibromas are pink to red nodules with a smooth, glistening surface, distributed bilaterally over the centrofacial areas, particularly in the naso-labial folds (in a butterfly fashion), into the cheeks and on the chin (Figs 9.2a and b). The upper lip is usually spared but the lesions may sometimes be found on the forehead or eyelids. Angiofibromas with a prominent vascular component are more obvious when the child is irritated or in warm weather. Early angiofibromas are red, due to an excessive vascular proliferation. Later, the lesions thicken and elevate, forming reddish-pink angiofibromas (Fig. 9.3).

Angiofibromas are a unique skin lesion in TSC with a clearly defined age of presentation. In a large majority of patients examined in the Children's Memorial Health Institute in Warsaw the facial angiofibromas appeared between the second and fifth year of age. In this age group the lesions became evident in 56 out of 79 (70.9%) examined children. In the remaining patients they appeared in 8 children below 2 years of age (in none during the first year of age), in 11 children aged 5 to 9 years, and in 4 children aged 9 to 14 years. Only 6 children over 5 years of age had no obvious facial angiofibromas (Jóźwiak et al. 1998b).

There are a few reports of angiofibromas becoming evident early. Webb et al. (1996) described the onset of facial angiofibromas in one child in the second year of life, and Rogers (1988) observed the lesions even in the neonatal period. The very beginning of the facial angiofibromas may be easily overlooked. In the first stage of their development, some parents of the affected children noted excessive centrofacial flushing, especially when the child cried.

As the child grows, the lesions may gradually enlarge and become more numerous, especially in the pubertal period. Sometimes they extend down the nasolabial folds or on to the chin (Fig. 9.4). In some patients the angiofibromas may not be seen until puberty or later in life; however, once developed, they persist for life. Facial angiofibromas can bleed or become painful after minor trauma.

Histopathology
Nickel and Reed (1962) demonstrated in their histopathologic study of 74 biopsy specimens that the sebaceous glands in the lesions of prepubescent patients with TSC are not pathologically enlarged, as one might expect if these patients indeed had adenomas of sebaceous glands, but may even be absent or atrophic. This was in

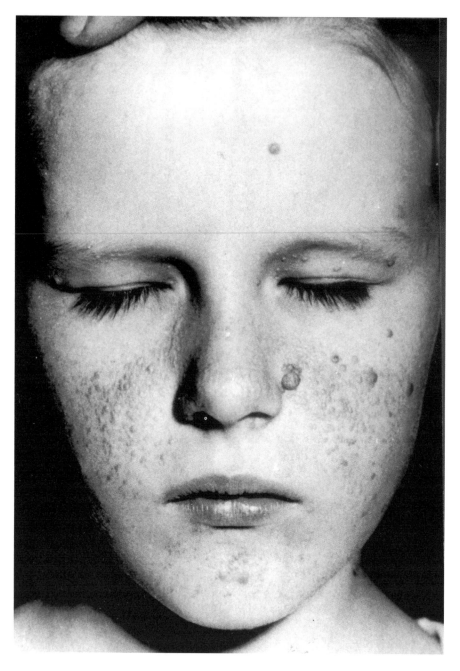

Fig. 9.2(a). Small papular angiofibromas distributed symmetrically over the centrofacial area and on the cheeks in a 9-year-old girl with TSC. Note a butterfly distribution of the lesions.

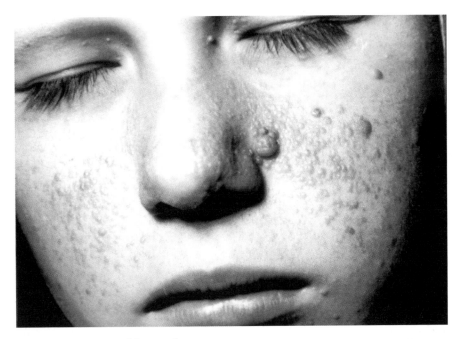

Fig. 9.2(b). Close view of the same lesions.

contrast to the previous opinion that the typical facial sign of TSC represented adenoma sebaceum. The term "angiofibroma" seems to be more proper and acceptable as there is hyperplasia of both connective tissue and vascular elements of the dermis. The multitude of vessels results in red colour of the lesions in some patients. Large angiofibromas may be polypoid and are characterized by the presence of dense fibrous tissue with collagen bundles often arranged in layers around adnexal structures. In perivascular areas multinucleated giant cells can be found. With increasing age the collagen becomes sclerotic and layered.

Diagnostic significance
Angiofibromas are a unique feature of TSC, and their diagnostic significance has never been questioned. In 1908 the facial angiofibromas (as "adenoma sebaceum") were included by Vogt (1908) in the diagnostic triad of TSC (with learning disability and epilepsy). In the recent classifications of diagnostic criteria from 1992 (Roach et al. 1992) and 1998 (Roach et al. 1998), multiple, bilateral lesions in characteristic distribution are regarded as primary or pathognomonic of TSC and do not require histopathological confirmation. As facial angiofibromas are usually not visible in children under 2 to 3 years of age their diagnostic significance is limited in the youngest children. However, their high frequency and specificity justify their diagnostic usefulness in older children and adults.

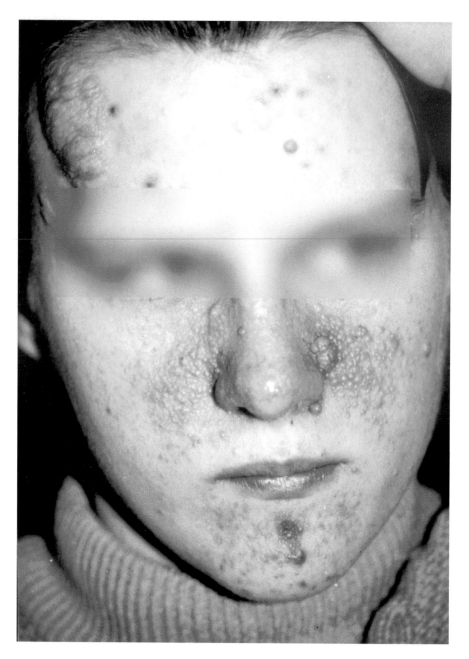

Fig. 9.3. The same patient as in Figs 9.2a and b at the age of 16 years. Apparent progression of facial angiofibromas. Note the large fibrous plaque on the forehead.

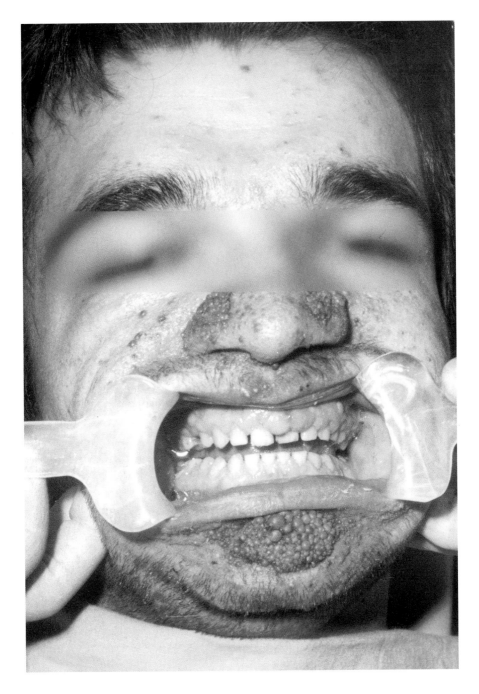

Fig. 9.4. Advanced facial angiofibromas on the face in a 17-year-old patient with TSC. Note prominent nodules on the chin and hypertrophied gingivas.

Some recent reports on multiple endocrine neoplasia (MEN) have raised the question of the relationship between MEN and facial angiofibromas. Darling et al. (1997) found multiple facial angiofibromas in 88% of their 32 patients with MEN type I. The relationship between TSC and MEN is not yet well established.

Differential diagnosis
Angiofibromas are not clinically diagnostic. They may be mistaken for a variety of other disorders, most commonly acne vulgaris, rosacea, multiple trichoepitheliomas, basal cell nevus syndrome, syringomas and other benign appendageal tumours, verruca vulgaris, and sarcoidosis. Multiple trichoepitheliomas, an autosomal dominant genodermatosis, share a central facial distribution of solid, flesh-coloured nodules, but tend to have a less prominent vascular component (Centurion et al. 2000). Multiple trichoepitheliomas ordinarily first appear during early childhood or at puberty, slowly enlarging and becoming more numerous over several years. Histologically, they show tumour islands composed of basophilic cells usually arranged in a lacelike or adenoid network. Often these cells also appear as solid aggregates, interspersed among horn cysts. These tumour islands show peripheral palisading of their cells and are surrounded by stroma with a moderate number of fibroblasts. When in doubt, a skin biopsy specimen is recommended.

Treatment
Various modalities have been used in the treatment of facial angiofibromas, including shave excision, cryosurgery, dessication, dermabrasion, carbon and argon laser (Janniger and Goldberg 1990, Verheyden 1996, Bittencourt et al. 2001). In patients with very large angiofibromas, the only available treatment is surgical removal of the lesions, dermabrasion, and/or laser destruction. Surgical excision is a reasonable option if only a few large lesions are present. It is usually performed under local anaesthesia in an outpatient setting, with good results and minimal scarring. If facial angiofibromas affect large areas of the face, dermabrasion is the treatment of choice. Argon laser therapy also seems to be very effective, although it is expensive and requires repeated courses of treatment. There are some new reports on the successful treatment of angiofibromas with the potassium titanyl phosphate laser (Finch et al. 1998).

There is no consensus about the most suitable time of the treatment. Some authors suggest removal of early angiofibromas, being convinced that such an approach should prevent the development of full-fledged, fibrous angiofibromas. However, as the lesions may continue to grow until adulthood, and since there is faster growth during puberty, the postponement of the treatment until then may be justified. The decision must be balanced by the serious psychosocial problems that are caused in adolescents with fair cognitive development and extensive angiofibromas. Cosmetic treatment of the lesions is strongly recommended in this group of children.

FOREHEAD FIBROUS PLAQUE

Good and Garb in 1943 were among the first to discover a relationship between forehead fibrous plaque and TSC (Good and Garb 1943). Clinically, it is distinct from the papular angiofibroma; however, histologically, the forehead fibrous plaque is classified as an angiofibroma.

Incidence

The incidence of the lesion is probably higher then previously thought. Webb et al. (1996) found forehead fibrous plaques in 36% of a mixed cohort of paediatric and adult patients. In our study, we could observe plaques in 20 out of 106 children (18.9%) (Jóźwiak et al. 1998b). They were evident in six children below 2 years of age, in four children aged 2 to 5, in seven aged 5 to 9, and in three aged 9 to 14 years. In some children, forehead fibrous plaques may appear in the neonatal period and represent the first skin lesion of TSC. There is a higher incidence of forehead plaques in the *TSC2* population than in the *TSC1* population (p < 0.01) (Dabora et al. 2001).

Clinical description

Forehead fibrous plaque is a yellowish-brown or flesh-coloured patch of raised skin of variable size and shape, from a few millimetres to several centimetres in diameter. The lesion is usually localized on the forehead or scalp, it is soft, medium or hard in consistency, and may have a smooth or rough surface. Single large or sometimes multiple lesions can be seen. Because of a lesser vascular component than facial angiofibromas, forehead fibrous plaque is not altered by changing colour in warm weather or when the child cries.

Unlike facial angiofibromas, forehead plaque may become evident at any age (Fryer et al. 1987, Jóźwiak et al. 1998b). In some patients it can be seen at birth. In newborns and infants it is hyperpigmented, flat and soft in consistency; it gradually grows and after many years becomes raised and solid. The larger lesions tend to calcify. An old suggestion that forehead fibrous plaques are more prominent in individuals with TSC and severe learning disability (Nickel and Reed 1962) has not been confirmed by Rogers (1988), nor in our experience (Jóźwiak et al. 1998b).

Histopathology

Histologically these lesions are classified as angiofibromas, although they have a less prominent vascular component. In specimens obtained from large fibrous plaques, hyalinization, sclerosis of collagen fibres and calcification may be seen.

Diagnostic significance

In the previous classification of diagnostic criteria for TSC from 1992 (Roach et al. 1992), the forehead fibrous plaques were regarded as secondary diagnostic features of TSC. The new edition of the classification in 1998 (Roach et al. 1998) reclassified them as major features, like facial angiofibromas. These two related lesions should be regarded as one entity for the diagnostic criteria.

Differential diagnosis
The differential diagnosis of forehead fibrous plaque includes a variety of disorders, some of which may only rarely be seen as plaques. These include the solitary mastocytoma, trichoepithelioma, granuloma faciale and sarcoidosis. A skin biopsy specimen is recommended.

Treatment
Forehead fibrous plaque can be treated by some laser techniques. As there is no non-scarring method for the removal of these lesions and they tend to recur following removal, some authors suggest that they are not removed, unless the lesions cause severe problems. Removal of large disfiguring forehead fibrous plaques may be necessary, especially in adolescents and adults with fair cognitive development.

PERIUNGUAL FIBROMAS
The first description of periungual or subungual fibromas in association with facial angiofibromas was reported by Kothe in 1903. The lesions are also known as Koenen's tumours, after Koenen's description in 1932 of ungual fibromas in 6 out of 9 members of a Dutch family with TSC.

Incidence
The incidence of periungual fibromas in unselected patients with TSC ranges from 17% (Lagos and Gomez 1967) to 52% (Nickel and Reed 1962). Periungual fibromas, common in adult patients with TSC, are much less frequent in children. Webb et al. (1996) found them in none of their children with TSC before the age of 5 years, but in 68% between the ages of 15 and 29 years. In our paediatric population of patients with TSC we have seen them in 16 out of 106 children (15.1%) – in one child aged 2 to 5 years, in three children aged 5 to 9, in eight aged 9 to 14, and in four over 14 years (Jóźwiak et al. 1998b).

Clinical description
Ungual or periungual fibromas are flesh or reddish in colour and usually arise from the bed under the nail plate or from the skin of the nail groove, more often around or under the toenails than on the fingers (Fig. 9.5). Their size ranges from several millimetres to about 1 cm. Very often periungual fibromas cause a longitudinal groove on the nail surface, which occasionally occurs without visible fibroma. It has been suggested that tight shoes may stimulate fibroma growth, especially on the lateral aspect of the fifth toe. The lesions usually appear around puberty and become more prevalent with increasing age. They tend to regrow after their removal.

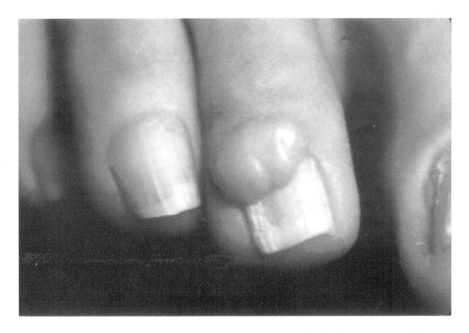

Fig. 9.5. Periungual fibroma arising from the nail bed. Longitudinal nail grooving is evident.

Histopathology
Histopathologic examination confirms that the lesions are fibromas or angiofibromas, resembling the changes found in facial angiofibromas and forehead plaques. Giant fibroblasts with a "glial appearance" may be seen in large periungual fibromas.

Diagnostic significance
Ungual or periungual fibromas are regarded as very characteristic or pathognomonic for TSC.

According to the last classification of diagnostic criteria by Roach et al. (1998), periungual fibromas are a major sign of TSC. Special attention should be paid to singular lesions, which may arise spontaneously or after trauma, and may not be related to TSC. Zeller et al. (1995) described seven patients with solitary ungual fibromas and without any other feature of TSC. Thus, these lesions cannot be considered diagnostic of TSC without other signs. Multiple lesions are probably a more reliable diagnostic sign than a single lesion. When associated with other major features of TSC, the diagnostic significance of both single and multiple periungual fibromas may be similar. Histopathological confirmation may be required only in a very few patients, when the ungual fibroma is the sole feature of TSC. As ungual fibromas usually appear around puberty, their diagnostic usefulness in small children is very limited. Nevertheless, we found them helpful in making the diagnosis even in these patients, when ungual fibromas were demonstrated in their apparently non-affected parents.

Differential diagnosis
The differential diagnosis includes epithelial inclusion cysts, verruca vulgaris, pyogenic granuloma and infantile digital fibromatosis (Rogers 1988). A history of trauma should be considered.

Treatment
Sometimes patients remove ungual fibromas themselves, especially when the lesions are large and produce difficulties in wearing shoes. Also, in some patients they can bleed and become a source of chronic infection. Excision of troublesome ungual fibromas is the easiest method of treatment, although recurrences are frequent. Some authors have suggested that laser treatment might be the most effective therapy for ungual fibromas (Pasyk and Argenta 1988, Berlin and Billick 2002).

HYPOMELANOTIC MACULES
Critchley and Earl (1932) were probably the first to describe, in 1932, "patches of abnormal whiteness" in their patients with TSC. Later, others also observed hypomelanotic macules in patients with TSC (Butterworth and Wilson 1941, Nickel and Reed 1962, Gold and Freeman 1965). Early presentation of hypomelanotic macules and their significance as the first visible sign of TSC were emphasized by Gold and Freeman (1965) and Harris and Moynahan (1966). One of the most comprehensive studies on the incidence of hypomelanotic macules in TSC and their diagnostic significance was undertaken by Fitzpatrick et al. (1968).

The very high frequency of the lesions in patients with TSC, and their early presentation, even in newborns and infants, have attracted much interest in recent years. One must consider the specificity of hypomelanotic macules for TSC, their incidence in the general population, and the necessary number of detected spots. Hypomelanotic macules play an important role in the diagnosis of TSC, especially in small children. Some authors have pinpointed their significance in the diagnosis of TSC in children with *TSC2/PKD1* gene mutation (Sperandio et al. 2000).

Incidence
The incidence of hypomelanotic macules in populations with TSC varies from 50% in one series (Harris and Moynahan 1966) to 97.2% in our experience (Jóźwiak et al. 1998b), or 100% in the group of children under 5 years of age examined by Webb et al. (1996). The true prevalence seems to be above 90%. It has been suggested that the lower incidence reported in the earlier studies might be related to the fact that at that time the diagnostic value of hypomelanotic macules had not been recognized, or the patients were not examined with the Wood's light.

Hypomelanotic macules were revealed in 103 out of 106 children (97.2%) examined in the Children's Memorial Health Institute in Warsaw. Their incidence increased from 89.6% in children below 2 years of age to 97.2% in children aged 14 to 18 (Jóźwiak et al. 2000).

Clinical description
Hypomelanotic macules in patients with TSC vary in shape from oval to lanceolate or "ash leaf-shaped" (Figs 9.6 and 9.7). Their margins are usually clearly delineated; their size ranges from several millimetres to several centimetres. They are asymmetrically distributed over the body surface, but predominate on the trunk, buttocks and extremities, and are rarely evident on the face. Hypomelanotic macules on the scalp may produce areas of hypopigmented hairs (poliosis). A white forelock may be an early sign of TSC (Desch 1996, Tunnessen et al. 1996). Sometimes the hypomelanotic areas may be seen along the lines of cleavage of the trunk following a dermatomal distribution. The number of macules varies from 1 to more than 40.

In the majority of patients with TSC, multiple hypomelanotic macules are easily visualized under normal lightning. In a few patients the lesions are visible only with ultraviolet light (Wood's lamp) – since they are deficient in melanin, hypomelanotic macules absorb less ultraviolet light emitted by the lamp than surrounding normal skin. In our clinical practice, we have been able to note the lesions under normal light

Fig. 9.6. Typical hypomelanotic macule of lance ovate shape and distinct borders seen in patient with TSC.

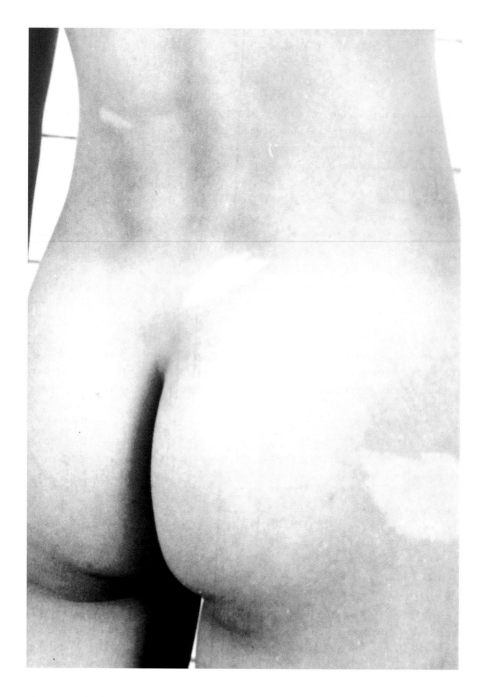

Fig. 9.7. Multiple hypomelanotic macules on the trunk and buttocks. Note lance ovate shape of the lesions.

in about 80 to 85% of children. We used a Wood's lamp only in children with apparently negative skin examination under normal light. Also, Norio et al. (1996) found the Wood's lamp of limited value in the majority of patients. However, the lamp may be helpful in the skin examination of relatives with TSC.

Usually, hypomelanotic macules are observed in neonates or infants. They are regarded as a first visible sign of TSC (Gold and Freeman 1965, Fitzpatrick et al. 1968). We observed hypomelanotic macules at birth in 66 children, and in 20 others the presentation was delayed until the first few months of age. In total, in our study, hypomelanotic macules have been observed in 95 children (89.6%) below 2 years of age. In another eight patients the appearance of these lesions was even more delayed: in six children they appeared between 2 and 5 years, and in two patients between 5 and 9 years (Jóźwiak et al. 1998b). Contrary to the widespread opinion that the number of hypomelanotic macules increases in childhood and they persist throughout life, Webb et al. (1996) found the lesions in 100% of children with TSC before the age of 5 years, but in only 58% of patients after 30 years of age. They suggest that some lesions may disappear with age. So far this hypothesis has not been confirmed.

Histopathology
Skin biopsy specimens taken from hypomelanotic macules of patients with TSC usually demonstrate a normal number of melanocytes, with reduction in the intensity of histochemical reaction compared with surrounding normal skin. Electron microscopic studies, showing reduced number, diameter and melanization of mela-nosomes in melanocytes in patients with TSC, may be necessary to differentiate a hypomelanotic macule from vitiligo, nevus anemicus, nevus depigmentosus, piebaldism or Vogt–Koyanagi–Harada syndrome (Jimbow et al. 1957, Krysicka-Janniger 1993, Schwartz and Janniger 1997).

Diagnostic significance
Because of their high incidence and very early presentation, hypomelanotic macules play an important role in the diagnosis of TSC. They may be the only skin lesions in infants and, if associated with infantile spasms, they strongly suggest a diagnosis of TSC. However, hypomelanotic macules by themselves are not sufficient for a diagnosis of TSC. Although they are found in 90 to 98% of patients with TSC, they are not specific for the disease and may be found in presumably healthy persons.

One of the earliest reports on the prevalence of hypopigmented macules in individuals without TSC was presented by Zaremba (1968). The author found that 3.3% of 1013 children from institutions for those with severe learning disability, presumably without TSC, had hypopigmented macules. Debard and Richardet (1975) reported that of 9737 infants examined at ages 1 to 18 months, 0.73% had hypopigmented macules. Of the 0.03% with three or more macules, two infants had TSC and one had neurofibromatosis. Screening of newborn infants for white spots, carried out by Alper and Holmes (1983), has shown that 0.8% of all infants have hypomelanotic macules. According to these authors, the prevalence rate is 0.4% for white infants and 2.4% for black infants (Alper and Holmes 1983).

Vanderhooft et al. (1996), in a general population study of 423 white people younger than 45 years of age, found 20 (4.7%) with at least one hypomelanotic macule (three had two lesions and one had three lesions). No one in the study had more than three macules. Although the individuals with hypomelanotic macules were not extensively evaluated for other evidence of TSC, none had other obvious signs of the disease.

The previous diagnostic criteria classified hypomelanotic macules as a tertiary feature of TSC (Roach et al. 1992). Taking into account the new data regarding the incidence of hypomelanotic macules in healthy populations, the latest consensus panel recommended that the presence of three or more hypomelanotic macules should be considered a major feature of TSC, while one or two such lesions should not be used to establish the diagnosis (Roach et al. 1998). Certainly, careful skin examination with a search for hypomelanotic macules may be very useful diagnostically in any infant or child with epilepsy or learning disability, or in immediate relatives of patients with TSC before genetic counselling.

Differential diagnosis

There are many hypopigmented spots that should be differentiated from hypomelanotic macules found in TSC patients. The type and number of white cutaneous alterations were evaluated by Norio et al. in a group of 100 medical students and 100 schoolchildren (Norio et al. 1996); 93% of the former and 79% of the latter had some whitish lesions, many of them scars; 20% of the adults and 12% of the children had roundish or oval macules larger than 10 mm in diameter, not known to be scars. This study and other reports on the incidence of hypopigmented macules in healthy populations indicate that conclusions about the diagnostic value of hypomelanotic macules in TSC cannot be drawn too hastily.

There are a few dermatological conditions which manifest with skin lesions mimicking the hypopigmentation in TSC. Hypomelanotic macules of TSC should be differentiated from other isolated white macules in vitiligo, nevus anemicus, nevus achromicus, hypomelanosis of Ito, piebaldism, pityriasis alba, tinea versicolor or Vogt–Koyanagi–Harada syndrome.

On superficial skin examination, patches of vitiligo might be confused with the hypopigmented macules of TSC. However, more careful examination with an application of the Wood's lamp demonstrates that the lesions in vitiligo are completely amelanotic rather than hypopigmented. The lesions are usually located symmetrically near natural orifices and joints. Usually they are not congenital. Biopsy specimens taken from the lesions show absolute absence of melanocytes and total loss of melanin (Krysicka-Janniger 1993, Krysicka-Janniger and Schwartz 1993, Schwartz and Janniger 1997).

The nevus anemicus is a congenital, non-progressive functional vascular developmental anomaly appearing as one or more patches of varying sizes and shapes distinctly paler than surrounding skin (Ahkami and Schwartz 1999). The shape is often corymbiform, with a pale patch surrounded by smaller satellite macules. The patches may be linear in configuration, or grouped. The disorder is most commonly seen on the trunk, particularly the chest and back. Diascopy (examination with a glass or clear plastic plate, usually a flat blade or microscope slide, pressed against the skin to permit observation of changes produced in the underlying skin after the blood vessels are emptied and skin is blanched) often renders its outline unrecognizable from its blanched surroundings, whereas it may be highlighted by the application of gentle friction which flushes the surrounding skin. Similarly, application of heat or cold produces erythema of adjacent normal skin, so that the non-erythematous nevus anemicus stands out prominently.

Nevus achromicus, sometimes also called *nevus depigmentosus* (which is a misnomer, as lesions are hypopigmented, not depigmented), is usually present at birth and may be clinically indistinguishable from hypomelanotic macules in TSC. The nevus is characterized by bizarre pattern or dermatomal distribution. The lesions vary from a few centimetres in diameter to extensive, covering large areas of the trunk and limbs. Electron microscopic studies reveal fewer melanosomes, which are normal in size and melanization. Melanin transportation to keratinocytes is significantly decreased, unlike in TSC, where this transportation is only slightly decreased (Jimbow et al. 1957).

Similar lesions appear in hypomelanosis of Ito, in which hypopigmented streaks are associated with multiple abnormalities. The disorder is now recognized as a heterogeneous group of conditions explained by genetic or chromosomal mosaicism. In some patients with only skin representation of hypomelanosis of Ito, this can be regarded as monosymptomatic expression of mosaic phenotypes, while in others multisystem presentation can be observed, with ocular, skeletal and neurological abnormalities.

Hypopigmented lesions in piebaldism, an autosomal dominant skin disease, are present at birth and remain unchanged throughout life. The main features are: white, triangular forelock of the scalp, a white macule in the centre of the chin, decreased areas of pigmentation on the trunk, mid-arm to wrist, and mid-thigh to calf. Electron microscopic examination reveals absolute absence of melanocytes.

In pityriasis alba, a common condition in childhood, hypopigmented areas are thought to result from xerosis. There may be seen on a minimal scale, usually not associated with erythema. In tinea versicolor, hypopigmented areas are associated with scale. A KOH preparation shows the characteristic hyphae and spores in a "spaghetti and meatball" pattern. Hypopigmented macules and poliosis (areas of hypopigmented hair) may be the features of Vogt–Koyanagi–Harada syndrome. The lesions are accompanied by dysacusia, chronic bilateral uveitis and neurological symptoms. Also, some inflammatory diseases (e.g. dermatomycosis) may be associated with areas of skin hypopigmentation.

SHAGREEN PATCHES

Hallopeau and Leredde (1895) gave the first description of shagreen patches in a patient with facial angiofibromas and seizures. Their original definition, cited by Rogers (1988), is very suggestive: "when the patient stands, one sees an elevated mass, divided by longitudinal folds; one can take this mass between the fingers, separate them from the deep layers; actually, it is a part of the skin".

Incidence

The incidence of shagreen patches in patients with TSC ranges from 21% (Gomez 1988c) to 68% (Nickel and Reed 1962), or 80% (Butterworth and Wilson 1941). The frequency of the lesions increases with age. Webb et al. (1996) found the lesions in 25% of children below 5 years of age, and in 54 to 55% of patients from other age groups: above 5 to 14, 15 to 29, and more than 30 years of age. In our patients, the incidence rose from 5.7% in children below 2 years of age, to 20.8% in children aged 2 to 5, to 34.9% in those aged 5 to 9, to 47.2% in those aged 9 to 14, and to 48.1% in those aged 14 to 18 (Jóźwiak 1995b, Jóźwiak et al. 2000).

Clinical description

Shagreen patches are firm yellowish-red or pink nodules slightly elevated above the surrounding skin, with surface resembling in texture the skin of an orange. Usually they are distributed asymmetrically on dorsal body surfaces and particularly on the lumbosacral skin (Figs 9.8a and b). They are rare on the skin of the chest, abdomen, shoulders or buttocks. In the majority of patients the lesions are multiple and small, from a few millimetres to 1 cm in size, and might easily be overlooked in smaller children. Appearing in clusters, in a few patients they become large lesions more then 10 cm in diameter. First appearance of the lesions usually takes place soon before or around puberty, but we observed several patients with shagreen patches present from early infancy. The youngest age at which the lesions were seen was 5 months. The number and size of the patches gradually increase with age until adulthood.

Histopathology

From a histopathological point of view, the shagreen patches consist of a single or a cluster of connective tissue hamartomas. Rogers (1988) delineates two main types of shagreen patches. In the first, more common, type, a band of superficial dermis is normal but its deeper layers are composed of a haphazard arrangement of collagen fibres. In the second type, a uniform hamartomatous proliferation of collagen

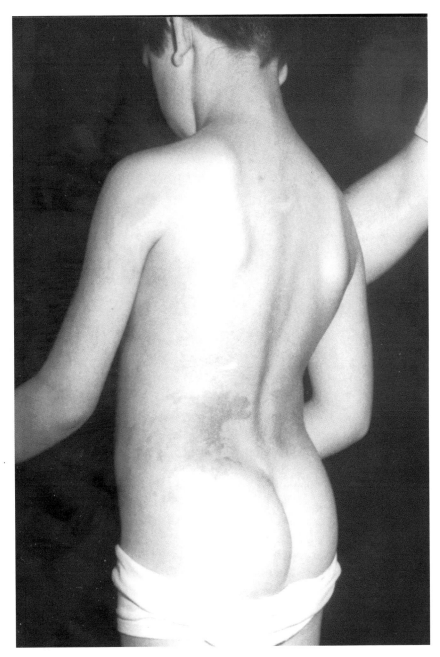

Fig. 9.8(a). A shagreen patch in a 10-year-old boy with TSC. Typical location of the plaque in the lumbosacral region. Note two hypomelanotic macules on the upper back.

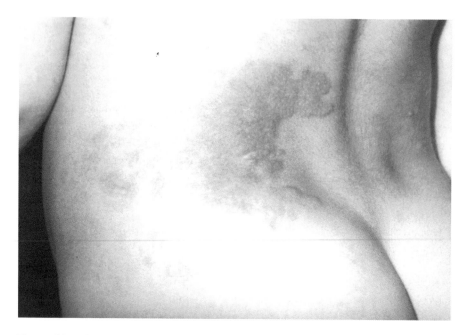

Fig. 9.8(b). A close view of the same lesion. The plaque is elevated with less evident lateral border and several small papules at the periphery.

throughout the whole section of dermis is seen. The general appearance of both types is one of excess collagen and elastic tissue in disproportion to the amount of muscle, adipose tissue, appendages and vascular structures (Rogers 1988).

Diagnostic significance
In the previous classification of diagnostic criteria for TSC (Roach et al. 1992), the shagreen patches were regarded as a secondary feature, less diagnostically useful than facial papulonodular angiofibromas or periungual fibromas. In the latest revision of the diagnostic criteria (Roach et al. 1998), shagreen patches are regarded as a major feature. Leaving out the question of their specificity, they represent the third most common skin feature, after hypomelanotic macules and angiofibromas, in patients with TSC, and may be very helpful in diagnosis even in children.

Differential diagnosis
The shagreen patch is difficult to differentiate both clinically and histopathologically from other connective tissue nevi. The differential diagnosis should include connective tissue nevi with osteopoikilosis (Buschke–Ollendorf syndrome). In both these conditions the lesions are located ventrally or dorsally, usually bilaterally and symmetrically, and appear earlier in childhood.

Treatment
Enlarging shagreen patches may require cosmetic treatment (Wendt and Watson 1991).

"CONFETTI-LIKE" LESIONS
This kind of hypopigmentation in TSC has been recognized as a diagnostic feature relatively late. The "confetti-like" lesions have been separated from other hypopigmentations of TSC only during the last two decades. We describe them separately, as, according to the latest classification, their diagnostic significance differs from the diagnostic value of hypomelanotic macules (Roach et al. 1998).

Incidence
There are very few data on the incidence of "confetti-like" lesions in TSC patients. Their true prevalence in the general population is also obscure. In our group of 106 children with TSC, we revealed "confetti-like" lesions in three children (2.8%), two aged 5 to 9 years and one 17-year-old (Jóźwiak et al. 1998b). Their prevalence in adults seems to be higher, as we found them also in 4 out of 20 affected parents (20%). Webb et al. (1996) reported "confetti-like" lesions in 28% of unselected patients with TSC, "often at a young age". Unfortunately the age of patients with the lesions was not specified.

Clinical description
"Confetti-like" macules are multiple, small white spots, 1–2 mm in diameter, often symmetrically distributed on the limbs, characteristically over the forearms and lower legs. According to Webb et al. (1996) they might easily be overlooked without the use of a Wood's lamp. In our experience they usually appear in the second decade or in adulthood.

Histopathology
Their histopathology seems to be similar to that of hypomelanotic macules.

Diagnostic significance
As they are very seldom studied in children, their diagnostic significance is mainly restricted to adolescents and adults. In the previous diagnostic criteria recommendations (Roach et al. 1992), the "confetti-like" lesions, like the hypomelanotic macules, were regarded as a tertiary feature of TSC. Recent recommendations (Roach et al. 1998) classify the "confetti-like" lesions as a minor feature of TSC (unlike hypomelanotic macules, which are regarded as a major feature).

Differential diagnosis

The "confetti-like" lesions should be differentiated from the skin lesions appearing after repeated sun exposure. In the elderly they may resemble idiopathic guttate hypomelanosis.

OTHER SKIN LESIONS NOT INCLUDED IN THE LIST OF DIAGNOSTIC CRITERIA FOR TSC

MOLLUSCUM FIBROSUM PENDULUM

Skin tags, particularly in axillae and groins, are frequently seen in normal elderly people, but are uncommon in children and adolescents. In individuals with TSC, multiple, soft, pedunculated growths (molluscum fibrosum pendulum) are commonly present on the neck, and rarely in axillae and groins (Fig. 9.9). Webb et al. (1996) reported the presence of the lesions in 6% of patients with TSC aged 13 to 28 years. We have found them in 24 out of 106 (22.6%) children with TSC examined in the Children's Memorial Health Institute in Warsaw, including four children below 5 years of age (Jóźwiak et al. 1998b). Such early presentation and particular location may be specific for TSC, but this cannot be assessed with a high level of confidence because of a lack of epidemiological studies evaluating specifically for this finding in healthy children. Comparatively low incidence of the lesions and lack of histological specificity resulted in an absence of the molluscum fibrosum

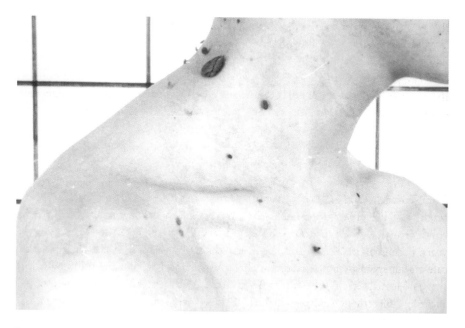

Fig. 9.9. Pedunculated growths (molluscum fibrosum pendulum) around the neck in a 12-year-old child with TSC.

pendulum on the list of diagnostic features of TSC. We believe that it should be regarded as a minor feature. The presence of multiple pedunculated fibromas on the neck in a child should alert the clinician to the possibility of TSC.

Café-au-lait Spots

Café-au-lait spots have been reported in some patients with TSC. When associated with TSC, these flat, hyperpigmented macules are usually single and have a diameter of 0.5 to 3 cm. They have well-demarcated borders and vary in shape from oval to round. They are asymmetrically distributed over the body surface, but predominate on the trunk, buttocks and extremities.

The incidence of café-au-lait spots in healthy subjects seems to be at least 10 to 15%. Crowe et al. (1956) revealed that 10% of the general population have one or more café-au-lait spots, and patients with six or more spots, most of which exceed 1.5 cm in diameter, nearly always have neurofibromatosis type I (NF-1). Vanderhooft et al. (1996) carefully examined the skin of 423 individuals younger than 45 years, representing the white general population, and found café-au-lait spots in 65 of them (15.4%). The prevalence of café-au-lait spots in healthy populations and TSC patients seems to be similar. In one of the first studies assessing the incidence of the spots in patients with TSC, Nickel and Reed (1962) found them in 7% of their patients. A similar incidence of these lesions was also reported by Lagos and Gomez (1967) in 1967. In another study, Bell and McDonald (1985) compared the prevalence of café-au-lait spots in normal subjects (16%) and in patients with TSC (15.4%), and did not reveal any statistically significant differences between the two groups.

The presence of café-au-lait spots in patients with TSC misled some authors to the concurrent diagnosis of neurofibromatosis type I and TSC. The true association of these two conditions seems to be exceptional, and is well documented in only two reports (Schull and Crowe 1953, Lee et al. 1994). Lee et al. (1994) described both entities in a 16-year-old male. His mother and sister demonstrated features of TSC, but NF-1 seemed to have resulted from a new mutation.

We have found the café-au-lait spots in 30 out of 106 children (28.3%) with TSC (Jóźwiak et al. 1998b). They were usually single and appeared in the first months of life. They occurred in 24 children below the age of 2 years, in two children aged 2 to 5 years, in three aged 5 to 9 years, and in one child of 14 to 18 years. Because of a similar incidence in the healthy population and in TSC patients, café-au-lait spots are not regarded as characteristic for TSC and are not included in the list of diagnostic criteria. In differential diagnosis, NF-1 should always be excluded. Electron microscopic study of the lesions reveals, in neurofibromatosis, giant pigment granules in melanocytes and keratinocytes (Jimbow et al. 1957).

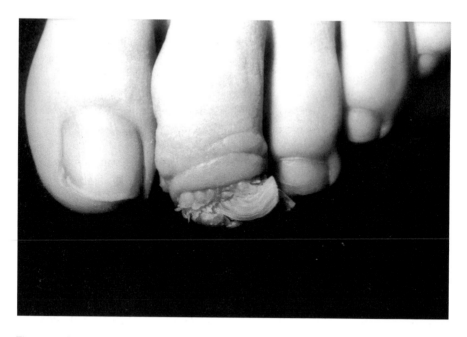

Fig. 9.10. Cutaneous horn arising from the nail bed of a child with TSC.

OTHER SKIN LESIONS

In children with TSC many other skin tumours have been reported, such as lipomas (Klein and Barr 1986), neurofibromas, cystoadenomas, angiokeratomas (Gil-Mateo et al. 1996), cutaneous horns, etc. (Fig. 9.10). Because of their low prevalence in the whole TSC population it is difficult to judge whether they represent a coincidental finding or are the result of a possible "dysplastic" nature of TSC. Nico et al. (1999) described two patients with the complete syndrome of TSC who had, in addition to characteristic facial angiofibromas, multiple angiofibromas in the genital area. Histopathological examination confirmed the diagnosis of angiofibroma. The true prevalence of these lesions in the TSC population is unknown.

MOLECULAR BASIS OF SKIN MANIFESTATIONS OF TSC

TSC is a hereditary disorder characterized by epilepsy, learning disability and hamartomatous lesions in multiple organs. It has been shown that the genes responsible for TSC, *TSC1* and *TSC2*, act as tumour suppressors, but the mechanism of hamartomatous growth in several tissues is not completely understood. Although TSC is clearly inherited as an autosomal dominant disease, there is a continuum of varied expressivity, from severely affected to apparent total nonpenetrance (Gomez 1988c, Jóźwiak and Michałowicz 1996).

Recent molecular studies seem to explain some mechanism of pathogenesis of lesions in TSC (Jóźwiak 1995a, Young and Povey 1998). The wide clinical variation seen in TSC, even within a given family, may be partially explained by Knudsen's two-hit model applied for many tumour suppressor genes. According to this hypothesis, the development of tumours must arise from two independent mutational events – a germline alteration on the tumour suppressor gene, inherited from an affected parent, and a second somatic mutation in the allele inherited from the unaffected parent. The earlier the second mutation arises, the more widespread its effect, and the more organs and tissues may be involved.

This "loss of heterozygosity" (LOH) caused by a second mutation on a homologic chromosome has been recently proved in angiomyolipomas, cortical tubers, giant cell astrocytomas, periungual fibromas and cardiac rhabdomyomas in patients with TSC (Sepp et al. 1996). Further studies should answer the question of whether loss of heterozygosity may be responsible for the appearance of other skin lesions in TSC. Unilateral facial angiofibromas may represent such clinical evidence. In the literature, several reports exist on the presence of unilateral facial angiofibromas (McGrae and Hashimoto 1996, Anliker et al. 1997, Garcia-Muret et al. 1998, Jóźwiak et al. 1998b, Silvestre et al. 2000, Del Pozo et al. 2002). Our patient demonstrated multiple unilateral facial angiofibromas without any other features associated with TSC (Fig. 9.11) (Jóźwiak et al. 1998b). The possibility that these patients are mosaics, with LOH resulting in unilateral angiofibromas, is very probable, but not proven.

Both protein products of the TSC genes, hamartin and tuberin, probably function as part of the same complex or as an adjacent step in the same pathway. Preliminary results of genotype-phenotype studies, indicating very little phenotypic difference between *TSC1* and *TSC2* mutations, may support this hypothesis (Jóźwiak et al. 1998a). The cellular pathway is likely to involve a small GTPase signalling molecule and might be important for endocytosis and cell growth.

Pathological studies of stroma of facial angiofibromas, ungual fibromas and shagreen patches indicated that the lesions contain polygonal cells with pointed prolongations reminiscent of a starfish. These lesions are larger than ordinary fibroblasts and have characteristics halfway between fibroblasts and histiocytes (Ishibashi et al. 1991). Ishibashi et al. (1991) found that they stain for neuron-specific enolase and, more strikingly, react with monoclonal antibody to glial fibrillary acidic protein (GFAP), thus expressing neural rather than fibroblastic features. When cultured in vitro, some of the cells have long cytoplasmic processes like glial cells.

Others have found neuronal markers in the cells obtained from angiofibromas and renal angiomyolipomas and called them N-cells. Johnson et al. (1991) proposed that N-cells may result from dedifferentiation of a normal occurring cell in the skin, possibly a fibroblast or a melanocyte, which regresses to a more primordial state, or from failure of certain dermal cells to achieve terminal differentiation. As the neuron-like cells express some neuronal and occasionally oligodendroglial markers, their inability to differentiate must have occurred before migration to the periphery.

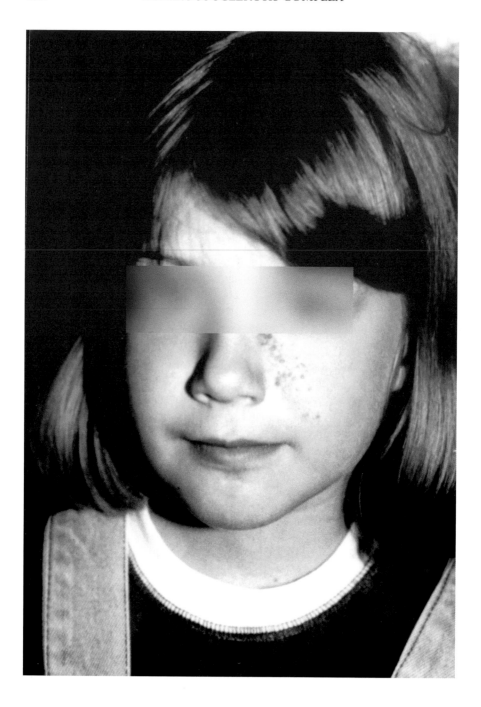

Fig. 9.11. Unilateral facial angiofibroma in a girl without any other stigmata of TSC.

The TSC hamartomas are essentially benign; they rarely progress to become malignant tumours. This benign nature of TSC lesions might be partially explained by the studies of Toyoshima et al. (1999). The authors revealed similar changes in cultured angiofibroma stroma cells from TSC to those observed in human senescent fibroblasts: a low proliferative capacity, an increase in cell size, increased binucleated cells in association with abnormal cytokinesis and increased senescent-associated beta-galactosidase. Growth of facial angiofibromas in TSC may be caused by a gain in enhanced sensitivity toward some of the potential mitogens, and forced multiplication without loss of the cellular senescent program. This may be the reason why TSC hamartomas rarely progress to malignancy and why the growths are limited to a finite size.

STOMATOLOGICAL MANIFESTATIONS
Although the first patients with TSC were described in 1880, it was not until the 1940s that oral involvement was well recognized. Up to now there has been little reference to the oral manifestations of TSC in the literature. These lesions include gingival fibromas or papillomas, fibromas of the tongue and palate, and enamel hypoplasia.

GINGIVAL AND ORAL FIBROMAS
Butterworth and Wilson in 1941 reported a few fibrous papules on the gingiva in the incisor and canine regions, and a large fibrous plaque on the dorsum of the tongue, in one of their patients (Butterworth and Wilson 1941). Fibromas of the upper lip were also mentioned by Good and Garb (1943).

Incidence
Nodular tumours of the oral cavity, fibromas or papillomas were found in 11% of 186 patients examined by Schuermann et al. (1966). The authors did not reveal any sex prevalence.

There is a lack of epidemiological studies on the incidence of these lesions in patients with TSC. We have found gingival hypertrophy in 17 (48.5%) and nodular fibromas in 7 (20%) out of 35 children with TSC (Jóźwiak 1995b).

Clinical description
The fibromas of the oral cavity occur most commonly on the gingiva, predominantly in the anterior segment of the upper jaw, but also on the tongue and palate. They have been noted in four of our patients under 5 years of age, and their incidence increases with age. Phenytoin medication, frequently used in epileptic patients with TSC, may additionally speed up the growth of the lesions. Hypertrophied gingiva may be very painful and cause episodes of haemorrhages (Mackler et al. 1972), resulting in inability to chew and eat. Large fibromas of the tongue may produce

macroglossia. Davis et al. (1964) reported two pedunculated haemangiomas on the tongue in one patient.

Histopathology
The microscopic study of the gingival lesions usually reveals extensive branching and fusing of spiked rete ridges of the epithelium, hyalinized fibrous connective tissue bands in the submucosa, and fibroblasts with large ovoid nuclei in the lamina propria area (Mackler et al. 1972). This picture is consistent with a fibrous hyperplasia of the gingiva.

Diagnostic significance
According to the recent modification of the diagnostic criteria for TSC, gingival fibromas should be regarded as a minor feature of TSC. Because of a lack of large epidemiological studies their true prevalence in the TSC population is still uncertain.

Treatment
Large gingival lesions may require a surgical incision. Gingivectomy and gingivoplasty may be performed if needed, usually under general anaesthesia.

ENAMEL HYPOPLASIA
Linear enamel hypoplasia in a patient with TSC was first noted by Carol (1921), but it was only in the 1970s that Witkop and Rao (1971) and Hoff et al. (1975) suggested that it might be a characteristic finding in TSC. The enamel defects in patients with TSC are thought to result from a disturbance in cell differentiation and possibly a defective interaction between odontoblasts and ameloblasts (Hoff et al. 1975). Depending on the quantity of disordered ameloblasts, small or crater-like structures are formed.

Incidence
There are few epidemiological studies evaluating the frequency of dental pits in the TSC population. Hoff et al. (1975) described the lesions in all six TSC patients as small pit- and crater-like defects. Enamel defects were found on all tooth surfaces of these patients. The total number of pits varied from 1 to 11, with an average of three pits per tooth surface. Lygidakis and Lindenbaum (1987) reported enamel defects in 25 out of 35 (71%) patients with TSC. They were less often found in children (62%) than in adults (77%). An even higher incidence of the lesion was reported by Mlynarczyk (1991). The author found enamel pitting in all 29 (100%) patients above 11 years of age, and in 16 out of 21 (76%) younger children. There was no evidence of sex preponderance.

Clinical description

Enamel pits are usually asymptomatic, but may expedite the development of caries in TSC patients. These defects are easily distinguishable from primary carious lesions because they are located away from the gingivae on the outer surfaces (an area rarely involved in caries). The incidence of lesions increases with age (Lygidakis and Lindenbaum 1987, Mlynarczyk 1991). They are easily detected in permanent teeth but in deciduous teeth the pits are smaller and less frequent, requiring very careful inspection. Gomez (1988b) divides the lesions into three categories: (1) small pits not visible without magnification and only 4 µm in diameter; (2) indentations up to 60 µm diameter; (3) crater-like structures corresponding to pits visible with the naked eye, with a diameter of approximately 100 µm.

Histopathology

On scanning electron microscopy the pits appear as crater-like structures filled with presumably organic material, and extend from the amelodential junction to the tooth surface.

Diagnostic significance

According to the latest revision of the diagnostic criteria, the enamel pits are regarded as minor features of TSC. They seem to be more diagnostic in adults because of their higher incidence and greater specificity in this age group.

Differential diagnosis

Enamel pits may be seen in 7% of adults and 20% of children in the normal population (Mlynarczyk 1991). Clinically similar enamel hypoplasia has been reported in patients with pitted amelogenesis imperfecta, epidermolysis bullosa dystrophica, pseudohypoparathyroidism, tricho-dento-osseous syndrome and D-dependent rickets.

Treatment

No treatment is required.

Recently, several odontogenic or intraoral tumours have been reported in patients with TSC: epithelial odontogenic tumour (Rubin et al. 1987), desmoblastic fibroma (Miyamoto et al. 1995), odontogenic myxoma (Harrison et al. 1997), and a large cavernous hemangioma (Lygidakis and Lindenbaum 1989).

REFERENCES

Ahkami RN, Schwartz RA (1999) Nevus anemicus. *Dermatology (Basel)* 198: 327–9.

Alper JC, Holmes LB (1983) The incidence and significance of birthmarks in a cohort of 4,641 newborns. *J Pediatr Dermatol* 1: 58–68.

Anliker MD, Dummer R, Burg G (1997) Unilateral agminated angiofibromas: a segmental expression of tuberous sclerosis? *Dermatology* 195: 176–8.

Balzer F, Ménétrier P (1885) Étude sur un cas d'adénomes sébacés de la face et du cuir chevelu. *Arch Physiol Norm Pathol* 6: 564–76.

Bell SD, McDonald DM (1985) The prevalence of café-au-lait patches in tuberous sclerosis. *Clin Exp Dermatol* 10: 562–5.

Berlin AL, Billick RC (2002) Use of CO_2 laser in the treatment of periungual fibromas associated with tuberous sclerosis. *Dermatol Surg* 28: 434–6.

Bittencourt RC, Huilgol SC, Seed PT, et al. (2001) Treatment of angiofibromas with a scanning carbon dioxide laser: a clinicopathological study with long-term follow-up. *J Am Acad Dermatol* 45: 731–5.

Bourneville DM (1880) Sclérose tubéreuse des circonvolutions cérébrales: idiotie et épilepsie hémiplégique. *Arch Neurol (Paris)* 1: 81–91.

Butterworth T, Wilson M (1941) Dermatologic aspects of tuberous sclerosis. *Arch Dermatol Syph (Chic.)* 43: 1–41.

Campbell AW (1905) Cerebral sclerosis, III: tuberose sclerosis. *Brain* 28: 382–96.

Carol WLL (1921) Beitrag zur Kenntnis des Adenoma Sebaceum (Pringle) und sein Verhaltnis zur Kranheit von Bourneville und von Recklinghausen. *Acta Derm Venereol (Stockh.)* 2: 186.

Centurion SA, Schwartz RA, Lambert WC (2000) Trichoepithelioma papulosum multiplex. *J Dermatol* 27(3): 137–43.

Critchley M, Earl CJC (1932) Tuberous sclerosis and allied conditions. *Brain* 55: 311–46.

Crowe FW, Schull WJ, Neel JV (1956) *Clinical, Pathological and Genetic Study of Multiple Neurofibromatosis*. Springfield, IL: Charles C Thomas.

Dabora SL, Jóźwiak S, Franz DN, et al. (2001) Mutational analysis in a cohort of 224 tuberous sclerosis patients indicates increased severity of TSC2 compared with TSC1 disease in multiple organs. *Am J Hum Genet* 68: 64–80.

Darling TN, Skarulis MC, Steinberg SM, et al. (1997) Multiple facial angiofibromas and collagenomas in patients with multiple endocrine neoplasia type I. *Arch Dermatol* 133: 853–7.

Davis RK, Baer P, Archard HO, Palmer JH (1964) Tuberous sclerosis with oral manifestations. *Oral Surg* 17: 395–400.

Debard A, Richardet JM (1975) Signification des taches achromiques chez le nourrisson [letter]. *Nouvelle Presse Med* 4: 2404.

Del Pozo J, Martinez W, Calvo R, et al. (2002) Unilateral angiofibromas. An oligosymptomatic and segmentary form of tuberous sclerosis. *Eur J Dermatol* 12: 262.

Desch LW (1996) White forelock could be early sign of tuberous sclerosis. *Arch Ped Adol Med* 150: 651.

Finch TM, Hindson C, Cotterill JA (1998) Successful treatment of adenoma sebaceum with the potassium titanyl phosphate laser. *Clin Exp Dermatol* 23: 201–3.

Fitzpatrick TB, Szabó G, Hori Y (1968) White leaf-shaped macules: earliest visible sign of tuberous sclerosis, *Arch Dermatol* 98: 1–6.

Fryer AE, Osborne JP, Schutt W (1987) Forehead plaque: a presenting skin sign in tuberous sclerosis. *Arch Dis Childh* 62: 292–3.

Garcia-Muret MP, Pujol RM, de Moragas JM (1998) Multiple and unilateral angiofibromas of the face: forme fruste of Bourneville tuberous sclerosis. *Ann Dermatol Venereol* 125: 325–7.

Gil-Mateo MP, Miquel FJ, Velasco AM, et al. (1996) Widespread angiokeratomas and tuberous sclerosis. *Br J Dermatol* 135: 280–2.

Gold AP, Freeman JM (1965) Depigmented nevi: the earliest sign of tuberous sclerosis. *Pediatrics* 35: 1003–5.

Gomez MR (1987) Tuberous sclerosis. In: Gomez MR (ed) *Neurocutaneous Diseases. A Practical Approach*. Boston: Butterworth, pp 30–52.

Gomez MR (1988a) Criteria for diagnosis. In: Gomez MR (ed) *Tuberous Sclerosis*. New York: Raven Press, pp 9–19.

Gomez MR (1988b) Liver, digestive tract, spleen, vascular and lymphatic systems. In: Gomez MR (ed) *Tuberous Sclerosis*. New York: Raven Press, pp 179–89.

Gomez MR (1988c) Varieties of expression of tuberous sclerosis. *Neurofibromatosis* 1: 330–8.

Good CH, Garb J (1943) Systemic nevi of the face, tuberous sclerosis, epilepsy and fibromatous growth on scalp. *Arch Dermatol Syph* 47: 197–215.

Hallopeau H, Leredde M (1895) Sur un cas d'adénomes sébacés à forme sclereuse. *Ann Dermatol Syph (Paris)* 6: 473–9.

Harris R, Moynahan EJ (1966) Tuberous sclerosis with vitiligo, *Br J Dermatol* 78: 419–20.

Harrison MG, O'Neill ID, Chadwick BL (1997) Odontogenic myxoma in an adolescent with tuberous sclerosis. *J Oral Pathol Med* 26: 339–41.

Hoff M, van Grunsven MF, Tonglebloed WL, Gravenmade EJ (1975) Enamel defects associated with tuberous sclerosis. *Oral Surg* 40: 261–9.

Ishibashi Y, Watanabe R, Nogita T, et al. (1991) Abnormal gene expressions of stroma cells in patients with tuberous sclerosis. In: Johnson WG, Gomez MR (eds) *Tuberous Sclerosis and Allied Disorders. Ann NY Acad Sci* 615: 228–42.

Janniger CK, Goldberg DJ (1990) Angiofibromas in tuberous sclerosis: comparison of treatment by carbon dioxide and argon laser. *J Dermatol Surg Oncol* 16: 317–20.

Jimbow K, Fitzpatrick TB, Szabo G, Hori Y (1957) Congenital circumscribed hypomelanosis: characterisation based on electron microscopic study of tuberous sclerosis, nevus depigmentosus and piebaldism. *J Invest Dermatol* 64: 50–62.

Johnson WG, Yoshidome H, Stenroos ES, Davidson MM (1991) Origin of the neuron-like cells in tuberous sclerosis tissue. In: Johnson WG, Gomez MR (eds) *Tuberous Sclerosis and Allied Disorders. Ann NY Acad Sci* 615: 211–19.

Jóźwiak S (1992) Diagnostic value of clinical features and supplementary investigations in tuberous sclerosis in children. *Acta Paediatr Hungarica* 32: 71–88.

Jóźwiak S (1995a) Oncogenesis in tuberous sclerosis complex. *The Cancer J* 8: 260–3.

Jóźwiak S (1995b) Stwardnienie guzowate u dzieci – analiza kliniczna. Praca na stopień doktora habilitowanego nauk medycznych. (Habilitation work) Warszawa.

Jóźwiak S, Michałowicz R (1996) Skąpoobjawowe występowanie stwardnienia guzowatego w dwóch rodowodach. *Neurol Neurochir Pol* 30: 917–23.

Jóźwiak S, Kwiatkowski D, Michałowicz R, et al. (1998a) Obraz kliniczny stwardnienia guzowatego w rodowodach TSC1 i TSC2. *Pediatria Pol* 73: 509–16.

Jóźwiak S, Schwartz RA, Krysicka-Janiger C, et al. (1998b) Skin lesions in children with tuberous sclerosis complex – their incidence, natural course and diagnostic significance. *Int J Dermatol* 37: 911–17.

Jóźwiak S, Schwartz RA, Krysicka Janniger C, Bielicka-Cymerman J (2000) Usefulness of diagnostic criteria of tuberous sclerosis in pediatric patients. *J Child Neurol* 15: 652–9.

Klein JA, Barr RJ (1986) Diffuse lipomatosis and tuberous sclerosis. *Arch Dermatol* 122: 1298–302.

Koenen J (1932) Eine familiäre hereditäre Form von tuberösen Sklerose. *Acta Psychiatr (Kbh)* 1: 813–21.

Kothe R (1903) Zur Lehre von den Talgdrüsengeschwüllsten. *Arch F Dermat u Syph* 68: 33–54.

Krysicka-Janniger C (1993) Childhood vitiligo. *Cutis* 51: 25–8.

Krysicka-Janniger C, Schwartz RA (1993) Tuberous sclerosis: recent advances for clinician. *Cutis* 51: 167–74.

Lagos JC, Gomez MR (1967) Tuberous sclerosis: reappraisal of a clinical entity. *Proc Mayo Clin* 42: 26–49.

Lee TC, Sung ML, Chen JS (1994) Tuberous sclerosis associated with neurofibromatosis: report of a case. *J Formos Med Assoc* 93: 797–801.

Lygidakis NA, Lindenbaum RH (1987) Pitted enamel hypoplasia in tuberous sclerosis patients and first-degree relatives. *Clin Genet* 32: 216–21.

Lygidakis NA, Lindenbaum RH (1989) Oral fibromatosis in tuberous sclerosis. *Oral Surg Oral Med Oral Pathol* 68: 725–8.

McGrae JD, Hashimoto K (1996) Unilateral facial angiofibromas – a segmental form of tuberous sclerosis? *Br J Dermatol* 134: 727–30.

Mackler SB, Shoulars HW, Burkes EJ (1972) Tuberous sclerosis with gingival lesions. *Oral Surg* 34: 619–24.

Miyamoto Y, Satomura K, Rikimaru K, Hayashi Y (1995) Desmoplastic fibroma of the mandible associated with tuberous sclerosis. *J Oral Pathol Med* 24: 93–6.

Mlynarczyk G (1991) Enamel pitting: a common symptom of tuberous sclerosis. *Oral Surg Oral Med Oral Pathol* 71: 63–7.

Nevin NC, Pearce WG (1968) Diagnostic and genetical aspects of tuberous sclerosis. *J Med Genet* 5: 273–80.

Nickel WR, Reed WB (1962) Tuberous sclerosis. *Arch Dermatol* 85: 209–26.

Nico MM, Ito LM, Valente NY (1999) Genital angiofibromas in tuberous sclerosis: two cases. *J Dermatol* 26: 111–14.

Norio R, Oksanen T, Rantanen J (1996) Hypopigmented skin alterations resembling tuberous sclerosis in normal skin. *J Med Genet* 33: 184–6.

Pasyk KA, Argenta LC (1988) Argon laser surgery of skin lesions in tuberous sclerosis. *Ann Plastic Surg* 20: 426–33.

Perusini G (1905) Über einen Fall von Sclerosis tuberosa hypertrophica. *Mschr Psychiatr Neurol* 17: 69–255.

Pringle JJ (1890) A case of congenital adenoma sebaceum. *Br J Dermatol* 2: 1–14.

Rayer POF (1835) *Traité théorique et pratique de maladies de la peau, 2nd edn.* Paris: Baillière.

Roach ES, Smith M, Huttenlocher P, et al. (1992) Diagnostic criteria: tuberous sclerosis complex. *J Child Neurol* 7: 221–4.

Roach ES, Gomez MR, Northrup H (1998) Tuberous Sclerosis Complex Consensus Conference: revised clinical diagnostic criteria. *J Child Neurol* 13: 624–8.

Rogers RS (1988) Dermatologic manifestations. In: Gomez MR (ed) *Tuberous Sclerosis.* New York: Raven Press, pp 111–31.

Rubin MM, Delgado EB, Cozzi GM, Palladino VS (1987) Tuberous sclerosis complex and a calcifying epithelial odontogenic tumour of the mandible. *Oral Surg Oral Med Oral Pathol* 64: 207–11.

Schuermann H, Greiter A, Horenstein O (1966) *Krankheiten der Mund-Schleimhaut und der Lippen.* Berlin: Urban Schwarzenberg.

Schull WJ, Crowe FW (1953) Neurocutaneous syndrome in the M kindred. A case of simultaneous occurrence of tuberous sclerosis and neurofibromatosis. *Neurology (Minneap.)* 3: 904–9.

Schwartz RA, Janniger CK (1997) Vitiligo. *Cutis* 60: 239–44.

Sepp T, Yates J, Green A (1996) Loss of heterozygosity in tuberous sclerosis hamartomas. *J Med Genet* 33: 962–4.

Silvestre JF, Banuls J, Ramon R, et al. (2000) Unilateral multiple facial angiofibromas: a mosaic form of tuberous sclerosis. *J Am Acad Dermatol* 43: 127–9.

Sperandio M, Weber L, Jauch A, et al. (2000) Cutaneous white spots in a child with polycystic kidneys: a clue TSC2/PKD1 gene mutation. *Nephrol Dial Transplant* 15: 909–12.

Toyoshima M, Ohno K, Katsumoto T, et al. (1999) Cellular senescence of angiofibroma stroma cells from patients with tuberous sclerosis. *Brain Dev* 21: 184–91.

Tunnessen WW, Simon NP, Simon NW (1996) White forelock could be early sign of tuberous sclerosis. *Arch Ped Adol Med* 150: 651–2.

Vanderhooft SL, Francis JS, Pagan RA, et al. (1996) Prevalence of hypopigmented macules in a healthy population. *J Pediatr* 129: 355–61.

Verheyden CN (1996) Treatment of the facial angiofibromas of tuberous sclerosis. *Plast Reconstr Surg* 98: 777–83.

Vogt H (1908) Zur Diagnostik der tuberösen Sklerose. *Z Erforsch Behandl jugendl Schwachsinns* 2: 1–12.

von Recklinghausen FD (1862) Ein Herz von einem Neugeborenen welches mehrere theils nach aussen, theils nach den Hohlen prominirende Tumouren (Myomen) trug. *Verh Ges Geburtsh Monatsschr Geburtsheilk* 20: 1–2.

Webb DW, Clarke A, Fryer A, Osborne JP (1996) The cutaneous features of tuberous sclerosis: a population study. *Br J Dermatol* 135: 1–5.

Wendt JR, Watson LR (1991) Cosmetic treatment of shagreen patches in selected patients with tuberous sclerosis. *Plast Reconstr Surg* 87: 780–2.

Witkop CJ Jr, Rao S (1971) Inherited defects in tooth structure. In: Bergsma D (ed) *Birth Defects: Original Articles Series. Orofacial Structures*. Baltimore: Williams and Wilkins, 169–81.

Young J, Povey S (1998) The genetic basis of tuberous sclerosis. *Mol Med Today* 7: 313–19.

Zaremba J (1968) Tuberous sclerosis: a clinical and genetical investigation. *J Ment Defic Res* 12: 63–80.

Zeller J, Friedman D, Clerici T, Revuz J (1995) The significance of a single periungual fibroma: report of seven cases. *Arch Dermatol* 131: 1465–6.

10
OPHTHALMOLOGICAL MANIFESTATIONS

Sergiusz Jóźwiak

The first descriptions of ocular pathology in TSC patients appeared in the medical literature at the beginning of the twentieth century (Campbell 1905, Berg 1913). However, it was not until van der Hoeve published a series of papers, between 1920 and 1937, that ocular findings became commonly accepted as an important part of TSC. The term "phakoma", used by van der Hoeve to describe the characteristic retinal lesions of TSC, soon gave its name to a whole group of disorders with similar retinal lesions, including neurofibromatosis and von Hippel-Lindau disease (van der Hoeve 1920).

It is thought that approximately half of patients with TSC demonstrate ocular pathology. Retinal hamartomas, retinal pigmentation and vascular changes, optic nerve atrophy, glaucoma, and coloboma of the iris, lens, choroid and retina are among the most frequent ophthalmological manifestations.

RETINAL FINDINGS

Detection of retinal lesions in TSC patients may be difficult. Many patients have severe central nervous system impairment which makes it difficult for them to recognize or report visual deficiency. Additionally, the lesions may be difficult to detect by fundoscopic inspection and, if the patient is unable to co-operate, sedation and indirect ophthalmoscopy may be required.

The incidence of retinal hamartomas, the most frequent retinal lesions in TSC, ranges from 4 to 76% (Critchley and Earl 1932, Nevin and Pearce 1968, Szreter et al. 1994, Robertson 1999), most often being about 40 to 50%. Application of fluorescein angiography may increase detectability of retinal hamartomas to 87% (Kiribuchi et al. 1986). They are more frequent in patients with *TSC2* gene mutations (Dabora et al. 2001). The incidence of the lesions increases slightly with increasing age of examined patients. In the group of children seen in the Children's Memorial Health Institute in Warsaw, we found them in 4 out of 49 children (8.2%) aged below 2 years, in 7 out of 41 children (17.1%) aged 2 to 5, in 7 out of 34 patients (20.6%) aged 5 to 9, in 5 out of 29 children (17.2%) aged 9 to 14, and in 5 out of 16 patients (31.3%) aged 14 to 18 years (Jóźwiak et al. 2000).

Three basic morphological forms of retinal hamartomas are recognized: (1) non-calcified; (2) calcified mulberry-like; (3) transitional type sharing morphologic characteristics of both previously mentioned types. There are few large studies evaluating the incidence of different forms of retinal hamartomas in patients with TSC (Szreter et al. 1994, Robertson 1999).

NON-CALCIFIED RETINAL HAMARTOMA

Non-calcified retinal hamartomas are the most common type of retinal lesions. In the largest group of 68 patients with retinal hamartomas, seen at the Mayo Clinic, non-calcified tumours were found in 39 individuals (57%) (Robertson 1999). We found them in 13 out of 19 (68%) patients with retinal hamartomas (Szreter et al. 1994). The lesions are relatively flat, smooth-surfaced, salmon, salmon-grey, or the same colour as the surrounding eye (Robertson 1999). They are translucent and poorly circumscribed, sometimes being noticed only because of a circular light reflex (Fig. 10.1). The tumours are slightly elevated. The visibility of the underlying tissue, which usually includes a vessel, may be decreased. As these lesions are frequently located superficially to retinal arteries, searching along vessels, from the disc toward the periphery, is the best method of detection. These hamartomas usually occur in the posterior pole of the fundus, and may be single or multiple. Because of their intensely vascular appearance, fluorescein angiography may be helpful in identification of these otherwise undetectable lesions (Kiribuchi et al. 1986).

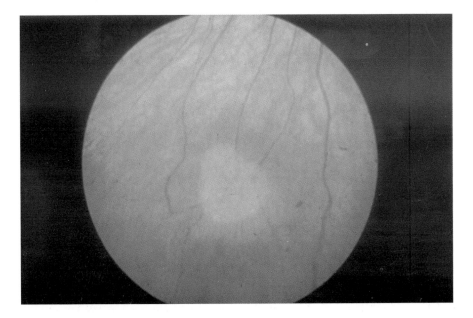

Fig. 10.1. Large, smooth-surfaced, semitransparent retinal hamartoma overlying retinal vessels. (Reproduced with permission of Professor Marek Prost, Ophthalmology Department, Children's Memorial Health Institute, Warsaw.)

Calcified Mulberry-like Hamartoma

These lesions are regarded as a more classical type of retinal hamartoma. They are composed of clusters of opaque, cystic or calcified nodules. Because of their elevated multinodular appearance, the lesions are frequently likened to grains of tapioca, salmon eggs or mulberries (Fig. 10.2). Usually the mulberry-like hamartomas are located at the disc margin, but they may also occur in the central part of the retina. The size of the lesions varies from 0.5 to 4 disc diameters, and they may be several millimetres thick (Robertson 1999). Sometimes, when located at the optic disc, the hamartomas may resemble drusen, but have a greater tendency to obscure underlying vessels. There are reports on periodic filling of cystic areas and emptying into the vitreous humour, resulting in vitreous haemorrhage and transient visual disturbances (Atkinson et al. 1973, Jost and Olk 1986). Occasionally, blood vessels may be present in the vicinity or in the mass of the tumour, which may suggest their role in hamartoma development. A high proportion of calcium within the tumour mass allows its sonographic and roentgenographic visualization (Nyboer et al. 1976). Calcified mulberry-like hamartomas are less frequent than non-calcified translucent ones, and were seen in 4 out of 19 (21%) of our patients with retinal hamartomas (Szreter et al. 1994), and in 34 out of 68 (50%) of patients examined by Robertson (Robertson 1999).

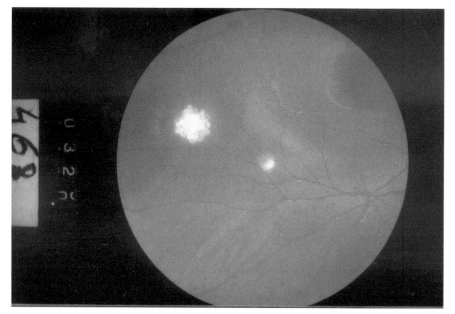

Fig. 10.2. Easily recognized elevated calcified multinodular lesion of mulberry-like type. Note additional small semitransparent retinal hamartoma with decreased visibility of the retinal vessels underlying the lesion, in the central part of the picture.

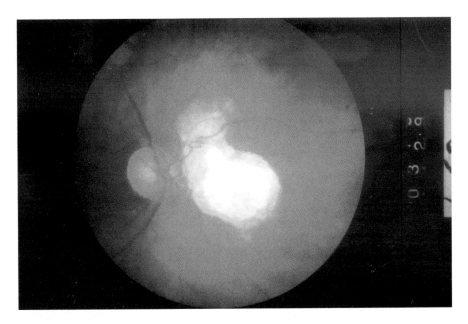

Fig. 10.3. Large elevated retinal hamartoma of mixed type with upper semitransparent part with visible underlying vessels and calcifications at the lower part of the lesion.

MIXED TYPE OF RETINAL HAMARTOMA

This third type of retinal tumour shares the features of both previously described types. Usually, the periphery of the tumour is flat and semitransparent, whereas its central part is calcified and nodular (Fig. 10.3). This type of retinal hamartoma is relatively rare in patients with TSC. It has been found in 2 out of 19 (10.5%) of our patients with retinal hamartomas (Szreter et al. 1994), and in 8 out of 68 (11.8%) patients in Robertson's series (Robertson 1999). In 40 to 50% of patients, retinal hamartomas may appear bilaterally. Frequently, the coexistence of different types of retinal hamartomas in one patient, or even in one eye, may be observed. We have not found any association between morphological type of tumour and other clinical signs of TSC (Szreter et al. 1994).

PIGMENTARY ABNORMALITIES

Retinal pigmentary disturbances with hypopigmentation or hyperpigmentation have been described in patients with TSC. Depigmented lesions of a "punched out" appearance are usually seen either near the posterior pole or halfway toward the periphery of the fundus (Robertson 1991). Sometimes the depigmented lesions may display a grey-white plaque-like centre, which obscures the choroidal vasculature. Depigmented lesions can measure up to half the diameter of the optic disc, and may be surrounded by a cuff of pigmentation (Robertson 1991). The histological correlate and frequency of the lesions remain unknown. Isolated hyperpigmentations resembling congenital retinal pigment epithelial hypertrophy have been documented in several reports (Szreter et al. 1994).

EVOLUTION OF RETINAL CHANGES

It is well known that retinal hamartomas may be found in patients at any age. There are many reports on early appearance of the lesions. They have been described in small children and even newborns (Shami et al. 1993). We have observed them in four children below 2 years of age. The youngest child was a 6-month-old girl (Szreter et al. 1994). In the majority of cases retinal hamartomas do not grow and remain stable even for several decades. The progression of lesions, both in number and size, has been documented in only a small number of patients with TSC.

Szreter at al. (1994) reported on 59 children with TSC who underwent two or more ophthalmological examinations. In 11 out of 19 patients with retinal hamartomas initial ophthalmological examination was within normal limits, in five children the lesions did not increase, and in three individuals the authors observed gradual progression of the hamartomas. In one girl, six small semitransparent retinal hamartomas appeared during a four-year follow-up period. An evolution of retinal hamartoma from pigmentary changes, through semitransparent lesion to mulberry-like hamartoma over a period of 13 years has been documented in another patient. None of the lesions decreased in size during the observation. Follow-up ranged from 1 year to 15 years, with an average of 5.2 years. Clear evidence of the evolution of a relatively flat, semitransparent lesion into an elevated, nodular calcified tumour over a period of 20 years has been documented also by Nyboer et al. (1976).

There is another well-documented and long-term prospective study of retinal hamartomas in patients with TSC (Zimmer-Galler and Robertson 1995). In this study, 16 TSC patients with diagnosed retinal hamartomas were re-examined 6 to 34 years after initial diagnosis. New fundus photographs of 37 hamartomas were compared with the previous ones. A progression of the lesions or new calcifications were documented in three patients. In a fourth patient a retinal hamartoma appeared to originate from a site that had been previously photographically documented to be normal (Zimmer-Galler and Robertson 1995).

Four stages of development of retinal hamartomas have been suggested by Szreter et al. (1994): (1) retinal pigmentary changes (relative hyperpigmentation); (2) semitransparent, salmon-grey retinal hamartoma; (3) partially calcified, mixed tumour; (4) calcified mulberry-like hamartoma. The transition from one stage to another may take many years or even decades and may never be observed in the majority of patients. Why calcified mulberry-like lesions may be found in small children, or even in infants, is still unclear. Further long-term studies are needed. There is one anecdotal description of spontaneous regression of retinal astrocytic hamartoma in the literature (Kiratli and Bilgic 2002).

HISTOPATHOLOGY

Histopathologically, retinal lesions are predominantly composed of an astrocytic proliferation, which in small lesions is limited to the superficial layers of the retina, the nerve fibre and ganglion layers. Occasionally, large hamartomas may involve the whole section of the retina or optic disc. Frequently, the superficial retinal blood vessels may be incorporated into the hamartoma. Occasionally, the tumours may be located in the outer layer of the retina (Margo et al. 1993). In such a location they may be misdiagnosed as a choroidal lesion invading the outer retina (Robertson 1999). The larger retinal hamartomas may contain areas of necrosis with hyalinization and focal calcification. They are frequently complicated by cystic degeneration with spaces filled with serous exudates or blood.

The origin of retinal hamartomas in TSC is thought to be identical to that of the central nervous system tumours – a proliferation of undifferentiated "glioneurocytes" with development of variable neuronal and glial features (Bender and Yunis 1982). The cells may be large and round, resembling ganglion cells or glia. Usually, they have one oval, but they sometimes have as many as five nuclei. The processes of these cells may extend to envelop blood vessels. The abundant cytoplasm and indistinct cell borders result in a frequently described syncytium appearance (Messinger and Clarke 1937, Nyboer et al. 1976).

Recent immunohistochemical studies have shown that, despite their astrocytic appearance, the tumour cells may demonstrate both glial and neuronal characteristics. Margo et al. (1993) reported immunoreactivity for γ-enolase (neuron-specific enolase), supporting the neuronal origin of the hamartoma. Other results have been obtained by Shields et al. (1996), who showed immunoreactivity for vimentin and glial fibrillary acidic protein (GFAP), supporting the diagnosis of an astrocytic tumour. Milot et al. (1999) found GFAP immunoreactivity in approximately 50% of the tumour cells.

DIAGNOSTIC SIGNIFICANCE AND DIFFERENTIAL DIAGNOSIS OF RETINAL HAMARTOMAS

As retinal hamartomas have been reported in infants and even in newborns, they may be very valuable diagnostic features of TSC, especially in this group of patients, preceding the appearance of other symptoms and signs of the disease by months or years. Sometimes they may be the sole manifestation of the disease (Walsh et al. 1938, Koch 1964).

Multiple retinal nodular hamartomas are regarded as characteristic for TSC and have recently been included in the major diagnostic criteria for the disease (Roach et al. 1998). However, we must be aware that retinal hamartomas are clinically indistinguishable from the ocular lesions of neurofibromatosis. Patients with clinical features of both entities have been reported (Kirby 1951, Lee et al. 1994). If retinal findings are the sole manifestation of TSC, a definite diagnosis should be postponed until the appearance of other features of the disease. An examination of family members may be of value (Elcioglu et al. 1998, Roach et al. 1999).

The multinodular, mulberry-like lesions may imitate drusen of the optic disc, but have a greater tendency to obscure underlying vasculature (Reese 1940). The mulberry-like hamartomas, especially those in the peripheral parts of the retina, also require differentiation from retinoblastoma (Balmer et al. 1993). In most cases the appearance of other TSC features allows this differentiation. The honey-comb appearance of regressing retinoblastoma should not be present with retinal hamartoma. In doubtful cases, close follow-up for the size changes indicative of retinoblastoma is necessary. Weekly re-examination has been suggested (Gass 1974). In case of rapid growth, such an approach allows early diagnosis of retinoblastoma and application of appropriate treatment. According to Robertson (1999), in the majority of cases there is no need for biopsy, and clinical and roentgenologic information is sufficient for the diagnosis of retinal hamartoma in TSC.

TREATMENT

The recognition of retinal hamartomas helps facilitate the diagnosis of TSC and genetic counselling, but fortunately, since the majority of retinal hamartomas are asymptomatic and their growth is rarely observed, most TSC patients with the retinal lesions do not require any treatment. According to the recommendations of the Tuberous Sclerosis Consensus Conference (Roach et al. 1999), patients whose initial evaluation reveals only minor lesions are less likely to benefit from repeated examinations. Moreover, ophthalmic examination can be difficult to perform without sedation in a severely intellectually impaired child. However, patients with large or progressive tumours, or lesions causing secondary exudative changes, need continuing eye care. In particular, the latter lesions should be studied angiograph-ically to determine the extent of the vascular component, which might be treated by photocoagulation (Seige 1976, Bloom and Mahl 1991). Large, progressive retinal hamartomas may be destroyed by the same method. A detection of papilledema should prompt urgent neurological consultation to exclude intracranial hypertension.

VISUAL LOSS

Visual loss is infrequent in patients with TSC. It may be associated with unusual locations and sizes of retinal hamartomas and their consequences: macula involve-ment, haemorrhage into the vitreous cavity, or retinal detachment. Kiribuchi et al. (1986) reported visual impairment in 3 out of 100 (3%) TSC patients – one patient had an optic disc hamartoma, another a huge tumour occupying one-third of the vitreous cavity with retinal detachment and optic disc atrophy, and the third patient had an endophytic hamartoma with vitreous haemorrhage and posterior vitreous detachment. Robertson (1999) reported a patient who had begun losing vision in his left eye at the age of 7 years and had been found to be practically blind at age 22. He had a large mulberry lesion extending from the temporal margin of the optic disc into the macular area. The development of the vitreous haemorrhage led to painful glaucoma and blindness.

Eye enucleation has been described in other patients (Atkinson et al. 1973, Nicholson and Green 1975). However, retinal hamartomas seem to be a less common cause of visual impairment than chronic papilledema caused by increased intracranial pressure (ICP). The increased ICP in TSC patients usually results from an obstruction of the foramina of Monro by subependymal giant cell astrocytoma. Only early surgical decompression may prevent the development of persistent visual loss. The frequency of this phenomenon in the TSC population is thought to be below 5%, but its effects on vision may be devastating (Dotan et al. 1991). Usually the symptoms of increased intracranial pressure (headache, nausea, vomiting, diplopia, lethargy) will alert the physician to the diagnosis. However, in intellectually impaired patients these signs and symptoms may easily be overlooked and undetected, leading to persistent optic atrophy. Dotan et al. (1991) reported four TSC patients with visual loss caused by brain tumours. Optic nerve atrophy secondary to brain tumours was observed in 3 out of 106 children with TSC treated in the Children's Memorial Health Institute in Warsaw between 1984 and 1994 (Jóźwiak 1995). Periodic ophthalmological examination or even brain neuroimaging studies are especially recommended in intellectually impaired patients with TSC.

NON-RETINAL MANIFESTATIONS OF TSC

Usually, primary non-retinal manifestations of TSC do not produce any significant complaints and are rarely reported. However, some non-retinal findings may be secondary to progressive, expanding retinal lesions (e.g. vitreous haemorrhage, cataract, coloboma of the choroid and retina) (Atkinson et al. 1973, Nicholson and Green 1975). Angiofibromas often involve the eyelids of TSC patients, and very small tumours are sometimes found on the conjunctiva (Luo 1940). Adenomas of the tarsal glands at the free edge of the eyelid, and ciliary poliosis, have also been described (DiTizio 1963).

Epicanthal folds seen in some TSC patients are thought to be incidental findings (Chao 1959). Russell et al. (1996) found abnormal sphenoid bone morphology in some TSC patients. The authors hypothesized that the abnormalities may reflect the severity of some ocular findings in the disease. Reported corneal changes include megalocornea, pannus, band keratopathy and posterior embryotoxon (Rumberg and Herzog 1966, Welge-Lussen and Latta 1976).

Different forms of abnormal eye mobility – nonparalytic strabismus, nystagmus, and paralysis of cranial nerves III and VI – have been observed (Nevin and Pearce 1968, Hered 1992, Szreter et al. 1994). Sector depigmentation of the iris, the ocular equivalent of skin depigmentations in TSC, has been documented in some reports

(Kranias and Romano 1977, Lucchese and Goldberg 1981, Szreter et al. 1994). Enophthalmos and phthisis of the globe have been seen in association with TSC, but are likely to be incidental findings (Luo 1940, Jordano et al. 1958).

REFERENCES

Atkinson A, Sanders MD, Wong V (1973) Vitreous haemorrhage in tuberous sclerosis. *Br J Opthalmol* 57: 773–9.

Balmer A, Gailloud C, Munier F, et al. (1993) Retinoblastoma. Unusual warning and clinical signs. *Ophthalmic Paediatr Genet* 14: 33–8.

Bender BL, Yunis EJ (1982) The pathology of tuberous sclerosis. *Pathol Ann* 17: 339–82.

Berg H (1913) Vererbung der tuberösen Sklerose durch zwei bzw. drei Generationen. *Z Ges Neurol Psychiatr* 19: 528–39.

Bloom SM, Mahl CF (1991) Photocoagulation for serous detachment of the macula secondary to retinal astrocytoma. *Retina* 11: 416–22.

Campbell AW (1905) Cerebral sclerosis. *Brain* 28: 382–96.

Chao DHC (1959) Congenital neurocutaneous syndromes in childhood. II. Tuberous sclerosis. *J Pediatr* 55: 447–59.

Critchley M, Earl CJC (1932) Tuberous sclerosis and allied conditions. *Brain* 55: 311–46.

Dabora SL, Jóźwiak S, Franz DN, et al. (2001) Mutational analysis in a cohort of 224 tuberous sclerosis patients indicates increased severity of TSC2 compared with TSC1 disease in multiple organs. *Am J Hum Genet* 68: 64–80.

DiTizio A (1963) Atypical eye changes in four cases of Bourneville's tuberous sclerosis. *Boll Oculist* 42: 32–52.

Dotan SA, Trobe JD, Gebarski SS (1991) Visual loss in tuberous sclerosis. *Neurology* 41: 1915–17.

Elcioglu N, Karatekin G, Elcioglu M, et al. (1998) Tuberous sclerosis: clinical evaluation in a family and implications for genetic counseling. *Genet Couns* 9: 131–8.

Gass JDM (1974) A stereoscopic presentation. In: Smith TL (ed) *Differential Diagnosis of Intraocular Tumours*. St Louis: Mosby, p 371.

Hered RW (1992) Tuberous sclerosis. *Arch Ophthalmol* 110: 410–11.

Jordano J, Galera H, Toro M, Carreras B (1958) Astrocytoma of the retina. *Br J Opthalmol* 58: 555–9.

Jost BF, Olk RJ (1986) Atypical retinitis proliferans, retinal telangiectasis, and vitreous hemorrhage in a patient with tuberous sclerosis. *Retina* 6: 53–6.

Jóźwiak S (1995) Stwardnienie guzowate u dzieci – analiza kliniczna. Praca na stopień doktora habilitowanego nauk medycznych. Warszawa.

Jóźwiak S, Schwartz RA, Krysicka Janniger C, Bielicka-Cymerman J (2000) The usefulness of diagnostic criteria of tuberous sclerosis in pediatric patients. *J Child Neurol* 15: 652–9.

Kiratli H, Bilgic S (2002) Spontaneous regression of retinal astrocytic hamartoma in a patient with tuberous sclerosis. *Am J Ophthalmol* 133: 715–16.

Kirby TJ (1951) Ocular phacomatoses. *Am J Med Sci* 222: 227–39.

Kiribuchi K, Uchida Y, Fukuyama Y, Maruyama H (1986) High incidence of fundus hamartomas and clinical significance of a fundus score in tuberous sclerosis. *Brain Dev* 8: 509–17.

Koch G (1964) The contribution of different techniques to classification. 1. Genetics. The genetics of cerebral tumours. *Acta Neurochir (Wien)* suppl. 10: 24–9.

Kranias GK, Romano PE (1977) Depigmented iris sector in tuberous sclerosis. *Am J Ophthalmol* 83: 758–9.

Lee TC, Sung ML, Chen JS (1994) Tuberous sclerosis associated with neurofibromatosis: report of a case. *J Formos Med Assoc* 93: 797–801.

Lucchese NJ, Goldberg MF (1981) Iris and fundus pigmentary changes in tuberous sclerosis. *J Pediatr Ophthalmol Strabismus* 18: 45.

Luo TH (1940) Conjunctival lesions in tuberous sclerosis. *Am J Ophthalmol* 23: 1029–34.

Margo CE, Barletta JP, Staman JA (1993) Giant cell astrocytoma of the retina in tuberous sclerosis. *Retina* 13: 155–8.

Messinger HC, Clarke BE (1937) Retinal tumours in tuberous sclerosis: review of the literature and report of a case with special attention to microscopic structure. *Arch Ophthalmol* 18: 1–11.

Milot J, Michaud J, Lemieux N, et al. (1999) Persistent hyperplastic primary vitreous with retinal tumour in tuberous sclerosis. Report of a case including tumoral immunohistochemistry and cytogenetic analysis. *Ophthalmology* 106: 630–4.

Nevin NC, Pearce WG (1968) Diagnostic and genetical aspects of tuberous sclerosis. *J Med Genet* 5: 273–80.

Nicholson DH, Green WR (1975) Tumours of the eye, lids, and orbit in children. In: Harley R (ed) *Pediatric Ophthalmology*. Philadelphia: WB Saunders, pp 957–62.

Nyboer JH, Robertson DM, Gomez MR (1976) Retinal lesions in tuberous sclerosis. *Arch Ophthalmol* 94: 1277–80.

Reese AB (1940) Relation of drusen of the optic nerve to tuberous sclerosis. *Arch Ophthalmol* 24: 187–205.

Roach ES, Gomez MR, Northrup H (1998) Tuberous Sclerosis Complex Consensus Conference: revised clinical diagnostic criteria. *J Child Neurol* 13: 624–8.

Roach ES, DiMario F, Kandt RS, Northrup H (1999) Tuberous Sclerosis Consensus Conference: recommendations for diagnostic evaluation. *J Child Neurol* 14: 401–7.

Robertson DM (1991) Ophthalmic manifestations of tuberous sclerosis. *Ann NY Acad Sci* 615: 17–25.

Robertson DM (1999) Ophthalmic findings. In: Gomez MR, Sampson JR, Whittemore VH (eds) *Tuberous Sclerosis Complex*. New York: Oxford University Press, pp 145–59.

Rumberg J, Herzog I (1966) Tuberous sclerosis. *NY State J Med* 66: 642–7.

Russell BG, Jensen H, Kjaer I (1996) Ocular findings and sphenoid bone morphology in tuberous sclerosis. *Acta Ophthalmol Scand* 74: 36–9.

Seige B (1976) Fotokoagulacja zmian siatkówkowych w chorobie Pringle'a. *Klin Oczna* 46: 919–22.

Shami MJ, Benedict WL, Myers M (1993) Early manifestation of retinal hamartomas in tuberous sclerosis. *Am J Ophthalmol* 115: 539–40.

Shields JA, Shields CL, Ehya H, et al. (1996) Atypical astrocytic hamartoma diagnosed by fine-needle biopsy. *Ophthalmology* 103: 949–52.

Szreter M, Jóźwiak S, Michałowicz R (1994) Objawy okulistyczne u dzieci ze stwardnieniem guzowatym. *Klin Oczna* 96: 315–17.

van der Hoeve J (1920) Eye symptoms in tuberous sclerosis of the brain. *Trans Ophthalmol Soc UK* 40: 329–34.

Walsh MN, Koch FLP, Brunsting HA (1938) The syndromes of tuberous sclerosis, retinal tumours, and adenoma sebaceum: report of a case. *Proc Mayo Clin* 13: 155–60.

Welge-Lussen L, Latta E (1976) Tuberosen sklerose mit Megalokornea und Iriskolobom. *Klin Mbl Augenheilk* 168: 557–63.

Zimmer-Galler IE, Robertson DM (1995) Long-term observation of retinal lesions in tuberous sclerosis. *Am J Ophthalmol* 119: 318–24.

11
RENAL INVOLVEMENT

Sergiusz Jóźwiak

Since description of the first patients with TSC, multiorgan presentation of the disease has become evident. Although almost every organ and tissue in the body has been reported to be involved, visceral, and especially renal, lesions are among the most frequently observed.

Many of the lesions, including angiomyolipoma (AML) of the kidney, lymphangiomyomatosis, splenic hemangioma and hepatic hamartoma, are vascular and mesenchymal malformations. The renal cysts and focal histiocytoid cells of the spleen consist of collections of distinctly abnormal but relatively uniform cells. All the lesions are either slow-growing or static.

RENAL LESIONS

In 1880 renal manifestations were first noted in patients with TSC. Bourneville was the first to recognize renal lesions in an individual with TSC, but he thought they were unrelated to the cerebral findings (Bourneville 1880). It is estimated that more than 80% of individuals with TSC may develop some form of renal manifestation during their lifetime. Renal involvement is second to neural involvement as a cause of morbidity and mortality in patients with TSC (Shepherd et al. 1991). Two renal abnormalities are regarded as very characteristic for TSC: AMLs and renal cysts. Both lesions may occur separately or together, and both are commonly bilateral and multiple. There may also be an increased risk of malignant renal tumours, especially renal cell carcinomas.

RENAL ANGIOMYOLIPOMA

AMLs are benign noncapsulated tumours consisting of fat, abnormal blood vessels and smooth muscle tissue in varying amounts. Because of their clinical characteristics, they are regarded as "tumorous malformations" rather than "true neoplasm" (Bjornsson et al. 1999).

Incidence

The incidence of renal AMLs in the general population has been estimated to be 1 to 2%, but only 1.8% of all AMLs are detected in patients with TSC (van Baal et al. 1989). In sporadic cases, however, they tend to be solitary and are found from 6 to 8 times more frequently in females than in males. The incidence of renal AMLs in patients with TSC is very high. The lesions are reported in 50 to 90% of patients (Weinblatt et al. 1987, Jóźwiak and Michałowicz 1991), with a slightly higher preponderance in females than in males (1.2:1) (Ewalt et al. 1998). Usually, renal AMLs are not seen in infants and small children, but their incidence increases with age. In a group of children examined in the Children's Memorial Health Institute in Warsaw, renal AMLs were noted in 4 out of 24 (16.7%) children below 2 years of age, 10 out of 24 (41.7%) aged 2 to 5 years, 23 out of 36 (63.9%) aged 5 to 9, 22 out of 34 (64.7%) aged 9 to 14, and 12 out of 13 (92.3%) aged 14 to 18 years (Jóźwiak et al. 2000). Large renal AMLs are much more frequent in patients with *TSC2* gene mutations (Dabora et al. 2001).

Clinical manifestations
In patients with TSC, renal AMLs are usually multiple and bilateral. In children the majority of tumours are 3 to 8 mm in diameter; their size increases with age of patient. Despite their frequent occurrence, the lesions rarely produce troublesome symptoms (Fig. 11.1).

Small angiomyolipomas are asymptomatic. Renal symptoms or signs of angiomyolipomas rarely appear before the third decade of life. Symptoms include

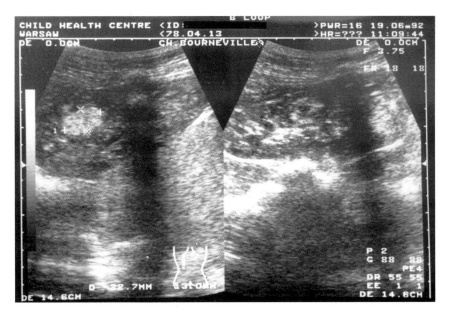

Fig. 11.1. Ultrasonography of the abdomen in a 17-year-old patient with TSC. Large hyperechogenic mass, 2 cm in diameter, presumably angiomyolipoma, is seen in the middle part of the left kidney. On the right are multiple smaller tumours. The patient remains symptom-free. (Reproduced with permission of Dr Marek Pędich, Children's Memorial Health Institute, Warsaw.)

flank pain, nausea and vomiting, hypertension, uremia and fever. There are also reports of sudden bleeding into the kidney from ruptured aneurysmatic vessels within the angiomyolipoma, followed by bleeding into the retroperitoneal space. However, bleeding or rupture seldom occur in children, and are usually related to larger tumours appearing in adolescents and adults. End-stage renal insufficiency caused by replacement of renal parenchyma by tumour masses may be observed in adult patients with multiple and large AMLs, and may necessitate renal transplantation (Neumann et al. 1995).

In the study of van Baal et al. (1989) the tumour size correlated well with the presence or absence of symptoms. Twenty-one of the 22 asymptomatic renal AMLs measured less than 4 cm in diameter. Seventeen of the 19 lesions in the symptomatic group were larger than 5 cm. The tumours that are larger in size appear to have greater propensity for growth than the smaller ones. There is an increased growth potential of renal AMLs in female patients (Ewalt et al. 1998).

Ultrasonography is the imaging method of choice for detection of AMLs. In doubtful cases computerized tomography or magnetic resonance imaging are necessary to assess the presence of intratumour components, which confirms diagnosis (Lemaitre et al. 1995) (Fig. 11.2).

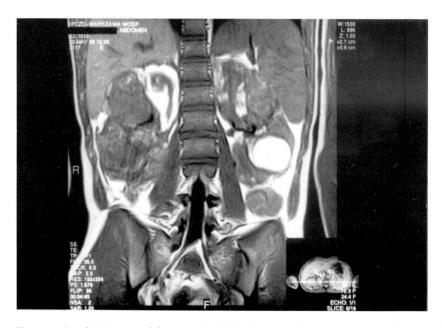

Fig. 11.2. Renal MRI in an adolescent with TSC. The renal architecture is distorted by multiple tumours. (Reproduced with permission of Dr Marek Pędich, Children's Memorial Health Institute, Warsaw.)

Histopathology

Renal angiomyolipomas, associated or not with TSC, have a characteristic appearance. On macroscopic examination these yellowish-white lesions, of firm consistency, are situated mainly in the cortical zone of the kidneys. They range in size from microscopic collections of abnormal cells to large masses exceeding 20 cm in diameter, which completely replace the kidney. Frequently they are accompanied by transparent serous lentoid cysts. The renal AMLs are circumscribed but not encapsulated and may bulge from the renal surface. Sometimes the tumours trangress the renal capsule and invade surrounding fat or the renal vein.

Microscopically, renal AMLs contain varying proportions of blood vessels, adipose tissue and smooth muscle cells, justifying the name "angiomyolipoma" (Fig. 11.3). Depending on which tissue predominates, the tumour may also be identified as myolipoma or angiomyoma. With age there is an increasing amount of fat within the lesions. The spindled muscle cells are frequently dysplastic, with large immature nuclei and occasional mitoses. There is a large number of moderate- to large-size blood vessels with characteristic thick, eccentric walls. The elastic lamina of the vessels is usually abnormal or incomplete, possibly explaining their propensity to rupture. Dysplastic appearance of smooth muscle cells with nuclear hyper-

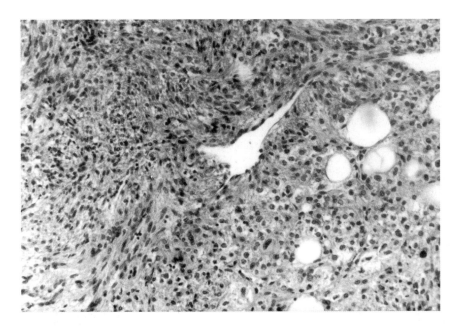

Fig. 11.3. Histologic section of renal angiomyolipoma of a patient with TSC. Mature adipose tissue with scarce large vessels and bundles of smooth muscles. (Hematoxylin and eosin, X 120.) (Reproduced with permission of Professor Bogdan Woźniewicz, Children's Memorial Health Institute, Warsaw.)

chromatism and mitoses may lead to erroneous diagnosis of malignancies. In every patient with multiple renal AMLs a search for other signs of TSC should be implemented and a diagnosis of malignancy should be excluded.

Recent developments in immunohistology support a thesis of neural crest origin of renal AMLs. The identification in renal AMLs of a group of distinctive epithelioid cells showing the co-expression of muscle and melanogenesis markers may confirm the thesis. The cells, named "perivascular epithelioid cells" (PECs), can also be found in other organs and outside angiomyolipoma. Usually, they are described as epithelioid cells arranged around vascular spaces. Recent studies have shown that this cell can modulate its appearance and give rise to various morphologic patterns, from a purely epithelial-like lesion to a purely spindle-cell one. The PECs in AMLs demonstrate the immunoreactivity with HMB45, HMSA-1 and Leu-7, antibodies originally described as specific for melanosomes and other cells of neural crest derivation (Bjornsson et al. 1995, Bonetti et al. 1997, Kimura et al. 1997). The immunoreactivity with actin and, less consistently, desmin was also reported (Bonetti et al. 1997). These cells are usually negative for vimentin, cytokeratins, and in most instances S-100 protein.

Some PEC lesions show loss of heterozygosity on *TSC1* or *TSC2* genes. This might be consistent with Knudson's hypothesis applicable to tumour suppressor gene function of the TSC genes; that is, loss of both copies of the gene, one through the germline and one through a somatic event in the lesion, is critical for the pathogenesis of TSC-associated renal AMLs (Jóźwiak 1995b). The hypothesis that a somatic mutation of TSC genes might be responsible for the development of PEC lesions should be considered (Bonetti et al. 1997). Analysis of renal AMLs from TSC patients indicates that loss of heterozygosity (LOH) for polymorphic markers near *TSC1* (9q34) or *TSC2* (16p13) occurs in 60% of the lesions (Henske et al. 1996). LOH on chromosome 16p13 has also been observed in some non-TSC-associated AMLs (Henske et al. 1995). These findings may confirm that AML originates from a single progenitor cell with pluripotential differentiation ability.

The clonality of AML has also been demonstrated by non-random X-chromosome inactivation (Green et al. 1996). In renal AMLs there is a much higher incidence (7:1) of LOH on chromosome 16p13 than on chromosome 9q34 (Henske et al. 1996). Such a preponderance can be explained by the more frequent distribution of *TSC2* mutations in the general population, more pronounced renal involvement leading to more frequent surgical intervention in *TSC2* patients, or both.

Diagnostic significance
Single renal AMLs may occur in the general population over the age of 30, predominantly in women; in an autopsy series, renal AMLs, lipomas or myomas were evident in as many as 12% of the population (Bernstein and Robbins 1991).

When multiple, renal AMLs should always be suspected to be TSC-associated, and a careful diagnostic evaluation should be performed. There are descriptions of patients with multiple renal AMLs and no other signs of TSC having children with the full clinical picture of the disease (Farrow et al. 1968). There are some characteristic features of renal AMLs unrelated to TSC. Van Baal et al. (1989) found that sporadic AMLs are rarely observed in children, but more often in females than in males, and are singular and larger than 5 cm in diameter.

According to the latest revision of the diagnostic criteria for TSC, multiple renal AMLs are regarded as a major feature (Roach et al. 1998).

Differential diagnosis
The differential diagnosis of renal AMLs mainly includes renal malignancies. In patients with the classic triad of flank pain, painless haematuria and palpable abdominal mass, the differentiation of a renal neoplasm from unilateral AML may be especially difficult. The presence of fever and weight loss, observed in 30% of cases of renal malignancies, is unusual in renal AMLs, unless retroperitoneal haemorrhage is the manner of presentation. There are few descriptions of renal AMLs with retroperitoneal lymph node involvement, suggesting the continuum between AML and renal cell carcinoma. Recent immunohistochemical reports have hypothesized that some AMLs may undergo transformation to malignant AMLs. Malignant AMLs histologically may resemble sarcomatoid renal cell carcinomas, but may be distinguished on the basis of cytokeratin staining (Al-Saleem et al. 1998). Immunostaining for HMB-45 may be useful in distinguishing AML from other tumours of the kidney and liver, especially from renal cell carcinoma and hepato-cellular carcinoma (Koide et al. 1998).

Treatment
All individuals with TSC should undergo regular monitoring of the kidneys to identify those with growing lesions. Most authors recommend prospective renal ultrasonography of AMLs every 2 to 3 years before puberty and yearly after puberty. Larger lesions, exceeding 4 cm in diameter, may require even more frequent examinations because of a high risk of rapid enlargement and bleeding (Bradshaw et al. 1998). Such an approach should allow identification of individuals who can be treated with arterial embolization or nephron-sparing surgery, preventing the patients from developing symptoms and life-threatening bleeding (Dickinson et al. 1998, Fazeli-Matin and Novick 1998, Lee et al. 1998, De Luca et al. 1999).

Arterial embolization is regarded by some authors as the treatment of choice in all renal AMLs that are symptomatic and measure more than 4 cm. There is an increasing number of reports about interventional selective embolization of haemorrhagic AMLs. Pain and fever lasting for several days after embolization may be observed in about 90% of patients. To reduce the symptoms associated with postembolization syndrome, a tapering dose of prednisone over a two-week period was applied by some authors (Bissler et al. 2002).

Reports of long-term follow-up of patients with AMLs treated by embolization are as yet limited (Hamlin et al. 1997). Total nephrectomies should be avoided because the disease is bilateral and progressive. Very large, bilateral AMLs may result in the development of renal failure, caused by destruction of the renal parenchyma, and require dialysis or renal transplantation (Clarke et al. 1999). Fortunately, this complication is relatively uncommon and observed only in adult patients.

Renal Cysts

Renal cysts are the second most frequent renal lesion in patients with TSC, after AMLs. As the *TSC2* gene at chromosome 16p13.3 lies immediately adjacent to the major gene for autosomal dominant polycystic kidney disease (*PKD1*), the presence of multiple, large renal cysts observed in some individuals with TSC may constitute a contiguous gene syndrome caused by deletion of both genes (Longa et al. 1997, Sampson et al. 1997, Torra et al. 1998).

Incidence

The incidence of renal cysts in TSC is lower than that of AMLs. Stillwell et al. (1987) observed renal cysts in 18% of 95 patients with TSC, aged 2 months to 54 years, who underwent careful radiographic evaluation. A higher incidence of renal cysts was reported by Cook et al. (1996), who detected them in 45 out of 139 patients (32%). The true prevalence of the lesions may be even higher, as in autopsy studies 53% of the individuals with TSC had renal cysts (Stillwell et al. 1987). In the group of 91 children examined by ultrasonography in the Children's Memorial Health Institute in Warsaw, renal cysts were detected in 14 children (15.4%). Their incidence increased with age, from 8.3% in children below 2 years of age, to 30.8% in children aged 14 to 18 (Jóźwiak 1995a). A higher incidence of the lesions in males than in females (1.5:1) was reported in some studies (Webb et al. 1993, Ewalt et al. 1998), but not documented in others (Cook et al. 1996).

In our experience with TSC patients we are able to clearly delineate two types of renal cysts, each with a different natural history, clinical presentation and outcome. The commoner type of cyst is small (2 mm to 1 cm), and appears as a single or a few cysts (usually fewer than five). These cysts are infrequent in small children; their incidence increases with age of examined patients. They usually accompany renal AMLs and are probably related to their formation. Spontaneous appearance or disappearance of the cysts, reported by Ewalt et al. (1998), may confirm such a relationship.

The second type of renal cyst is large (1 to 5 cm in diameter), usually bilateral and numerous, resembling lesions found in polycystic kidney disease (PKD) (Fig. 11.4). These cysts are much less common in TSC patients, and are usually evident

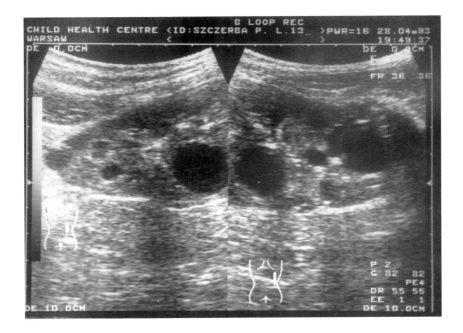

Fig. 11.4. Multiple large cysts and small hyperechogenic nodules in the right kidney of a patient with TSC. (Reproduced with permission of Dr Marek Pędich, Children's Memorial Health Institute, Warsaw.)

in infants and small children, preceding the appearance of other stigmata of the disease. Their incidence does not increase with age. We have found such lesions in 2 out of more than 110 children examined by ultrasonography in our institution (unpublished data).

Clinical manifestations
Small and sporadic cysts observed in the majority of patients with TSC are usually asymptomatic, but children with mutations in the *PKD1* gene and large, multiple cysts may demonstrate severe hypertension and moderate azotemia from the neonatal period or early infancy (Neumann et al. 1998).

As renal function in both groups of patients is influenced by gradual formation of renal AMLs, the replacement of renal parenchyma by enlarging masses may result in renal failure, usually much earlier in the group with the *PKD1* gene mutation. Such evolution of renal lesions in TSC patients is confirmed by the clinical data, indicating that most, if not all, of the adult patients with renal failure have coexisting multiple AMLs (Jóźwiak and Michałowicz 1991, Webb et al. 1993, Cook et al. 1996). Compression of the adjacent parenchyma by the enlarging cyst is thought to be an additional incapacitating factor.

In children with very severe cystic disease from early childhood, cysts are thought to be present from early beginning in the kidneys, even if they may be too small to be detectable by conventional imaging techniques. Enlargement of dilated abnormal nephrons may lead to progression of cystic disease without the recruitment of new cysts from previously normal nephrons. Other clinical manifestations of polycystic disease in TSC patients include palpable flank masses (mainly in children with *PKD1* gene mutation), flank pain and haematuria.

Cysts may be differentiated from AMLs by sonographic evidence of thin-walled, anechoic areas with posterior enhancement. Computed tomography helps to differentiate cysts from AMLs, demonstrating the difference in density between the relatively radiolucent fatty tissue of AMLs and the more radiodense fluid of cysts.

Histopathology
Formation of cysts is thought to result from tubular epithelial hyperplasia within the nephron (Saguem et al. 1992). On gross examination, cysts are present in the cortical region of the kidney, more commonly in the more superficial areas, and later extend into the medulla. Usually they tend to be clustered within a segmental area, with multiple lesions adjoining each other and ending abruptly at normal renal parenchyma. Histologically the cystic lesions are highly distinctive. They consist of the cystic spaces lined by cells resembling tubular epihelium, with abundant eosinophilic cytoplasm and large hyperchromatic nuclei. Mitoses may be observed. The cells may pile up on one another and protrude into the lumen of the cyst. This piling up of eosinophilic, epithelial cells is distinctly unusual in other renal cystic diseases. The finding of these lesions in a renal biopsy is probably diagnostic of TSC (Bender and Yunis 1982).

Diagnostic significance
According to the latest revision of the diagnostic criteria for TSC, renal cysts are regarded as a minor feature of TSC (Roach et al. 1998).

Differential diagnosis
The differential diagnosis should mainly include renal cysts observed in PKD not associated with TSC, or in von Hippel-Lindau disease. Such differentiation is easier in adolescents and adults with other stigmata of TSC, but may be difficult in infants and small children.

Treatment
The presence of small scattered renal cysts in patients with TSC is of little clinical importance. Patients with severe cystic disease and associated hypertension may require surgical decompression and sometimes nephrectomy. Conservative treatment of hypertension with antihypertensive drugs leaves the patient with a risk of

developing progressive renal insufficiency. Patients with end-stage renal impairment have been successfully treated by dialysis and by renal transplantation (Clarke et al. 1999).

RENAL LYMPHANGIOMATOUS CYSTS
This kind of cystic lesion has been identified in a limited number of patients with TSC. In the group of 403 TSC individuals on file at the Mayo Clinic only three patients had the characteristic combination of peri- and intrarenal cysts (Bjornsson et al. 1999). Renal failure and hypertension are frequent manifestations. Renal CT is the imaging method of choice. The lymphangiomatous cysts are lined with flat endothelial cells which differentiates them from the TSC-associated cysts lined with epithelial cells. The solid portions of the cysts consist of compact proliferations of spindle cells. The cytoplasma of the spindle cells demonstrates consistent expression of HMB-45 marker. A similar immunohistochemical profile is also present in AMLs and lymphangioleiomyomatosis.

RENAL CELL CARCINOMA
There are different types of renal neoplasms described in patients with TSC (leiomyosarcomas, fibroplastic sarcomas, angiosarcomas, liposarcomas, angiofibroliposarcomas, clear cell sarcomas, clear cell carcinomas, oncocytomas)(Gastoł et al. 1996, Tsujimura et al. 1996, Peccatori et al. 1997). A child with fatal outcome of renal clear cell sarcoma has been diagnosed in our institution (Gastoł at al. 1996) (Figs 11.5a–c). However, renal cell carcinomas (RCCs) have been the most frequently diagnosed in this group of patients.

Incidence
There are more than 30 reports of RCC in individuals with TSC, suggesting that TSC sufferers have a tendency to develop renal cell carcinomas. However, available epidemiological statistics and a meta-analysis of the literature do not confirm this relationship (Tello et al. 1998). Additional studies are needed.

Clinical manifestations
Costovertebral pain, a palpable mass and haematuria are regarded as the three classic diagnostic features of malignant renal tumours. Unfortunately, they may be noted in only 10% of patients with malignant tumours. In most patients the tumour may remain silent until it attains a large size. At this time, it gives rise to generalized constitutional symptoms, such as fever, weakness and weight loss (Gastoł et al. 1996). Moreover, in TSC patients the existing manifestations of the renal tumour may be easily explained by the presence of renal AMLs. Therefore, in many individuals with TSC, RCCs may be discovered in asymptomatic state by incidental radiological studies or during periodic sonographic investigation. RCC may produce

a diversity of paraneoplastic syndromes, ascribed to abnormal hormone production, including polycythemia, hypercalcemia, hypertension, Cushing syndrome, amyloidosis and hepatic dysfunction.

Most of the patients with TSC-associated RCC are younger by several decades than patients with sporadic RCC (Weinblatt et al. 1987, Bjornsson et al. 1999). There is a sex predilection for women with RCC among TSC patients, with a 6:1 female to male ratio (Weinblatt et al. 1987).

Histopathology

In most cases of TSC-associated RCC their histological appearance is indistinguishable from the usual and most frequent variant of RCC. Three out of seven cases reported by Bjornsson et al. (1999) had anaplastic carcinomas, with two of the three displaying both sarcomatoid and clear cell features within the same tumour. Such a proportion of sarcomatoid features is much higher than in sporadic carcinomas.

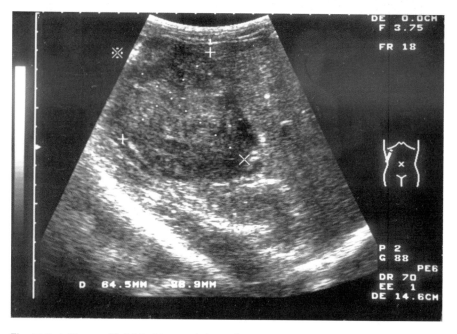

Fig. 11.5. A 10-year-old child with a renal clear cell sarcoma and TSC. The initial complaint was relapsing fever.
Fig. 11.5(a). Large tumour 6 × 9 cm in the right kidney on ultrasonography.

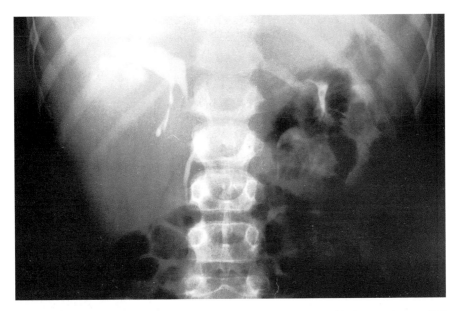

Fig. 11.5(b). Excretory urogram showing pyelocalyceal distortion caused by large oval mass which moved the kidney up and to midline. Apparent slight urinary retention. Right ureter moved to the median line. (Reproduced with permission of Dr Marek Pędich, Children's Memorial Health Institute, Warsaw.)

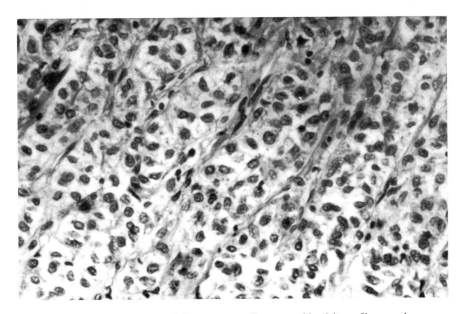

Fig. 11.5(c). Rows of round to oval clear-staining cells separated by delicate fibrovascular stroma. (Hematoxylin and eosin, ×250.) (Reproduced with permission of Professor Bogdan Woźniewicz, Children's Memorial Health Institute, Warsaw.)

Immunohistologically, TSC-associated RCCs differ distinctly from sporadic RCCs. Four of the seven tumours reported by Bjornsson et al. (1999) immuno-stained positively for a melanocyte-associated marker, HMB-45. None of 10 sporadic RCCs from a control group stained with this marker, and all stained with cytokeratin markers, which tended to be negative in TSC-associated tumours. Despite immunohistological similarity to renal AMLs and HMB-45 positivity, TSC-associated RCCs are clinically aggressive. The majority of patients with this type of tumour died of metastatic disease several months to two years after diagnosis (Bjornsson et al. 1995, Al-Saleem et al. 1998).

In a case of renal AML with malignant transformation, reported by Kawaguchi et al. (2002), the atypical epithelioid cells were immunoreactive for p53, whereas the foci of the typical AML were negative. Examination of the microdissected paraffin-embedded tissues revealed p53 mutations in the malignant epithelioid areas in the AML but not in the renal parenchyma or typical AML areas. Two out of five tumours analysed by Bjornsson et al. (1995) for loss of heterozygosity (LOH) demonstrated LOH on chromosome 9q34, and one on chromosome 16p13, supporting the hypothesis that TSC genes play a pathogenetic role in the development of these tumours.

Recent immunohistological studies of TSC-associated RCCs led some authors to conclude that a large proportion of these tumours may represent an unusual, monotypic, epithelioid variant of AML, rather than true RCC (Pea et al. 1998). This AML type seems to be a malignant tumour with potential for invasion and metastases. Similar carcinoma-like monotypic epithelioid AMLs have also been reported in patients without evidence of TSC (Martignoni et al. 1998).

Differential diagnosis
RCC should be differentiated from other renal masses: cysts, and benign and malignant renal tumours. The diagnosis may be especially difficult in TSC patients with coexisting multiple AMLs. Although hyperechoic renal masses that exhibit acoustic shadowing on sonographic examination are very likely to be AMLs, reliable confirmation may be difficult (Siegel et al. 1996). Renal CT or angiography may give additional data. The presence of calcification in any renal mass is infrequent in benign AMLs and is regarded as a strong indicator of malignancy. Recent immunohistochemical studies highlight the potential diagnostic confusion between malignant epithelioid AMLs and RCCs, with immunocytochemical staining for HMB-45 and cytokeratin aiding in the distinction (Pea et al. 1998, Al-Saleem et al. 1998).

Treatment
Categorical treatment recommendations for RCC in TSC are difficult because of the small number of patients. However, metastatic RCC with fatal outcome is common enough to mandate aggressive treatment, including nephrectomy.

Various malformations, including large kidneys, dilatation of the renal pelvis, double ureters, supranumerary kidneys and a single kidney have been reported in association with TSC.

REFERENCES

Al-Saleem T, Wessner LL, Scheithauer BW, et al. (1998) Malignant tumours of the kidney, brain, and soft tissues in children and young adults with the tuberous sclerosis complex. *Cancer* 83: 2208–16.

Bender BL, Yunis EJ (1982) The pathology of tuberous sclerosis. *Pathol Ann* 17: 339–82.

Bernstein J, Robbins TO (1991) Renal involvement in tuberous sclerosis. *Ann NY Acad Sci* 615: 36–49.

Bissler JJ, Racadio J, Donnelly LF, Johnson ND (2002) Reduction of postembolization syndrome after ablation of renal angiomyolipoma. *Am J Kidney Dis* 39: 966–71.

Bjornsson J, Nascimento A, Gulino S (1995) The expression of neural crest-associated markers in normal kidney and renal angiomyolipomas and carcinomas in patients with and without tuberous sclerosis. *Mod Pathol* 8: 72A.

Bjornsson J, Henske EP, Bernstein J (1999) Renal manifestations. In: Gomez MR, Sampson JR, Whittemore VH (eds) *Tuberous Sclerosis Complex*. New York: Oxford University Press, pp 181–93.

Bonetti F, Pea M, Martignoni G, et al. (1997) The perivascular epithelioid cell and related lesions. *Adv Anat Pathol* 4: 343–58.

Bourneville DM (1880) Sclérose tubéreuse des circonvolutions cérébrales: idiotie et épilepsie hémiplégique. *Arch Neurol (Paris)* 1: 81–91.

Bradshaw N, Brewer C, Fitzpatrick D, et al. (1998) Guidelines and care pathways for genetic diseases: the Scottish collaborative project on tuberous sclerosis. *Eur J Human Genet* 6: 445–58.

Clarke A, Hancock E, Kingswood C, Osborne JP (1999) End-stage renal failure in adults with the tuberous sclerosis complex. *Nephrol Dial Transplant* 14: 988–91.

Cook JA, Oliver K, Mueller RF, Sampson J (1996) A cross sectional study of renal involvement in tuberous sclerosis. *J Med Genet* 33: 480–4.

Dabora SL, Jóźwiak S, Franz DN, et al. (2001) Mutational analysis in a cohort of 224 tuberous sclerosis patients indicates increased severity of TSC2 compared with TSC1 disease in multiple organs. *Am J Hum Genet* 68: 64–80.

De Luca S, Terrone C, Rossetti SR (1999) Management of renal angiomyolipoma: report of 53 cases. *B J U Int* 83: 215–18.

Dickinson M, Ruckle H, Beaghler M, Hadley HR (1998) Renal angiomyolipoma: optimal treatment based on size and symptoms. *Clin Nephrol* 49: 281–6.

Ewalt DH, Sheffield E, Sparagana SP, et al. (1998) Renal lesion growth in children with tuberous sclerosis complex. *J Urol* 160: 141–5.

Farrow GM, Harrison EG, Utz DC, Jones DR (1968) Renal angiomyolipoma: a clinicopathologic study of 32 cases. *Cancer* 22: 564–70.

Fazeli-Matin S, Novick AC (1998) Nephron-sparing surgery for renal angiomyolipoma. *Urology* 52: 577–83.

Gastoł P, Jóźwiak S, Dura W (1996) Clear cell sarcoma of the kidney in a girl with tuberous sclerosis. *Surg Child Int* 4: 126–7.

Green JE, Adams GW, Shawker TH, et al. (1990) Hypertension and renal failure in a patient with tuberous sclerosis. *South Med J* 83: 451–4.

Green AJ, Sepp T, Yates JRW (1996) Clonality of tuberous sclerosis hamartomas shown by non-random X-chromosome inactivation. *Hum Genet* 97: 240–3.

Hamlin JA, Smith DC, Taylor FC, et al. (1997) Renal angiomyolipomas: long-term follow-up of embolization for acute haemorrhage. *Can Assoc Radiol J* 48: 191–8.

Henske EP, Neumann HPH, Scheithauer BW, et al. (1995) Loss of heterozygosity in the tuberous sclerosis (TSC2) region of chromosome band 16p13 occurs in sporadic as well as TSC-associated renal angiomyolipomas. *Genes Chrom Cancer* 13: 295–8.

Henske EP, Scheithauer BW, Short WP, et al. (1996) Allelic loss is frequent in tuberous sclerosis kidney lesions but rare in brain lesions. *Am J Hum Genet* 59: 400–6.

Jóźwiak S (1995a) Stwardnienie guzowate u dzieci – analiza kliniczna. Praca na stopień doktora habilitowanego nauk medycznych. (Habilitation work) Warszawa.

Jóźwiak S (1995b) Oncogenesis in tuberous sclerosis complex. *The Cancer J* 8: 260–3.

Jóźwiak S, Michałowicz R (1991) Zmiany w nerkach i wątrobie chorych na stwardnienie guzowate – aspekty diagnostyczne i kliniczne. *Pol Tyg Lek* 46: 787–9.

Jóźwiak S, Schwartz RA, Krysicka Janniger C, Bielicka-Cymerman J (2000) The usefulness of diagnostic criteria of tuberous sclerosis in pediatric patients. *J Child Neurol* 15: 652–9.

Kawaguchi K, Oda Y, Nakanishi K, et al. (2002) Malignant transformation of renal angiomyolipoma: a case report. *Am J Surg Pathol* 26: 523–9.

Kimura N, Watanabe M, Date F, et al. (1997) HMB-45 and tuberin in hamartomas associated with tuberous sclerosis. *Mod Pathol* 10: 952–9.

Koide O, Matsuzaka K, Tanaka Y (1998) Multiple giant angiomyolipomas with a polygonal epithelioid cell component in tuberous sclerosis: an autopsy case report. *Pathol Int* 48: 998–1002.

Lee W, Kim TS, Chung JW, et al. (1998) Renal angiomyolipoma: embolotherapy with a mixture of alcohol and iodized oil. *J Vasc Interv Radiol* 9: 255–61.

Lemaitre L, Robert Y, Dubrulle F, et al. (1995) Renal angiomyolipoma: growth followed up with CT and/or US. *Radiology* 197: 598–602.

Longa L, Scolari F, Brusco A, et al. (1997) A large TSC2 and PKD1 gene deletion is associated with renal and extrarenal signs of autosomal dominant polycystic kidney disease. *Nephrol Dial Transplant* 12: 1900–7.

Martignoni G, Pea M, Bonetti F, et al. (1998) Carcinomalike monotypic epithelioid angiomyolipoma in patients without evidence of tuberous sclerosis: a clinicopathologic and genetic study. *Am J Surg Pathol* 22: 663–72.

Neumann HPH, Bruggen V, Berger DP, et al. (1995) Tuberous sclerosis complex with end-stage renal failure. *Nephrol Dial Transplant* 10: 349–53.

Neumann HP, Schwarzkopf G, Henske EP (1998) Renal angiomyolipomas, cysts, and cancer in tuberous sclerosis complex. *Semin Pediatr Neurol* 5: 269–75.

Pea M, Bonetti F, Martignoni G, et al. (1998) Apparent renal cell carcinomas in tuberous sclerosis are heterogenous: the identification of malignant epithelioid angiomyolipoma. *Am J Surg Pathol* 22: 180–7.

Peccatori I, Pitingolo F, Battini G, et al. (1997) Pulmonary lymphangioleiomyomatosis and renal papillary cancer: incomplete expression of tuberous sclerosis? *Nephrol Dial Transplant* 12: 2740–3.

Radin R, Ma Y (2001) Malignant epithelioid renal angiomyolipoma in a patient with tuberous sclerosis. *J Comput Assist Tomogr* 25: 873–5.

Roach ES, Gomez MR, Northrup H (1998) Tuberous Sclerosis Complex Consensus Conference: revised clinical diagnostic criteria. *J Child Neurol* 13: 624–8.

Saguem MH, Laarif M, Remai S, et al. (1992) Diffuse bilateral glomerulocystic disease of the kidneys and multiple cardiac rhabdomyomas in a newborn: relationship with tuberous sclerosis and review of the literature. *Pathol Res Pract* 188: 367–73.

Sampson JR, Maheshwar MM, Aspinwall R, et al. (1997) Renal cystic disease in tuberous sclerosis: role of the polycystic kidney disease 1 gene. *Am J Hum Genet* 61: 843–51.

Shepherd CW, Gomez MR, Lie JT, Crowson CS (1991) Causes of death in patients with tuberous sclerosis. *Mayo Clin Proc* 66: 792–6.

Siegel CL, Middleton WD, Teefey SA, McClennan BL (1996) Angiomyolipoma and renal cell carcinoma: US differentiation. *Radiology* 198: 789–93.

Stillwell TJ, Gomez MR, Kelalis PP (1987) Renal lesions in tuberous sclerosis. *J Urol* 138: 477–81.

Tello R, Blickman JG, Buonomo C, Herrin J (1998) Metaanalysis of the relationship between tuberous sclerosis complex and renal cell carcinoma. *Eur J Radiol* 27: 131–8.

Torra R, Badenas C, Darnell A, et al. (1998) Facilitated diagnosis of the contiguous gene syndrome: tuberous sclerosis and polycystic kidneys by means of haplotype studies. *Am J Kidney Dis* 31: 1038–43.

Tsujimura A, Miki T, Sugao H, et al. (1996) Renal leiomyoma associated with tuberous sclerosis. *Urol Int* 57: 192–3.

van Baal JG, Fleury P, Brummelkamp WH (1989) Tuberous sclerosis and the relation with renal angiomyolipoma. A genetic study on the clinical aspects. *Clin Genet* 35: 167–73.

Webb DW, Super M, Colin I, et al. (1993) Tuberous sclerosis and polycystic kidney disease. *Br Med J* 306: 1258–9.

Weinblatt ME, Kahn E, Kochen J (1987) Renal cell carcinoma in patients with tuberous sclerosis. *Pediatrics* 80: 898–903.

12

CARDIAC AND VASCULAR INVOLVEMENT

Sergiusz Jóźwiak

Tuberous sclerosis complex (TSC) is a disorder characterized by hamartomas of many cutaneous and visceral organs. Cardiac involvement in TSC patients is usually related to a type of cardiac hamartoma, rhabdomyoma, with all its consequences: dysrhythmias, cardiac failure and death (Bussani et al. 2001). Cardiovascular problems are the most frequent cause of death among children with TSC below 10 years of age (Shepherd et al. 1991). Cardiac rhabdomyomas represent the earliest detectable hamartoma in TSC and, interestingly, are the only lesion in TSC which may regress with age. Their incidence in patients with TSC had been underestimated until non-invasive detection of the tumours by sector echocardiography became possible.

The frequent appearance of cardiac tumours in patients with TSC has been known for many years. In 1862 von Recklinghausen first described the association of cardiac masses with intracerebral sclerotic areas in a newborn who died soon after birth. Since then many cases of similar association have been reported.

INCIDENCE OF CARDIAC RHABDOMYOMAS

Rhabdomyoma is the most common primary cardiac tumour in infancy and childhood, whilst myxoma is the most frequent in adulthood. It is currently thought that the majority of children with documented cardiac rhabdomyomas have TSC. In an autopsy series of 36 patients with cardiac rhabdomyomas, 11 (31%) had a diagnosis of TSC (Fenoglio et al. 1976). Webb et al. (1993) identified 12 children (80%) with TSC in another paediatric group of 15 patients with cardiac rhabdomyomas.

In a review of all cases of cardiac rhabdomyomas published up until 1990, Harding and Pagon (1990) found that at least 172 out of 335 cases (51%) were associated with TSC. Data regarding TSC manifestations in an additional 117 cases were insufficient to confirm the diagnosis of TSC, but if one includes these 117 possible TSC cases, 86% of cardiac rhabdomyomas could be related to TSC.

The highest proportion of TSC associated with cardiac rhabdomyomas was reported by Bosi et al. (1996), who documented 30 cases of TSC in 33 patients (91%) with cardiac rhabdomyomas. The true prevalence of TSC in patients with cardiac rhabdomyomas may be close to 100%, as very often the tumours are the first manifestation of the disease, and are diagnosed in newborns and very small infants, when the majority of symptoms of TSC cannot be noted. The question of whether patients with multiple cardiac rhabdomyomas may be regarded as definite TSC cases is still unanswered (Uzun et al. 1997).

Conversely, cardiac rhabdomyomas are found in 47 to 67% of all patients with TSC. We found them in 46 out of 98 (47%) examined children (unpublished data). A similar incidence was reported by Smith et al. (1989), who detected cardiac tumours in 28 out of 60 patients. A higher incidence of rhabdomyomas among TSC patients was reported by Webb et al. (1993), 60%; Gibbs (1985), 64%; and Muhler et al. (1994), 67%.

These tumours represent the earliest detectable hamartoma in TSC, frequently evident in the neonatal period or even prenatally (Michałowicz et al. 1989, Kadar et al. 1998, Gushiken et al. 1999). The incidence of cardiac rhabdomyomas in TSC depends on the age of examined patients. There are many case or anecdotal reports, but only a few large studies evaluating the frequency of these tumours according to age.

It is commonly accepted that the tumours are more frequent in children, especially infants, than in adults. Smith et al. (1989) noted cardiac tumours in 64% (9/14) of patients under the age of 6 years, 47% (8/17) of those aged 6 to 12, 67% (8/12) of those aged 12 to 18, and in 18% (3/17) of adult patients.

In a study of 47 children examined between 1984 and 1991 in the Children's Memorial Health Institute in Warsaw, the highest frequency of cardiac tumours was noted in children with TSC below the age of 2 years (Fig. 12.1). We found them in 10 of the 11 children (91%) in that age group (Jóźwiak et al. 1994). There was a lower incidence of cardiac tumours in children aged between 2 and 9 years (21%), and another rise in their frequency in children aged between 9 and 18 years (58%), especially in girls (Jóźwiak et al. 1994).

Similar results were recently obtained in a larger group of our patients (Jóźwiak et al. 2000). Cardiac rhabdomyomas were noted on echocardiographic examination in 20 out of 24 (83.3%) children below 2 years of age, in 3 out of 14 (21.4%) aged 2 to 5, in 4 out of 19 (21.1%) aged 5 to 9, in 7 out of 17 (41.2%) aged 9 to 14, and in 3 out of 4 (75%) aged 14 to 18. Our data suggest that there is a second peak of higher incidence of cardiac rhabdomyomas in children at puberty. However, the groups observed were too small for significant statistical analysis.

There are contradictory data concerning the prevalence of cardiac tumours in males and females. Harding and Pagon (1990), in a review of cases of cardiac rhabdomyomas published until 1990, found a higher incidence in males than in females – 1.55:1 (161/104). Smith et al. (1989) reported a 1:1 (14/14) ratio of males and females with cardiac rhabdomyomas; and our unpublished data indicate an even lower ratio – 0.76:1 (16/21).

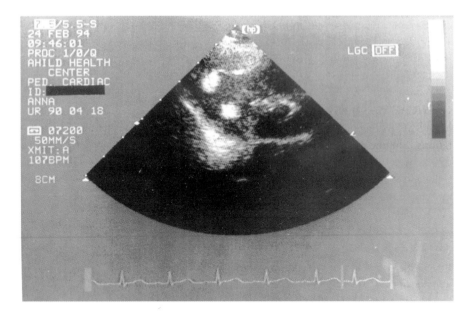

Fig. 12.1. Three-year-old child with TSC, with two large tumours in the right ventricle on echocardiographic examination. The patient remains symptom-free. (Reproduced with permission of Professor Wanda Kawalec, Children's Memorial Health Institute, Warsaw.)

In a large proportion of patients with cardiac rhabdomyomas, the tumours are multiple. In the Fenoglio et al. (1976) series of 36 patients with rhabdomyomas, only 3 (8%) had solitary tumours.

The lesions may be detected in any of the cardiac chambers. In the majority of patients with TSC the tumours are 5 to 15 mm in diameter. They appear with similar frequency, or slightly more frequently on the left side of the heart than on the right (Fenoglio et al. 1976, Bass et al. 1985, Bosi et al. 1996), and more commonly in the ventricles than in the atria (Fenoglio et al. 1976, Jóźwiak et al. 1994). In a large study of 47 patients with TSC and cardiac rhabdomyomas, Nir et al. (1995) noted tumours in the left ventricle in 32 patients (68%), in the left ventricular (LV) septum in 38%, in the LV apex in 38%; and in the right ventricle in 31 patients (66%), in the right ventricular (RV) septum in 38%, and in the RV apex in 32%. Eighteen patients (38%) had tumours located in the left ventricle only, while 14 patients (30%) had tumours in the right ventricle only, and 15 patients (32%) had tumours in both the left and right ventricles. Right atrial tumours were present in three patients (6%).

Relatively infrequently the cardiac rhabdomyomas protrude into the cardiac cavities in patients with TSC (Jóźwiak et al. 1994). Fenoglio et al. (1976) found solely intramural lesions in 9 out of 11 (82%) patients with pathologically confirmed cerebral TSC, while 16 out of 25 patients (64%) with rhabdomyoma but without evidence of TSC had one or more intracavitary tumours. These data may support a hypothesis that a TSC patient (with intramural tumours) has a better prognosis than patients with cardiac rhabdomyomas from the general population, who have obstructing intracavitary tumours resulting in cardiac failure and early death.

CLINICAL MANIFESTATIONS

Most TSC patients with cardiac rhabdomyomas do not exhibit any clinical manifestations (Smythe et al. 1990, Jóźwiak et al. 1994, DiMario et al. 1996, Quek et al. 1998). If cardiac symptoms occur, they are largely a consequence of tumour size or location within the heart. These symptoms and signs may be explained by one or more of three mechanisms: obstruction of inflow or outflow tract, secondary to an obstructing intracavitary tumour; myocardial involvement with secondary deterioration of ventricular function; and cardiac rhythm abnormalities (Mair et al. 1999).

The majority of cardiac manifestations in patients with TSC are related to the neonatal period and early infancy, although they may be noted at any age – from intrauterine life to late adulthood (Groves et al. 1992, Lopez Minguez et al. 1999). Intrauterine arrhythmia, fetal hydrops or multiple cardiac tumours, detected by fetal ultrasound screening, may be the first symptoms leading to the diagnosis of tuberous sclerosis before delivery.

Large obstructing intracavitary tumours may compromise ventricular function or disturb cardiac rhythm, producing severe symptoms and death, especially in newborns and infants. There are a few reports of sudden deaths of infants with TSC and cardiac rhabdomyomas (De Leon et al. 1988, Bordarier et al. 1994, Jóźwiak et al. 1994, Grellner and Henssge 1996). Cardiac rhabdomyomas arising from the intraventricular septum or located in the vicinity of cardiac valves may result in valvular dysfunction and congestive heart failure. These children may demonstrate tachypnea, cyanosis and tachycardia. Chest radiography may reveal cardiomegaly (Fig. 12.2).

Congestive heart failure develops in 2 to 4% of children with cardiac rhabdomyomas (Jóźwiak et al. 1994, Nir et al. 1995). Only one out of 47 patients reported by Nir et al. (1995) had symptoms of heart failure. Interestingly, a cardiac murmur may be heard in a relatively small proportion of patients. We detected it in 3 out of 22 (14%) children with cardiac masses (Jóźwiak et al. 1994). In the Smith et al. (1989) series of 60 patients with TSC only one infant presented a detectable cardiac murmur on first clinical examination.

The majority of descriptions in the literature of patients with cardiac rhabdomyomas leading to heart failure are related to masses in the left heart. One of our patients with multiple rhabdomyomas located mainly in the left ventricular outflow tract died at the age of 3 months (Jóźwiak et al. 1994). Five out of six infants with TSC and symptomatic cardiac rhabdomyomas, reported by Webb et al. (1993), died due to cardiac failure; all six had large left ventricular lesions. The surviving

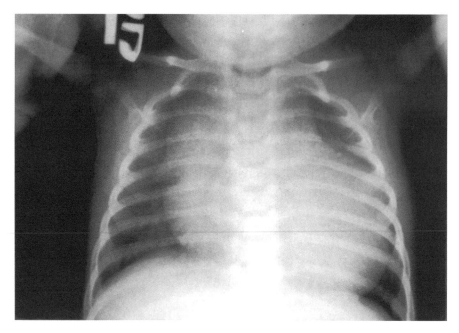

Fig. 12.2. Chest roentgenograph of a newborn with TSC and multiple cardiac tumours showing marked cardiomegaly.

child required a period of ventilatory support and had mitral valve replacement at 18 months for a lesion involving the valve. Kuehl et al. (1970) and Shaher et al. (1972) also described rhabdomyomas of the left ventricular outflow tract resulting in severe subvalvular aortic stenosis. Because of congestive heart failure some of these patients had to undergo surgical removal of the obstructing masses (Shaher et al. 1972, Smythe et al. 1990).

There are also a few reports documenting the presence of rhabdomyomas in the right ventricular outflow tract (Bosi et al. 1996). The outcome of these tumours may also be fatal, but there is an increasing number of reports of their successful surgical removal in newborns during the first days of life (Lababidi et al. 1984, Foster et al. 1994).

Congestive heart failure is uncommon among patients with only intramural lesions. Myocardial involvement and replacement of the ventricular muscle by non-contractile tumour tissue may mimic a cardiomyopathy. In a few patients with large intramural lesions myocardial dysfunction may result in cardiac decompensation and death (van der Hauwaert 1971). Fortunately, a much better scenario may be observed in the majority of patients. Intramural lesions rarely produce clinical signs. The prognosis for this group of patients is better than for patients with intracavitary tumours. In our retrospective studies of children with TSC we had six patients in whom the diagnosis of cardiomyopathy was established in the first months of life. On subsequent echocardiographic studies the diagnosis was abandoned, probably because of the regression of the tumour.

Until now there has been insufficient information on the incidence and importance of cardiac rhythm abnormalities in infants and children with TSC (Figs 12.3 and 12.4). Very few studies exist that assess arrhythmias prospectively. Most do so using the standard rather than the more diagnostic 24-hour electrocardiogram (Fig. 12.5). The possibility that cardiac tumours may interfere with a normal conduction pathway was first suggested by Wegman and Egbert (1935), who reported multiple rhabdomyomas invading the conducting system in a girl who had tachycardia with rates up to 200 beats per minute. In 1945, Duras observed frequent extrasystoles in a patient with severe learning disability and "adenoma sebaceum". In 1968, Taylor reported a "palpitation" in a patient with diagnostic features of TSC. Since then, many different types of cardiac rhythm abnormalities have been described in patients with TSC: atrial or ventricular tachycardia, complete heart block, ventricular fibrillation and Wolff–Parkinson–White syndrome.

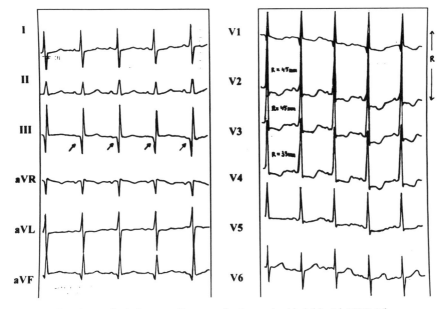

Fig. 12.3. Routine 12-lead electrocardiogram of a 2-month-old child with TSC. There are very deep Q waves in III lead (small arrows) and features of ventricular hypertrophy. R waves in precordial leads (V2–V4) are very high (33–45 mm), exceeding double the normal values for age (15–16 mm), which confirms significant hypertrophy, especially of the right ventricle. Echocardiographic examination documented multiple cardiac tumours. The largest pedunculated tumour occupied almost the whole right ventricular cavity. (Reproduced with permission of Anna Turska-Kmieć, MD, Children's Memorial Health Institute, Warsaw.)

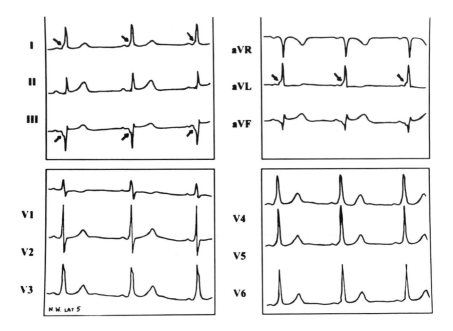

Fig. 12.4. Routine 12-lead electrocardiogram of a 5-year-old girl with TSC, showing preexcitation pattern of Wolf–Parkinson–White type: marked shortening of atrio-ventricular conduction time with lack of PQ segment and abnormal QRS disfigured by the presence of slur on the upstroke of the R wave or on the downstroke of an S wave (delta wave). (Arrows indicate delta wave.) Echocardiographic study documented multiple cardiac tumours in both ventricules and intraventricular myocardium. (Reproduced with permission of Anna Turska-Kmieć, MD, Children's Memorial Health Institute, Warsaw.)

There is a common opinion that the rhythm abnormalities in patients with TSC are caused by intramural rhabdomyomas interrupting the conduction pathways and leading to ectopic electrical foci or an accessory electrical circuit producing preexcitation (Wolff–Parkinson–White syndrome). The higher incidence of preexcitation among TSC patients than in the general population (0.15%) may support the thesis. Nir et al. (1995) documented Wolff–Parkinson–White syndrome in at least 2 out of 23 patients (9%) with rhabdomyoma who had electrocardiograms.

Although uncommon, rhythm abnormalities are responsible for dysrhythmic deaths in some patients with TSC. Such outcomes may involve children with coexisting rhabdomyomas. Case et al. (1991) described a 9-month-old girl with multiple cardiac tumours who presented with supraventricular and ventricular arrhythmia, and who, despite surgical removal of tumours and pacemaker placement, died of congestive heart failure.

Special attention should be paid to those children with cardiac rhabdomyomas receiving carbamazepine treatment because of epileptic seizures. Weig and Pollack

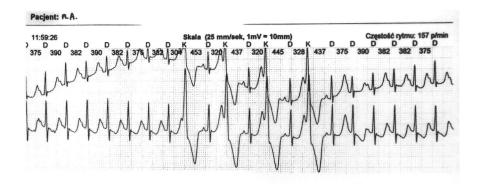

Fig. 12.5. 24-hour electrocardiogram of an infant with TSC, demonstrating premature ventricular complexes (marked with K). D symbols indicate dominating normal sinus rhythm with a rate of 157 beats per minute. Numbers correspond to intervals (in milliseconds) between succeeding excitations. (Reproduced with permission of Anna Turska-Kmieć, MD, Children's Memorial Health Institute, Warsaw.)

(1993) reported a 13-month-old boy with a single 2 to 3 mm mass in the intra-ventricular septum who developed second-degree atrioventricular block on this medication. After discontinuation of this therapy repeat EKG was normal, without conduction disturbances or ectopy.

Although dysrhythmias occur more often in patients with rhabdomyomas, sudden unexplained deaths suggestive of arrhythmic origin have been reported in children without detectable cardiac tumours. Nir et al. (1995) observed a patient who had a normal echocardiogram at 11 months of age, who died suddenly 1.5 years later and was then found to have multiple cardiac rhabdomyomas at autopsy. Such cases raise questions about the resolution limitations of echocardiography, a method unable to detect small tumours.

There are many descriptions of patients with TSC and rhythm abnormalities without detectable rhabdomyomas. Muhler et al. (1994) reported a few premature ventricular contractions in 10 out of 13 patients with heart tumours, but also in 2 out of 6 patients without confirmed cardiac rhabdomyomas. In addition, one of our patients with a normal echocardiographic examination had electrocardiographic evidence of Wolff–Parkinson–White syndrome, which disappeared during follow-up. It is very probable that in these patients small cardiac tumours, undetectable on echocardiography, form an abnormal conduction tissue producing preexcitation. Recent pathological studies have indicated that some of the cells in cardiac rhabdomyomas are structurally similar to Purkinje cells and may function as an accessory conducting bundle (Mehta 1993).

A possible relationship between cardiac rhabdomyomas and cerebral stroke in young children with TSC has been raised in a few papers (Kandt et al. 1985, Konkol et al. 1986). It is very unlikely that fragments from cardiac rhabdomyomas are the origin of these strokes, by embolization of the cerebral arteries, as the proposed rhabdomyomatous emboli have never been described angiographically or in post-mortem examinations of brains of patients with TSC. It is much more probable that a TSC-related defect of the cerebral artery wall leads to its dissection and thrombotic occlusion (Gomez 1989).

NATURAL HISTORY AND FOLLOW-UP

A high incidence of cardiac rhabdomyomas in infants and young children with TSC, and a relatively low incidence in adults, observed by some authors, gave rise to speculation on the possible regression of these tumours. Regression of the tumours had been described in the mid-1980s in a few case reports (Kandt et al. 1985, Alkalay et al. 1987), and subsequently in larger studies (Farooki et al. 1991, Jóźwiak et al. 1994, Nir et al. 1995, Bosi et al. 1996, DiMario et al. 1996). In our longitudinal study of 12 children we found complete resolution of the cardiac rhabdomyomas in 4 patients, regression in 2, and in 6 children the size of the tumours remained unchanged (Jóźwiak et al. 1994) (Fig. 12.6a and b). In the largest study, tumour regression was seen in 15 out of 26 patients (58%), and in 11 (42%) there was no change in tumour size or number (Nir et al. 1995).

The most rapid regression rate appears to occur in the first years of life. In the Nir et al. (1995) series, tumours regressed in a majority of patients (70%) seen initially before the age of 4 years, but only in a few patients (17%) seen initially after this age. Additionally, O'Callaghan et al.'s (1998) longitudinal study of patients with Wolff–Parkinson–White syndrome demonstrated that, in 5 out of 10 children, rhythm abnormalities disappeared on follow-up, which may confirm their association with cardiac rhabdomyomas.

A high incidence of rhabdomyomas in newborns and infants, their regression in early childhood, and a second peak in puberty in girls, observed in our patients (unpublished data), may suggest that enlargement of the tumours is related to oestrogen level. Further longitudinal prospective studies are needed.

Natural evolution of cardiac rhabdomyomas may also be influenced by ACTH treatment. Hishitani et al. (1997) documented a rapid enlargement of cardiac rhabdomyomas in two children receiving corticotropin therapy for infantile spasms.

HISTOPATHOLOGICAL STUDIES

Almost all cardiac tumours found in TSC patients are rhabdomyomas, and this type of heart tumour is the most frequent in the paediatric age group. Association of primary pericardial mesothelioma with TSC has been reported in only one patient by Naramoto et al. (1989).

On gross examination, cardiac rhabdomyomas have a grey or yellowish-white colour, measure a few millimetres to several centimetres in diameter, and are well

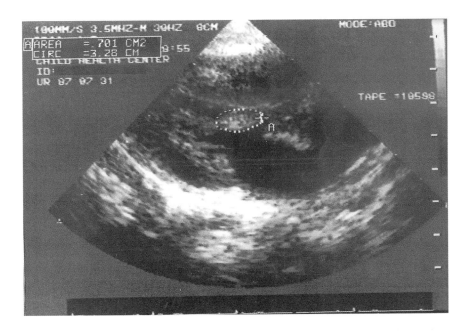

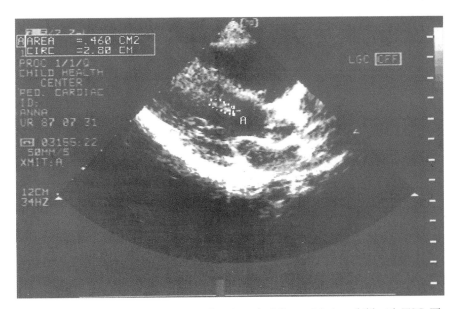

Fig. 12.6. Intramyocardial tumour protruding into the left ventricle in a child with TSC. The tumour has decreased in size in succeeding examinations carried out at age 2 (a) and 6 years (b). For comparison, area and circumference of the tumour are given in the left upper part of the figure. (Reproduced with permission of Professor Wanda Kawalec, Children's Memorial Health Institute, Warsaw.)

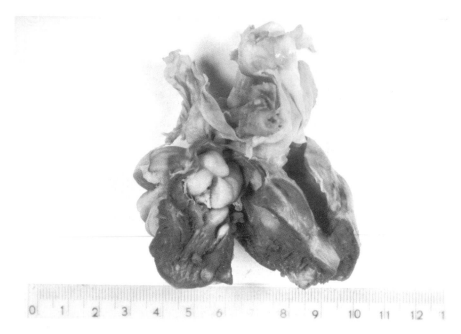

Fig. 12.7. Cut surface of the heart of a newborn with a family history of TSC, who died soon after birth. At autopsy a large cardiac tumour, which almost completely occupied the cavity of the right atrium, and several small tumours in the myocardium were found. (Reproduced with permission of Professor Bogdan Woźniewicz, Children's Memorial Health Institute, Warsaw.)

demarcated from the surrounding myocardium (Fig. 12.7). Cardiac rhabdomyomas are unencapsulated. The tumour cells range in size from 80 to 200µ and are larger than surrounding myocardial cells. Rhabdomyomatous nodules form a spongy tissue containing syncytial giant cells which have one or more nuclei surrounded by protoplasm with numerous extensions spread out like a fan. The tumour cells are typically characterized by a "chicken-wire" appearance and by so-called "spider cells" (Mair et al. 1999) (Figs 12.8 and 12.9).

The fact that cardiac rhabdomyomas do not undergo malignant sarcomatous transformation, and tend to regress on follow-up, supports the hypothesis that cardiac rhabdomyoma represents a fetal hamartoma rather than a true neoplasm (Jóźwiak 1995).

DIAGNOSIS

In a minority of patients the diagnosis of cardiac rhabdomyomas is available in the presence of cardiovascular symptoms and signs, described in the initial part of the chapter. Despite the frequent presence of tumours, most children are asymptomatic. Until recently, these hamartomas were diagnosed at necropsy. In the last two decades the introduction of sector echocardiography has allowed non-invasive detection

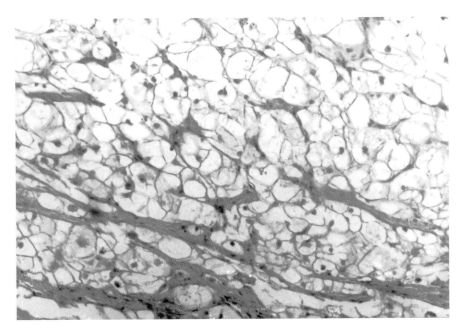

Fig. 12.8. Cardiac rhabdomyoma. Well-differentiated, large, rounded and polygonal cells with abundant acidophilic cytoplasm containing variable amounts of lipid and glycogen. (Hematoxylin and eosin, ×250.) (Reproduced with permission of Professor Bogdan Woźniewicz, Children's Memorial Health Institute, Warsaw.)

of tumours, frequently in asymptomatic patients. In our series of 22 children in whom cardiac rhabdomyomas were detected echocardiographically, only one child demonstrated symptoms of congestive heart failure, and three had a cardiac murmur (Jóźwiak et al. 1994).

Echocardiography has become the diagnostic procedure of choice for cardiac rhabdomyomas. A recent Tuberous Sclerosis Consensus Conference recommended an echocardiogram for patients of any age with symptoms of a cardiac rhabdomyoma (Roach et al. 1999). In our opinion, such examination should be carried out at least once in all patients with TSC, especially in early infancy. There are many reports of sudden deaths in asymptomatic children, with multiple cardiac rhabdomyomas revealed at autopsy (Grellner and Henssge 1996). Echocardiography, together with electrocardiographic examination, enables identification of children with potential risk of congestive heart failure or sudden death.

One should always be aware that, because of echocardiographic resolution limitations, very small tumours may be missed. Nir et al. (1995) reported a patient who had a normal echocardiogram at 11 months of age, and died suddenly 1.5 years later. At autopsy, multiple cardiac rhabdomyomas were found. The question of

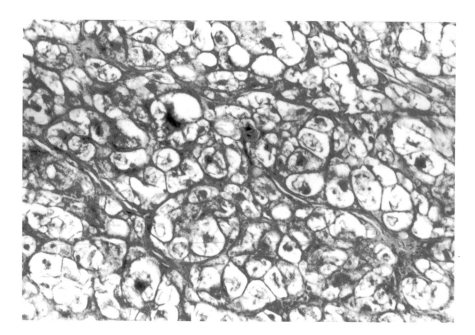

Fig. 12.9. Typical "spider cells" of rhabdomyoma with centrally located nucleus and peripheral threads of sarcoplasm. (Hematoxylin and eosin, ×250.) (Reproduced with permission of Professor Bogdan Woźniewicz, Children's Memorial Health Institute, Warsaw.)

whether a child who has a normal echocardiogram should have another echocardiogram on follow-up is still open.

There are preliminary studies on the effectiveness of electrocardiogram-gated MRI for detecting cardiac rhabdomyomas in patients with TSC (Fig. 12.10). Shiraishi et al. (1988) found MRI to be superior to echocardiography in the diagnosis and characterization of apical intracardiac tumours. They recommended two-dimensional echocardiography for the initial evaluation of cardiac masses in children with a predisposition to TSC. For further evaluation, electrocardiogram-gated MRI has been suggested.

According to the latest revision of diagnostic criteria for TSC, if detected, single or multiple cardiac rhabdomyomas are regarded as major diagnostic features (Roach et al. 1998). Some authors have postulated that all rhabdomyomas, even without any other evidence of TSC, should be considered as *formes frustes* of TSC (Elliott and Mac Geachy 1962). However, so far there is insufficient evidence for such an assumption.

The diagnostic significance of cardiac rhabdomyomas is especially high in newborns and small infants. Cardiac rhabdomyomas discovered prenatally or at birth are rarely associated with other manifestations of TSC (Jóźwiak 1992). In

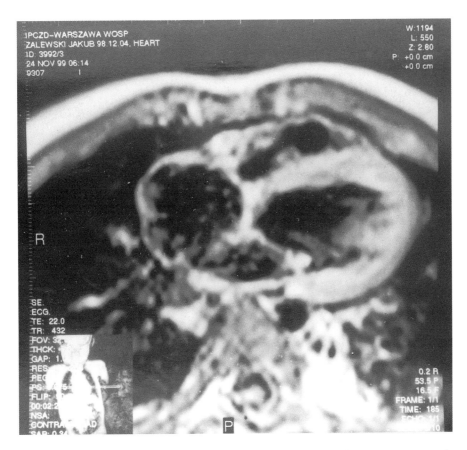

Fig. 12.10. Cardiac MRI of an infant with TSC. An intramyocardial and intracavitary tumour is seen in the right atrium. (Reproduced with permission of Dr Marek Pędich, Children's Memorial Health Institute, Warsaw.)

infants, the skin lesions of TSC may not be found even with a Wood's light. CT of the brain is seldom informative in early infancy. Echocardiography appears to be the most useful single diagnostic test in this age group. In our study, cardiac tumours were detected with echocardiography in 83% of patients below 2 years of age (Jóźwiak et al. 2000). Early death, insufficient follow-up or incomplete evaluation may result in failure to diagnose TSC in this group of young patients. However, the absence of other physical and laboratory findings of TSC in a newborn with cardiac rhabdomyoma does not exclude the diagnosis of TSC.

The introduction of high-resolution echocardiography resulted in an increase in the number of reports of cardiac rhabdomyomas diagnosed in utero (Goh et al. 1995, Itoh et al. 1996, Guschmann et al. 1997, Gushiken et al. 1999, Czechowski et al. 2000). Some of the tumours have been diagnosed at 22 weeks gestation

(Goh et al. 1995). Prenatal echocardiography should be offered to each family with a member (parent or child) affected with TSC. Early detection of cardiac tumours allows therapeutic abortion to be considered, in families willing to terminate the pregnancy, and enables early planning of treatment, if the child is going to be born.

Prenatal ultrasound screening for cardiac tumours and fetal ECG are not sensitive enough to detect all fetuses with TSC. The absence of visible cardiac lesions does not exclude the presence of the disease.

TREATMENT

The tendency of cardiac rhabdomyomas toward spontaneous resolution, particularly in infancy and early childhood, dictates a conservative approach in the majority of patients. According to the latest recommendations, periodic echocardiography of all asymptomatic patients is unnecessary (Roach et al. 1999). Occasionally asymptomatic children may require follow-up echocardiography – when the initial study raises specific concerns about the size or location of a rhabdomyoma, or in patients considered to be at relative risk of tumour enlargement, e.g. patients on ACTH treatment.

In patients with congestive heart failure, treatment with digitalis, diuretics and salt restriction may be utilized. Cardiac rhythm disturbances are usually treated with antidysrhythmic drugs. In children with dysrhythmia refractory to medication, a cardiac pacemaker or division of the abnormal conduction pathway may be considered.

Surgical excision of tumours in infancy is justified only in the presence of a life-threatening haemodynamic condition. These patients, frequently newborns, usually have multiple obstructing masses. The operative risk depends on the number, size and location of the tumours, but in this group of patients is very high. However, the prognosis for survival without surgical intervention in these critically ill children is very poor. In such cases, limited tumour resection, in order to avoid perioperative morbidity, may be sufficient, as the residual tumour mass will very probably involute. In infants with large multiple cardiac rhabdomyomas producing severe heart failure, cardiac transplantation may be a rational option (Demkow et al. 1995).

VASCULAR ANOMALIES

An association of arterial aneurysms and tuberous sclerosis has been reported in a number of patients. Such a coincidence, and usually at an early age, led Davidson (1974) to suggest a congenital defect of the arterial wall in the condition. This idea was taken up by Beall and Delaney (1983), who discussed the similarities between TSC and two other entities with high incidence of intracranial aneurysms and arteriopathy: polycystic kidney disease and fibromuscular dysplasia. In addition, Blumenkopf and Huggins (1985) suggested a common embryological aberration in polycystic kidney disease and TSC. Now, with the discovery of close localization of the *TSC2* gene and the *PKD1* gene on chromosome 16, the similarities might be explained by deletions of these contiguous genes.

There are at least 13 patients with TSC and aortic aneurysms described in the literature (Gomez 1999). Most of them were children under the age of 5 years. Of these 13 patients, 4 had aneurysms of the descending thoracic aorta and 9 of its abdominal part. In some cases an aortic aneurysm was an occasional finding. More often an aneurysm led to unexpected rupture, resulting in the sudden death of the patient (Shepherd et al. 1991).

In several reports aortic aneurysm was accompanied by other vascular lesions. Paraf and Bruneval (1996) described a 2.5-year-old girl who, in addition to having an abdominal aortic aneurysm, underwent a right nephrectomy for multiple renal angiomyolipomas and cysts. Microscopic examination of the aortic aneurysm and the right renal artery showed fibromuscular dysplasia.

Ng et al. (1988) reported a man who, in addition to having an abdominal aortic aneurysm, had dilatation of the left renal artery, consistent with its dysplasia. He underwent resection of the aortic aneurysm but died due to bleeding from the site of the anastomosis. The vascular walls of the resected aorta and its aneurysm were severely disrupted by fibrous tissues and calcifications. The smooth muscle and the elastic lamellae of the media were absent.

When medium-sized arterioles of internal organs were involved, most TSC cases demonstrated thickening of the medial layer, absent or deficient elastic tissue, hyalinization, and narrowing of vessel lumen.

There have been, to our knowledge, only seven patients described with TSC and intracranial or extracranial aneurysms (Gomez 1999). Six of them were between 6 and 26 years of age and one man was a 53-year-old. In most cases there were aneurysms of the internal carotid, and in a few there were aneurysms of anterior cerebral, middle cerebral or posterior communicating arteries.

REFERENCES

Alkalay AL, Ferry DA, Lin B, et al. (1987) Spontaneous regression of cardiac rhabdomyoma in tuberous sclerosis. *Clin Pediatr* 26: 532–5.

Bass JL, Breningstall GN, Swaiman KF (1985) Echocardiographic incidence of cardiac rhabdomyoma in tuberous sclerosis. *Am J Cardiol* 55: 1379–82.

Beall S, Delaney P (1983) Tuberous sclerosis with intracranial aneurysms. *Arch Neurol* 40: 826–7.

Blumenkopf B, Huggins MJ (1985) Tuberous sclerosis and multiple intracranial aneurysms: case report. *Neurosurgery* 17: 797–800.

Bordarier C, Lellouch-Tubiana A, Robain O (1994) Cardiac rhabdomyoma and tuberous sclerosis in three fetuses: a neuropathological study. *Brain Develop* 16: 467–71.

Bosi G, Lintermans JP, Pellegrino PA, et al. (1996) The natural history of cardiac rhabdomyoma with and without tuberous sclerosis. *Acta Paediatr* 85: 928–31.

Bussani R, Rustico MA, Silvestri F (2001) Fetal cardiac rhabdomyomatosis as a prenatal marker for the detection of latent tuberous sclerosis. An autopsy case report. *Pathol Res Pract* 197: 559–61.

Case CL, Gillette PL, Crawford FA (1991) Cardiac rhabdomyoma causing supraventricular and lethal ventricular arrhythmia in an infant. *Am Heart J* 122: 1484–6.

Czechowski J, Langille EL, Varady E (2000) Intracardiac tumour and brain lesions in tuberous sclerosis. A case report of antenatal diagnosis by ultrasonography. *Acta Radiol* 41: 371–4.

Davidson S (1974) Tuberous sclerosis with fusiform aneurysms of both internal carotid arteries manifested by unilateral visual loss and papilledema. *Bull Los Angeles Neurol Soc* 39: 128–32.

De Leon GA, Zaeri N, Foley CM (1988) Olfactory hamartomas in tuberous sclerosis. *J Neurol Sci* 87: 187–94.

Demkow M, Sorenson K, Whitehead BF, et al. (1995) Heart transplantation in an infant with rhabdomyoma. *Pediatr Cardiol* 16: 204–6.

DiMario FJ Jr, Diana D, Leopold H, Chameides L (1996) Evolution of cardiac rhabdomyoma in tuberous sclerosis complex. *Clin Pediatr (Phila)* 35: 615–19.

Duras FP (1945) Cardiac manifestations in a case of tuberous sclerosis. *Br Heart J* 7: 37–40.

Elliott GB, Mac Geachy WG (1962) The monster Purkinje-cell nature of so called "congenital rhabdomyoma of heart": a forme fruste of tuberous sclerosis. *Am Heart J* 63: 636–43.

Farooki ZQ, Ross RD, Paridon SM, et al. (1991) Spontaneous regression of cardiac rhabdomyoma. *Am J Cardiol* 67: 897–9.

Fenoglio JJ, McAllister HA, Ferrans VJ (1976) Cardiac rhabdomyoma: a clinicopathologic and electron microscopic study. *Am J Cardiol* 38: 241–51.

Foster ED, Spooner EW, Farina MA, et al. (1994) Cardiac rhabdomyoma in the neonate: surgical management. *Ann Thorac Surg* 37: 249–53.

Gibbs JL (1985) The heart and tuberous sclerosis: an echocardiographic and electrocardiographic study. *Br Heart J* 54: 596–9.

Goh RH, Lapalliainen RE, Mohide PT, Caco CC (1995) Multiple cardiac masses diagnosed with prenatal ultrasonography in the fetus of a woman with tuberous sclerosis. *Can Assoc Radiol J* 46: 461–4.

Gomez MR (1989) Strokes in tuberous sclerosis: are rhabdomyomas a cause? *Brain Dev* 11: 14–19.

Gomez MR (1999) Liver, digestive tract, spleen, arteries, thymus, and lymphatics. In: Gomez MR, Sampson JR, Whittemore VH (eds) *Tuberous Sclerosis Complex*. New York: Oxford University Press, pp 228–39.

Grellner W, Henssge C (1996) Multiple cardiac rhabdomyoma with exclusively histological manifestation. *Forensic Sci Int* 78: 1–5.

Groves AM, Fagg NL, Cook AC, Allan LD (1992) Cardiac tumours in intrauterine life. *Arch Dis Child* 67: 1189–92.

Guschmann M, Entezami M, Becker R, Vogel M (1997) Intrauterine rhabdomyoma of the heart. A case report. *Gen Diagn Pathol* 143: 255–9.

Gushiken BJ, Callen PW, Silverman NH (1999) Prenatal diagnosis of tuberous sclerosis in monozygotic twins with cardiac masses. *J Ultrasound Med* 18: 165–8.

Harding CO, Pagon RA (1990) Incidence of tuberous sclerosis in patients with cardiac rhabdomyoma. *Am J Med Genet* 37: 443–6.

Hishitani T, Hoshino K, Ogawa K, et al. (1997) Rapid enlargement of cardiac rhabdomyoma during corticotropin therapy for infantile spasms. *Can J Cardiol* 13: 72–4.

Itoh S, Tanaka C, Nakamura Y, et al. (1996) Prenatal management of fetal cardiac tumours. Two case reports. *Fetal Diagn Ther* 11: 361–5.

Jóźwiak S (1992) Diagnostic value of clinical features and supplementary investigations in tuberous sclerosis in children. *Acta Paediatr Hung* 32: 71–88.

Jóźwiak S (1995) Oncogenesis in tuberous sclerosis complex. *The Cancer J* 8: 260–3.

Jóźwiak S, Kawalec W, Dłużewska J, et al. (1994) Cardiac tumours in tuberous sclerosis: their incidence and course. *Eur J Pediatr* 153: 155–7.

Jóźwiak S, Schwartz RA, Krysicka Janniger C, Bielicka-Cymerman J (2000) The usefulness of diagnostic criteria of tuberous sclerosis in paediatric patients, *J Child Neurol* 15: 652–9.

Kadar K, Buzas E, Geczi E, Lozsadi K (1998) Rhabdomyomas as a first manifestation of childhood tuberous sclerosis. *Orv Hetil* 139: 2013–15.

Kandt RS, Gebarski SS, Goetting MG (1985) Tuberous sclerosis with cardiogenic cerebral embolism: magnetic resonance imaging. *Neurology* 35: 1223–5.

Konkol RJ, Walsh EP, Power T, Bresnen MJ (1986) Cerebral embolism resulting from an intracardiac tumour in tuberous sclerosis. *Pediatr Neurol* 2: 108–10.

Kuehl KS, Perry LW, Chandra R, Scott LP (1970) Left ventricular rhabdomyoma: a rare cause of subaortic stenosis in the newborn infant. *Pediatrics* 46: 464–8.

Lababidi Z, Wu JR, Walls J, Curtis J (1984) Neonatal cyanosis caused by cardiac rhabdomyomas. *Am Heart J* 108: 624–7.

Lopez Minguez JR, Urbano Galvez JM, Gonzalez Fernandez R, et al. (1999) Atrial fibrillation and the Wolff-Parkinson-White syndrome in a 68-year-old patient with tuberous sclerosis. *Rev Esp Cardiol* 52: 207–10.

Mair DD, Edwards WD, Seward JB (1999) Cardiac manifestations. In: Gomez MR, Sampson JR, Whittemore VH (eds) *Tuberous Sclerosis Complex*. New York: Oxford University Press, pp 194–206.

Mehta AV (1993) Rhabdomyoma and ventricular preexcitation syndrome. *Am J Dis Childh* 147: 669–71.

Michałowicz R, Jóźwiak S, Ignatowicz R (1989) Stwardnienie guzowate a guzy nowotworowe serca u dzieci. *Ped Pol* 64: 559–62.

Muhler EG, Turniski-Harder V, Engelhardt W, von Bernuth G (1994) Cardiac involvement in tuberous sclerosis. *Br Heart J* 72: 584–90.

Naramoto A, Itoh N, Nakano M, Shigematsu H (1989) An autopsy case of tuberous sclerosis associated with primary pericardial mesothelioma. *Acta Pathol Japonica* 39: 400–6.

Ng SH, Ng KK, Pai SCh, Tsai ChCh (1988) Tuberous sclerosis with aortic aneurysm and rib changes: CT demonstration. *J Comput Assist Tomogr* 12: 666–8.

Nir A, Tajik AJ, Freeman WK, et al. (1995) Tuberous sclerosis and cardiac rhabdomyoma. *Am J Cardiol* 76: 419–21.

O'Callaghan FJK, Clarke AC, Joffe H, et al. (1998) Tuberous sclerosis complex and Wolff–Parkinson–White syndrome. *Arch Dis Child* 78: 159–62.

Paraf F, Bruneval P (1996) Dysplasie fibromusculaire arteérielle et sclérose tubéreuse de Bourneville. *Ann Pathol* 16: 203–6.

Quek SC, Yip W, Quek ST, et al. (1998) Cardiac manifestations in tuberous sclerosis: a 10-year review. *J Paediatr Child Health* 34: 283–7.

Roach ES, Gomez MR, Northrup H (1998) Tuberous Sclerosis Complex Consensus Conference: revised clinical diagnostic criteria. *J Child Neurol* 13: 624–8.

Roach ES, DiMario F, Kandt RS, Northrup H (1999) Tuberous Sclerosis Consensus Conference: recommendations for diagnostic evaluation. *J Child Neurol* 14: 401–7.

Shaher RM, Mintzer J, Farina M, et al. (1972) Clinical presentation of rhabdomyoma of the heart in infancy and childhood. *Am J Cardiol* 30: 95–103.

Shepherd CW, Gomez MR, Crowson CS (1991) Causes of death in patients with tuberous sclerosis. *Mayo Clin Proc* 66: 792–6.

Shiraishi H, Yanagisawa M, Kuramatsu T, et al. (1988) Cardiac tumour in a neonate with tuberous sclerosis: echocardiographic demonstration and magnetic resonance imaging. *Eur J Pediatr* 148: 50–2.

Smith HC, Watson GH, Patel RG, Super M (1989) Cardiac rhabdomyomata in tuberous sclerosis: their course and diagnostic value. *Arch Dis Child* 64: 196–200.

Smythe JF, Dyck JD, Smallhorn JF, Freedom RM (1990) Natural history of cardiac rhabdomyoma in infancy and childhood. *Am J Cardiol* 66: 1247–9.

Taylor TR (1968) Tuberous sclerosis presenting as cardiac arrhythmia. *Br Heart J* 30: 132–4.

Uzun O, McGawley G, Wharton GA (1997) Multiple cardiac rhabdomyomas: tuberous sclerosis or not? *Heart* 77: 388.

van der Hauwaert LG (1971) Cardiac tumours in infancy and childhood. *Br Heart J* 33: 125–32.

von Recklinghausen F (1862) Ein Herz von einem Neugeborenen, welches mehrere theils nach aussen, theils nach den Höhlen prominirende Tumouren (Myomen) trug. *Monatschr Geburtsk Frauenkr* 20: 1–2.

Webb DW, Thomas RD, Osborne JP (1993) Cardiac rhabdomyomas and their association with tuberous sclerosis. *Arch Dis Child* 68: 367–70.

Wegman ME, Egbert DS (1935) Congenital rhabdomyoma of the heart associated with arrhythmia. *J Pediatr* 6: 818–24.

Weig SG, Pollack P (1993) Carbamazepine-induced heart block in a child with tuberous sclerosis and cardiac rhabdomyoma: implications for evaluation and follow up. *Ann Neurol* 34: 617–19.

13
HEPATIC, LUNG, SPLENIC AND PANCREATIC INVOLVEMENT

Sergiusz Jóźwiak and Paolo Curatolo

HEPATIC INVOLVEMENT

Until recently, hepatic hamartomas had been rarely reported in patients with TSC, probably in part due to their usually asymptomatic course. Their benign nature, coexistence with renal angiomyolipomas (AMLs) and angiomyolipomatous appearance in relatively few pathological studies suggest that the vast majority (if not all) of hepatic hamartomas are AMLs.

INCIDENCE

In 1992 we found 28 patients with TSC and liver involvement in the literature (Jóźwiak et al. 1992). Most of the reported hepatic hamartomas were found incidentally on postmortem examination (Viamonte et al. 1966, Grasso et al. 1982), by selective angiography (Compton et al. 1976, Marsidi and Wise 1983), by computed tomography (Newmark et al. 1982), or by ultrasonography (Fleury et al. 1987). There are now a few larger studies evaluating the incidence of the lesions in TSC patients. Compton et al. (1976) demonstrated vascular tumours of the liver with coeliac angiography in 5 out of 8 patients. In our study, hepatic hamartomas were demonstrated by ultrasonography in 12 out of 51 (23.5%) examined children (Jóźwiak et al. 1992).

As the incidence of the lesions increases with age, they are even more common in adult patients. Fleury et al. (1987) examined by ultrasonography 36 individuals with TSC, aged 6 to 48 years, and noted hepatic hamartomas in 13% (3 out of 23) of the children under 16 years of age, and in 23% (3 out of 13) of the older patients. We documented hepatic hamartomas in 2 out of 20 (10%) children who were 5 years of age or younger (an 8-month-old girl and a 5-year-old boy), in 5 out of 20 (25%) children aged between 5 and 10, and in 5 out of 11 (45%) over the age of 10 (Jóźwiak et al. 1992) (Fig. 13.1).

Hepatic hamartomas are more common in girls than in boys (2:1–5:1) (Jóźwiak et al. 1992, Sheffield et al. 1998).

CLINICAL MANIFESTATIONS

Hepatic hamartomas in TSC do not usually cause hepatic dysfunction or other symptoms or signs. The serum levels of liver enzymes are normal. These tumours are

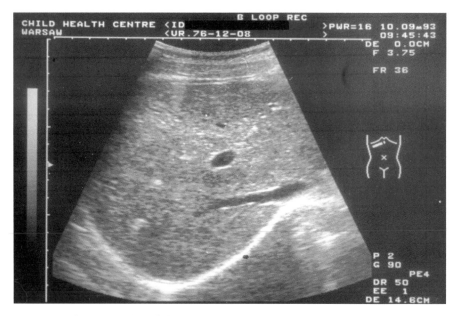

Fig. 13.1. Ultrasonography of the liver in a 12-year-old patient with TSC. Several small hyperechogenic areas in the hepatic parenchyma. (Reproduced with permission of Dr Marek Pędich, Children's Memorial Health Institute, Warsaw.)

found incidentally or during periodic follow-up of TSC patients. Sonographically the liver lesions are highly echogenic, round to ovoid in shape, and sharply demarcated from the surrounding normal parenchyma. Contrast-enhanced CT is able to provide greater detail by demonstrating low-density areas that represent fatty tissue. In addition, magnetic resonance imaging may demonstrate a hyperintense signal on T2-weighted images, indicating better than ultrasonography areas of fat in the tumour. Frequently these tumours are multiple and localized in both liver lobes. The average size of the lesion is 0.5 to 1.0 cm.

There are only two symptomatic hepatic hamartomas reported in the literature, presenting with flank pain, spontaneous haemorrhage or rapid growth (Kristal and Sperber 1989, Huber et al. 1996). Both of them proved to be hepatic AMLs. In contrast to renal lesions, hepatic AMLs grow more slowly, and were not mentioned as a possible cause of death in a large study of 355 patients with TSC (Shepherd et al. 1991).

Usually, renal AMLs precede development of hepatic AMLs in TSC patients, and are frequent coexisting lesions. They were noted in 9 out of 12 children with hepatic AMLs in our series (Jóźwiak et al. 1992), and in all 16 individuals with hepatic lesions reported by Sheffield et al. (1998).

Histopathology

There are only a few reports of pathological studies of liver lesions in TSC patients. Although hepatic AML is the most common type of hepatic hamartoma, occasionally other hamartomas have been documented, such as lipomesenchymal tumour, neurilemmoblastoma, or lipoma (Jóźwiak et al. 1992).

On gross examination, hepatic AMLs are yellow to light tan, depending on the amount of fat tissue. Histologically, these neoplasms are characterized by an admixture of mature fat cells, blood vessels and smooth muscle cells, with occasional foci of extramedullary hematopoiesis. There are aneurysmatic dilatations of thick-walled blood vessels, which may facilitate spontaneous bleeding.

The vascular nature of hepatic hamartomas has been suggested in several angiographic (Viamonte et al. 1966, Compton et al. 1976, Newmark et al. 1982, Marsidi and Wise 1983) and ultrasonographic (Fleury et al. 1987) studies. Interestingly, hemangioma, the most common benign tumour of the liver, has not been recognized in any of the histopathologically confirmed cases (Jóźwiak et al. 1992). We suspect that hepatic angiographic findings in TSC represent a vascular expression rather than a true hemangioma.

Tang et al. (2002) reported a preferential loss of one of the two human androgen receptor gene (HUMARA) alleles, indicating a clonal proliferation with involvement of different alleles, in a patient with multiple hepatic AMLs with absence of other stigmata of TSC.

Recent immunohistochemical studies have demonstrated that hepatic lesions in TSC patients may represent monotypic epithelioid AMLs with pronounced presence of epithelioid PEC (Bonetti et al. 1997). Positive HMB-45 staining has been proposed as a defining criterion of hepatic AML (Tsui et al. 1999).

Diagnostic Significance

Hepatic AMLs representing non-renal hamartomas are regarded as a minor feature of TSC (Roach et al. 1998).

Differential Diagnosis

The benign course of hepatic AMLs in TSC seems to be distinctly different from the clinical presentation of isolated hepatic AMLs. In a review of 52 cases of hepatic AMLs (including three patients with TSC), abdominal pain was reported in 37% of patients, followed by malaise and upper abdominal mass or hepatomegaly (Nonomura et al. 1994).

Treatment

As almost all hepatic AMLs are asymptomatic, no specific treatment is required. Only symptomatic AMLs may necessitate appropriate management.

LUNG INVOLVEMENT

In 1918, Lutembacher described cystic and nodular lesions in the lungs of a 36-year-old woman with TSC who had progressive dyspnea before she died from bilateral pneumotorax. This patient also had renal tumours, presumably AMLs. Von Stössel (1937) observed "muscular cirrhosis of the lungs" in a 43-year-old woman dying from respiratory failure. In 1966, Cornog and Enterline used the term "lymphangiomyoma" in describing a typical smooth muscle proliferation of multifocal origin seen in the lungs and lymph nodes. They noticed the striking preponderance of female affected subjects and the similarity of the histologic findings to those detected as lung involvement in TSC. Recently, it has become clear that the lung involvement in TSC is a lymphangioleiomyomatosis (LAM), a devastating and progressive interstitial lung disease that mostly affects young women. This disorder is characterized by the proliferation of atypical smooth muscle cells throughout the peribronchial, perivascular, and perilymphatic regions of the lung.

INCIDENCE

In past years, the incidence of lung involvement was estimated to be between 1 and 2.3% of all TSC patients (Jao et al. 1972, Castro et al. 1995). Recently, Costello et al (2000) reported that out of 78 women with definite TSC seen at the Mayo Clinic in Rochester from 1977 to 1998, 20 (26%) had evidence of LAM. Furthermore, 8 out of 14 women (57%) with no respiratory symptoms who underwent chest computed tomography had characteristic findings of LAM (Costello et al. 2000). Therefore, the frequency of lung involvement in women with TSC may be even higher than previously suspected, supporting the recommendation for computed tomographic scans of the chest for all women with TSC (Roach et al. 1999).

CLINICAL MANIFESTATIONS

The average age at onset of pulmonary symptoms in women is approximately 30 years. The characteristic clinical features of this disease are slowly worsening shortness of breath, and recurrent pneumothoraces. Other clinical features include cough, chest pain, hemoptysis, chyloptisis and chylothorax (Chu et al. 1999, Urban et al. 1999). The prognosis of LAM is considered poor, and respiratory failure is often severe and generally progressive (Hancock and Osborne 2002). Pulmonary lesions were the prevalent cause of death in TSC patients, especially those over the age of 40 (Shepherd et al. 1991). In older series, the median survival time from diagnosis to death was five years (Dwyer et al. 1971). Currently, with effective anti-estrogen hormonal therapy and the possibility of lung transplantation, most TSC patients with lung involvement live longer, with the average time since the onset of LAM among survivors approaching 10 years (Taylor et al. 1990, Urban et al. 1992).

Among individuals with pulmonary TSC, 80% had adenoma sebaceum, 60% had renal AMLs, and 25% had retinal phakomas (Dawson 1954). LAM also occurs in women who do not have neurologic, dermatologic, or retinal signs or symptoms of TSC (sporadic LAM). Sporadic LAM is rare, with fewer than 1000 women currently known to be affected in the United States. Clinical, radiological and histopathological features of sporadic LAM are nearly identical to those observed in patients with TSC-associated pulmonary LAM, supporting the hypothesis that they share common pathogenetic mechanisms (Chan et al. 1993). Furthermore, 60% of women with sporadic LAM also have renal AMLs (Chu et al. 1999), leading to speculation that sporadic pulmonary LAM and TSC are related diseases (Bonetti and Chiodera 1996). Smolarek et al. (1998) observed that 54% of AMLs from women with sporadic LAM have loss of heterozygosity in the *TSC2* region of chromosome 16p13. Recently, Carsillo et al. (2000) reported the identification of somatic *TSC2* mutations in 5 out of 7 AMLs from sporadic LAM patients, strongly supporting a direct role of *TSC2* mutations in the pathogenesis of AMLs in sporadic pulmonary LAM patients. The reasons that LAM occurs almost exclusively in women, whereas sporadic AMLs occur in both men and women, remain unknown. The fact that not all women had cystic lung disease may indicate that only certain types of TSC mutations are associated with LAM.

HISTOPATHOLOGY

Pulmonary LAM has a distinctive gross appearance. On macroscopic examination, the lungs appear voluminous and may be twice as heavy as normal lungs. A multitude of cysts, varying in size from a few millimetres to several centimetres, take the place of the normal fine lacy parenchymal pattern, having an appearance similar to a sponge. These cysts are generally empty, but sometimes may contain either chylous or serous fluid (Lie 1991). Microscopically, LAM is characterized by diffuse infiltration of the pulmonary interstitium by smooth muscle cells and cystic distortion of the lung architecture. Generally, the lungs cysts appear unlined. The interstitium between adjacent cyst walls consists of a proliferation of immature-looking smooth muscle cells with poorly defined interdigitating lymphatic spaces. These foci of spindle-cell proliferation can occur independently of the lung cysts throughout the parenchyma, as well as in extrapulmonary tissues (Shepherd et al. 1991, Castro et al. 1995).

Pulmonary nodular lesions observed in TSC patients are morphologically comparable to pulmonary LAM. However, according to current understanding of the pathogenesis of pulmonary hamartomatous lesions, the multifocal micronodular pneumocyte hyperplasia associated with TSC should be considered as a distinct type of lung lesion, whether it occurs with or without LAM (Maruyama et al. 2001).

DIAGNOSIS

Sometimes, the correct clinical diagnosis could be postponed until several years after the onset of symptoms. In fact, the insidious lung involvement in patients without the usual signs and symptoms characteristic of TSC may delay the diagnosis until the respiratory insufficiency becomes an irreversible cause of morbidity and mortality. This is because ordinary chest radiography is unable to detect early interstitial lung disease, including LAM (Muller et al. 1990). However, with progressive LAM, chest radiography may reveal evidence of pulmonary involvement, detecting diffuse reticular or reticulonodular infiltrates usually accompanied by hyperinflation. Computed tomography of the chest is able to confirm the diagnosis by detecting the characteristic diffuse cystic changes throughout the lung parenchyma, even when chest radiographs and pulmonary function results are normal (Fig. 13.2). Cystic changes can be observed particularly well when CT imaging is completed using a high-resolution algorithm.

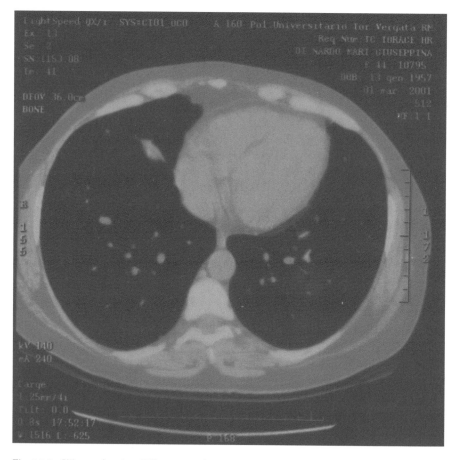

Fig. 13.2. CT scan showing diffuse cystic changes involving the lung parenchyma.

TREATMENT

Exacerbations of LAM can occur during pregnancy, and both improvement of symptoms and stabilization of the disease can be observed with treatments that decrease endogenous estrogen production (Sullivan 1998, Johnson and Tattersfield 1999). These findings suggest that steroid hormones may play a major role in the pathogenesis of LAM. Lung transplantation is considered the only effective therapy for end-stage LAM (Boehler et al. 1996). As a result of current treatment regimes, most patients now live longer.

SPLEEN INVOLVEMENT

Since the initial description of splenic hamartoma by Rokitansky in 1861, about 140 cases of true hamartomas have been reported in the literature (Hayes et al. 1998), but there are only 11 patients with TSC (Cares 1958, Morales 1961, Colonna et al. 1966, van Heerden and Longo 1967, Tsakraklides et al. 1974, Darden et al. 1975, Östör and Fortune 1978, Bender and Yunis 1981, Asayama et al. 1998, Gomez 1999). According to Bender and Yunis (1982), there are two types of splenic abnormalities seen in TSC patients: hemangiomatous malformations and histiocytoid cells.

HEMANGIOMATOUS MALFORMATIONS

Five patients with hemangiomatous malformations have been described. Three of them demonstrated symptoms of an enlarging abdominal mass (van Heerden and Longo 1967, Darden et al. 1975, Asayama et al. 1998). Only the patient reported by Asayama et al. (1998) manifested repeated bleeding within the spleen. This patient had TSC diagnosed in infancy, and on abdominal CT multiple bilateral renal AMLs and splenic mass were noted. During the follow-up of 62 months the splenic tumour increased in size and a splenectomy was performed. A large subcapsular haematoma of the spleen was documented, which was considered to be caused by repeated bleeding from a small AML.

Patients reported by van Heerden and Longo (1967) and Darden et al. (1975) were first seen with enlarging splenic masses and abdominal pain. The tumours were removed at surgery. In two other patients splenic hamartomas were asymptomatic and found incidentally on postmortem examination (Cares 1958, Gomez 1999).

All of the spleens involved weighed more than 350 g and contained one or more deep-red, multinodular masses, measuring 5 to over 10 cm in diameter. The lesions were usually well demarcated and occasionally had a partial fibrous capsule. Microscopically, they had distorted splenic architecture with markedly dilated sinusoids lined by a single layer of endothelial cells. These tumours showed no malpighian corpuscles.

Hemangiomatous hamartomas bear a superficial resemblance to renal AMLs, but muscle and fat have not been demonstrated. A splenic AML was recognized in only one patient (Asayama et al. 1998).

HISTIOCYTOID CELLS

This type of splenic lesion seems to be quite subtle and has never been reported to cause any clinical manifestations. All lesions were diagnosed on pathological examination in infants with TSC. Six patients with similar lesions have been identified (Morales 1961, Tsakraklides et al. 1974, Östör and Fortune 1978, Bender and Yunis 1981).

On gross examination the involved spleens were unremarkable. By light-microscopy there were occasional clusters of abnormal cells in the red pulp. The clusters were unencapsulated and uncircumscribed, mingled with normal splenic cells, and did not compress surrounding tissue (Bender and Yunis 1982). The largest clusters were approximately 1 mm in diameter (Bender and Yunis 1981).

The origin of histiocytoid cells is unclear. They appear to be seen only in neonates, suggesting a transient nature.

SPLENIC SARCOMA

There is only one patient described with splenic sarcoma and TSC (Colonna et al. 1966). As this is a single case, it is difficult to say whether any causative relationship between TSC and this kind of splenic tumour exists.

PANCREATIC INVOLVEMENT

The pancreas seems to be rarely involved in patients with TSC. However, the true prevalence of pancreatic hamartomas remains unknown because of infrequent examination of this organ. Kawamura was probably the first to report a pancreatic tumour in an individual with TSC (Kawamura 1913). Different types of pancreatic tumours have been documented in patients with TSC: AML (Maziak et al. 1996), non-hormone-producing islet cell tumours (Ilgren and Westmoreland 1984, Verhoef et al. 1999), insulinomas (Gutman and Leffkowitz 1959, Davidson 1960, Davoren 1992) Langerhans cell histiocytosis (Drut 1990) and adenocarcinoma (Lack et al. 1983).

Patients with pancreatic tumours demonstrated a vast variety of clinical manifestations: abdominal pain, behavioural changes with episodes of agitation or lethargy, hypoglycaemia or epilepsy. In some patients the tumours were asymptomatic, and were revealed at autopsy or incidentally on abdominal ultrasonography (Perou and Gray 1960, Maziak et al. 1996) (Fig. 13.3). In one 34-year-old patient we demonstrated a large pancreatic tumour on routine abdominal ultrasonographic examination (Fig. 13.4). She had no clinical manifestations and serum glucose level was normal. She refused any additional examinations, but, several years later, she developed abdominal symptoms, became cacchexic and died. At autopsy a large malignant non-hormone-producing islet cell pancreatic tumour was recognized. Recently, Verhoef et al. (1999) documented LOH in a non-hormone-producing islet cell pancreatic tumour in a 12-year-old boy with TSC, which may confirm a direct relationship of this tumour to TSC.

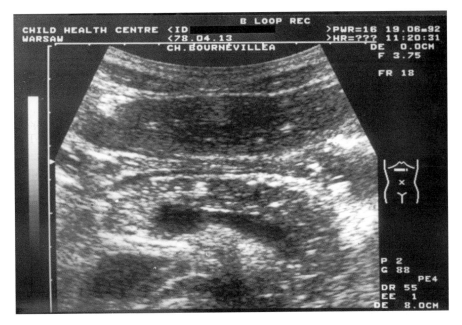

Fig. 13.3. Several hyperechogenic areas in the pancreatic parenchyma in a 16-year-old boy with TSC. The patient remains symptom-free. (Reproduced with permission of Dr Marek Pędich, Children's Memorial Health Institute, Warsaw.)

Because of relatively frequent malignant transformation of pancreatic tumours in TSC patients, surgical incision is usually recommended.

COLORECTAL INVOLVEMENT

The incidence of colorectal lesions in TSC patients has been evaluated in only two small studies (Devroede et al. 1988, Gould et al. 1990). Devroede et al. (1988) found colorectal polyps in 6 out of 12 (50%) patients with TSC. Gould et al. (1990) documented their presence in an even higher percentage of patients (78%). In all, apart from one patient reported by Devroede et al. (1988) in whom the polyps produced pain on defecation, the polyps were asymptomatic. Usually, they were small, 2–4 mm in diameter, sessile and occasionally filiform in appearance. Histological examination did not identify any adenomatous tissue, malignant or premalignant changes. The histology was described as representing microhamartomatous polyp formation.

As the colorectal polyps do not produce any clinical manifestations, special treatment is not necessary.

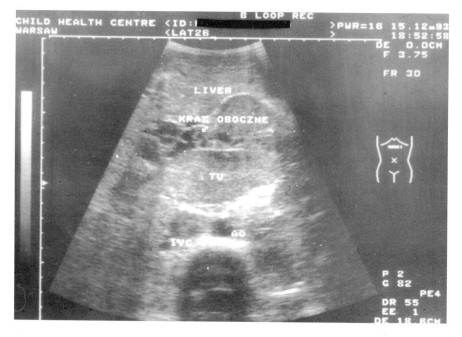

Fig. 13.4. Pancreatic tumour in a woman with TSC. The tumour infiltrates the pancreas and inferior vena cava with secondary formation of collateral circulation. Tu, tumour; Ao, aorta; IVC, inferior vena cava; Kraz oboczne, collateral circulation. (Reproduced with permission of Dr Marek Pędich, Children's Memorial Health Institute, Warsaw.)

LYMPH NODE INVOLVEMENT

Lymph nodes may demonstrate proliferation of vascular and smooth muscle cells, similar to that seen in the lungs. In most cases lymph node involvement is associated with involvement of lungs and kidneys (Monteforte and Kohnen 1974).

REFERENCES

Asayama Y, Fukuya T, Honda H, et al. (1998) Chronic expanding hematoma of the spleen caused by angiomyolipoma in a patient with tuberous sclerosis. *Abdom Imaging* 23: 527–30.

Bender BL, Yunis EJ (1981) Splenic involvement in tuberous sclerosis. Report of three cases. *Virchows Arch [Pathol Anat]* 391: 363–9.

Bender BL, Yunis EJ (1982) The pathology of tuberous sclerosis. *Pathol Ann* 17: 339–82.

Boehler A, Speich R, Russi E, Weder W (1996) Lung transplantation for lymphangioleiomyomatosis. *N Engl J Med* 335:1275–80.

Bonetti F, Chiodera P (1996) Lymphangioleiomyomatosis and tuberous sclerosis: where is the border? *Eur Respir J* 9: 399–401.

Bonetti F, Pea M, Martignoni G (1997) The perivascular epithelioid cell and related lesions. *Adv Anat Pathol* 4: 343–58.

Cares RM (1958) Tuberous sclerosis complex. *J Neuropathol Exp Neurol* 17: 247–54.

Carsillo T, Astrinidis A, Henske EP (2000) Mutations in the tuberous sclerosis complex gene TSC2 are a cause of sporadic pulmonary lymphangioleiomyomatosis. *PNAS* 97: 6085–90.

Castro M, Shepherd CW, Gomez MR, Lie JT, Ryu JH (1995) Pulmonary tuberous sclerosis. *Chest* 107: 189–95.

Chan J, Tsang W, Pau M, Tang M, Pang S, Fletcher C (1993) Lymphangiomyomatosis and angiomyolipoma: closely related entities characterized by hamartomatous proliferation of HMB-45-positive smooth muscle. *Histopathology* 22: 445–55.

Chu SC, Horiba K, Usuki J, et al. (1999) Comprehensive evaluation of 35 patients with lymphangioleiomyomatosis. *Chest* 115: 1041–52.

Colonna P, Dimitrov I, Tordjmann G, et al. (1966) Sarcome de la rate au cours d'une sclérose tubéreuse de Bourneville. *Presse Méd* 74: 447–8.

Compton WR, Lester PD, Kyaw MM, Madsen JA (1976) The abdominal angiographic spectrum of tuberous sclerosis. *Am J Radiol* 126: 807–13.

Cornog JL Jr, Enterline HT (1966) Lymphangiomyoma, a benign lesion of chyliferous lymphatics synonymous with lymphangiopericytoma. *Cancer* 19: 1909–30.

Costello LC, Hartman TE, Ryu JH (2000) High frequency of pulmonary lymphangioleiomyomatosis in women with tuberous sclerosis complex. *Mayo Clin Proc* 75: 591–4.

Darden JW, Teeslink R, Parrish RA (1975) Hamartoma of the spleen: a manifestation of tuberous sclerosis. *Am Surg* 41: 564–6.

Davidson SI (1960) A case of tuberous sclerosis with hypoglycemia attacks. *Dapim Refuiim* 19: 70–3.

Davoren PM (1992) Insulinoma complicating tuberous sclerosis. *J Neurol Neurosurg Psychiatry* 55: 1209.

Dawson J (1954) Pulmonary tuberous sclerosis and its relation to other forms of the disease. *Q J Med* 22: 113–45.

Devroede G, Lemieux B, Massé S, et al. (1988) Colonic hamartomas in tuberous sclerosis. *Gastroenterology* 94: 182–8.

Drut R (1990) Multivisceral dysplastic lesions in a patient with tuberous sclerosis and Langerhans cell histiocytosis. *Pediatr Pathol* 10: 633–9.

Dwyer JM, Hickie JB, Garvan J (1971) Pulmonary tuberous sclerosis: report of three patients and a review of the literature. *Q J Med* 40: 115–25.

Fleury P, Smits N, van Baal S (1987) The incidence of hepatic hamartomas in tuberous sclerosis. Evaluation by ultrasonography. *RöFo* 146: 694–6.

Gomez MR (1999) Liver, digestive tract, spleen, arteries, thymus and lymphatics. In: Gomez MR, Sampson JR, Whittemore VH (eds) *Tuberous Sclerosis Complex*. New York: Oxford University Press, pp 228–39.

Gould SR, Steward JB, Temple LN (1990) Rectal polyposis in tuberous sclerosis. *J Ment Def Research* 34: 465–73.

Grasso S, Manusia M, Sciacca F (1982) Unusual liver lesion in tuberous sclerosis. *Arch Pathol Lab Med* 106: 49.

Gutman A, Leffkowitz M (1959) Tuberous sclerosis associated with spontaneous hypoglycemia. *Br Med J* ii: 1065–8.

Hancock E, Osborne J (2002) Lymphangioleiomyomatosis: a review of the literature. *Respir Med* 96: 1–6.

Hayes TC, Bitton HA, Mewborne EB, et al. (1998) Symptomatic splenic hamartoma: case report and literature review. *Pediatrics* 101: E10.

Hsu TH, O'Hara J, Mehta A, et al. (2002) Nephron-sparing nephrectomy for giant renal angiomyolipoma associated with lymphangioleiomyomatosis. *Urology* 59: 138.

Huber C, Treutner KH, Steinau G, Schumpelick V (1996) Ruptured hepatic angiolipoma in tuberous sclerosis complex. *Langenbecks Arch Chir* 381: 7–9.

Ilgren EB, Westmoreland D (1984) Tuberous sclerosis: unusual association in four cases. *J Clin Path* 37: 272–8.

Jao J, Gilbert S, Messer R (1972) Lymphangiomyoma and tuberous sclerosis. *Cancer* 29: 1188–92.

Johnson SR, Tattersfield AE (1999) Decline in lung function in lymphangioleiomyomatosis: relation to menopause and progesterone treatment. *Am J Respir Crit Care Med* 160: 628–33.

Jóźwiak S, Michałowicz R (1991) Zmiany w nerkach i wątrobie chorych na stwardnienie guzowate – aspekty diagnostyczne i kliniczne. *Pol Tyg Lek* 46: 787–9.

Jóźwiak S, Pędich M, Rajszys P, Michałowicz R (1992) Incidence of hepatic hamartomas in tuberous sclerosis. *Arch Dis Childh* 67: 1363–5.

Kawamura R (1913) Ein Fall mit mehreren Gewebsmissbildungen. Darűnter einen Pankreasmitbildung. *Zbl Allg Pathol Anat* 24: 801–8.

Kristal H, Sperber F (1989) Hepatic angiomyolipoma in a tuberous sclerosis patient. *Isr J Med Sci* 25: 412–14.

Lack EE, Cassady JR, Levey R, Vawter GF (1983) Tumours of the exocrine pancreas in children and adolescents. A clinical and pathological study of eight cases. *Am J Surg Pathol* 7: 319–27.

Lie JT (1991) Cardiac, pulmonary, and vascular involvement in tuberous sclerosis. *Ann NY Acad Sci* 615: 58–70.

Lutembacher R (1918) Dysembryomes metatypiques des reins: carcinose submiliaire aigue du poumon avec emphyseme generalisé et double pneumothorax. *Ann Med* 5: 435–50.

Marsidi PJ, Wise HA (1983) Tuberous sclerosis and angiomyolipomatous kidney conditions. *Ohio State Med J* 79: 449–53.

Maruyama H, Ohbayashi C, Hino O, Tsutsumi M, Konishi Y (2001) Pathogenesis of multifocal micronodular pneumocyte hyperplasia and lymphangioleiomyomatosis in tuberous sclerosis and association with tuberous sclerosis genes TSC1 and TSC2. *Pathol Int* 51: 585–94.

Maziak DE, Kesten S, Rappaport DC, Maurer J (1996) Extrathoracic angiomyolipomas in lymphangioleiomyomatosis. *Eur Respir J* 9: 402–5.

Monteforte WJ, Kohnen PW (1974) Angiomyolipoma in a case of lymphangiomyomatosis syndrome: relationships to tuberous sclerosis. *Cancer* 34: 317–21.

Morales JB (1961) Congenital rhabdomyoma, tuberous sclerosis and splenic histiocytosis. *Arch Pathol* 71: 485–93.

Muller NL, Chiles C, Kullnig P (1990) Pulmonary lymphangioleiomyomatosis: correlation of CT with radiographic and functional findings. *Radiology* 175: 335–9.

Newmark H, Bhagwanani DG, Rishi US, et al. (1982) Tuberous sclerosis evaluated by computerized tomography. *Computed Radiol* 6: 287–93.

Nonomura A, Mizukami Y, Kadoya M (1994) Angiomyolipoma of the liver: a collective review. *J Gastroenterol* 29: 95–105.

Östör AG, Fortune DW (1978) Tuberous sclerosis initially seen as hydrops fetalis: report of a case and review of the literature. *Arch Pathol Lab Med* 102: 34–9.

Perou ML, Gray PT (1960) Mesenchymal hamartomas of the kidney. *J Urol* 83: 240–61.

Roach ES, Gomez MR, Northrup H (1998) Tuberous Sclerosis Consensus Conference: revised clinical diagnostic criteria. *J Child Neurol* 13: 624–8.

Roach ES, DiMario FJ, Kandt RS, Northrup H, National Tuberous Sclerosis Association (1999) Tuberous Sclerosis Consensus Conference: recommendations for diagnostic evaluation. *J Child Neurol* 14: 401–7.

Sheffield EG, Sparagana SP, Batchelor LL, et al. (1998) The incidence and natural history of hepatic angiomyolipomas in tuberous sclerosis complex in the pediatric population. Abstracts of World Congress on Tuberous Sclerosis, Göteborg, p. S12.

Shepherd CW, Gomez MR, Lie JT, Crowson CS (1991) Causes of death in patients with tuberous sclerosis. *Mayo Clin Proc* 66: 792–6.

Smolarek TA, Wessner LL, McCormack FX, Mylet JC, Menon AG, Henske EP (1998) Evidence that lymphangiomyomatosis is caused by TSC2 mutations: chromosome 16p13 loss of heterozygosity in angiomyolipomas and lymphnodes from women with lymphangiomyomatosis. *Am J Hum Genet* 62: 810–15.

Sullivan EJ (1998) Lymphangioleiomyomatosis: a review. *Chest* 114: 1689–1703.

Tang LH, Hui P, Garcia-Tsao G, et al. (2002) Multiple angiomyolipomata of the liver: a case report. *Mod Pathol* 15: 167–71.

Taylor JR, Ryu J, Colby TV, Raffin TA (1990) Lymphangioleiomyomatosis: clinical course in 32 patients. *N Engl J Med* 323: 1254–60.

Tsakraklides V, Burke B, Mastri A, et al. (1974) Rhabdomyomas of heart: a report of four cases. *Am J Dis Child* 128: 639–46.

Tsui WM, Colombari R, Portmann BC, et al. (1999) Hepatic angiomyolipoma: a clinico-pathologic study of 30 cases and delineation of unusual morphologic variants. *Am J Surg Pathol* 23: 34–48.

Urban T, Kutten F, Gompel A, et al. (1992) Pulmonary lymphangiomyomatosis: follow-up and long-term outcome with antiestrogen therapy: a report of eight cases. *Chest* 102: 472–6.

Urban T, Lazor R, Lacronique J, et al., Groupe d'Etudes et de Recherche sur les Maladies "Orphelines" Pulmonaires (GERM "O" P) (1999) Pulmonary lymphangioleiomyomatosis: a study of 69 patients. *Medicine (Baltimore)* 78: 321–37.

van Heerden JA, Longo MF (1967) The abdominal mass in a patient with tuberous sclerosis: surgical implications and report of a case. *Arch Surg* 93: 576–86.

Verhoef S, van Diemen-Steenvoorde R, Akkersdijk WL, et al. (1999) Malignant pancreatic tumour within the spectrum of tuberous sclerosis complex in childhood. *Eur J Pediatr* 158: 284–7.

Viamonte M, Ravel R, Politano V, Bridges B (1966) Angiographic findings in a patient with tuberous sclerosis. *Am J Radiol* 98: 723–33.

Von Stössel E (1937) Über muskuläre Cirrhose der Lunge. *Beitr Klein Tuberk* 90: 432–42.

14
MOLECULAR GENETICS

David J Kwiatkowski, Mary Pat Reeve, Jeremy P Cheadle and
Julian R Sampson

INTRODUCTION

Over the past decade there has been considerable progress in understanding the molecular genetics of tuberous sclerosis complex (TSC). In this chapter, we review this progress, from cloning and characterizing *TSC1* and *TSC2*, the genes responsible for TSC, through to gaining insights into the functions of their protein products, hamartin and tuberin, and the identification and engineering of animal models. We also present a comprehensive compilation and analysis of all reported *TSC1* and *TSC2* mutations (http://expmed.bwh.harvard.edu/ts/), consider their diagnostic implications and review genotype/phenotype relationships (Cheadle et al. 2000).

IDENTIFICATION AND CHARACTERIZATION OF THE TSC GENES
CLINICAL GENETICS OF TSC

TSC is an autosomal dominant genetic disorder in which sporadic cases account for about two-thirds of all patients, and reflect the occurrence of new mutations. Within families there is a wide variation in the extent and degree of clinical manifestations, indicating that there is no rigid correlation between specific TSC gene mutation and clinical outcome. However, there are no well-documented cases of non-penetrance of this disease when patients are evaluated in a comprehensive manner (complete physical examination including skin and retina, imaging studies of brain and kidneys). The birth incidence of TSC is generally considered to be about 1 in 10,000, although one study gave an indirect estimate as high as 1 in 6000 (Sampson et al. 1989a, Osborne et al. 1991). TSC affects all ethnic groups without apparent clustering, which we infer is due to a fairly uniform rate of new mutations in the TSC genes across all human populations.

LINKAGE STUDIES AND HETEROGENEITY

Linkage of TSC to 9q34 was reported in 1987 (Fryer et al. 1987), and this locus has been denoted *TSC1*. Subsequent studies provided strong evidence for locus heterogeneity (Northrup et al. 1987, Sampson et al. 1989b, Janssen et al. 1990, Northrup et al. 1992, Sampson et al. 1992) and led to the identification of a second locus at 16p13.3, denoted *TSC2* (Kandt et al. 1992). Among families large enough to permit linkage analysis, approximately half show linkage to 9q34 and half to 16p13, and there is no linkage evidence for a third locus (Janssen et al. 1994, Povey et al. 1994).

MAPPING AND IDENTIFICATION OF *TSC1*

Initial definition of the 1.5 Mb *TSC1* candidate region on chromosome 9q34 was achieved by identification of key meiotic recombination events in large *TSC1* families (Haines et al. 1991, Nellist et al. 1993). Many microsatellite markers from this region were then identified and a cosmid, PAC and BAC contig assembled (Kwiatkowski et al. 1993, Povey et al. 1994, van Slegtenhorst et al. 1995, Au et al. 1996, Hornigold et al. 1997). Two putative recombinants in unaffected individuals provisionally narrowed the candidate region to 900 kb between the markers D9S2127 and DBH. Large deletions or other rearrangements of the region were sought in patients with TSC, but no abnormalities were detected.

The *TSC1* region proved to be gene rich with over 30 genes identified in or mapped to the critical region by a variety of techniques. Many of these were assessed as positional candidates for *TSC1* without identification of mutations (van Slegtenhorst et al. 1997). In collaboration with investigators at the Whitehead Institute Genome Center, complete genomic sequencing of the region was initiated and GRAIL2 and BLAST were employed to predict further putative exons and genes. Systematic amplification and mutation screening of exons, using heteroduplex analysis on a panel of 20 unrelated familial TSC cases linked to 9q34 and 40 sporadic TSC cases, revealed mobility shifts corresponding to small truncating mutations in the 62nd exon screened (van Slegtenhorst et al. 1997). This exon corresponded to previously identified cDNA clones and a combination of 5'RACE, RT-PCR (using primers from predicted exons) and isolation of other cDNA clones defined the remainder of the open reading frame encoding a novel predicted protein product. Comparison of cDNA and genomic sequences revealed 23 exons, the first two of which were untranslated. The 8.6 kb full-length transcript had a 4.5 kb 3'UTR and was predicted to encode a 1164 aminoacid/130 kDa protein that was called hamartin (van Slegtenhorst et al. 1997) (Table 14.1).

SEQUENCE ANALYSIS OF *TSC1*

Hamartin is generally hydrophilic and has a single potential transmembrane domain at aminoacids 127–144 and a predicted 266 aminoacid coiled-coil region beginning at residue 730. Database searches revealed a possible yeast *Schizosaccharomyces pombe* homolog of *TSC1* encoding a hypothetical 103 kDa protein, but there were no strong matches with vertebrate proteins (van Slegtenhorst et al. 1997).

INTERSPECIES COMPARISONS OF *TSC1*

Orthologues of the *TSC1* gene have been characterized in the rat (Satake et al. 1999) and *Drosophila* (Ito and Rubin 1999). The deduced aminoacid sequence of the rat

TABLE 14.1
Similarities and differences between *TSC1* and *TSC2*. Y2H, yeast two-hybrid system.

	TSC1	*TSC2*
Localization	9q34	16p13.3
Positional cloning	No large rearrangements	Aided by cytogenetic
	Large-scale genomic sequencing	rearrangements and large genomic deletions
Structure	23 exons – 8.6 kb transcript	41 exons – 5.5 kb transcript
	Alternate splicing in the 5′UTR	Exons 25, 26 and 31 alternatively spliced
Mutations	Small truncating mutations	Large deletions/rearrangements
		Small truncating mutations
		Missense mutations
Occurrence	10–15% of sporadic cases	70% of sporadic cases
Phenotype	Less severe in multiple respects: learning disability, brain, skin, kidney, retina	More severe in multiple respects Contiguous gene deletion syndrome with *PKD1*
LOH in hamartomas	Rare (may reflect frequency)	Frequent
Expression	Widely expressed at low levels	Widely expressed at low levels
Product	Hamartin	Tuberin
Function(s)	With tuberin, functions to regulate mTOR/S6K	With hamartin, functions to regulate mTOR/S6K
	Regulates cell adhesion through interaction with ezrin and Rho (?)	GTPase activating protein (?) Role in the cell cycle (?)
Subcellular localization	Cytoplasmic, ? cortical	Cytoplasmic, ? Golgi-associated
Proteins	Stoichiometric binding to tuberin	Stoichiometric binding to hamartin
	Binds to ERM proteins	
Animal models	Knockout mice	Eker rat
	Drosophila	Knockout mice
		Drosophila (*gigas*)

TSC1 product consists of 1163 residues and shows approximately 86% identity with human hamartin. The *Drosophila TSC1* orthologue is encoded by 1100 aminoacids and is 22% identical (46% similar) to human hamartin. The predicted transmembrane and coiled-coil regions are conserved between rat, human and *Drosophila*, as is a further stretch of 133 aminoacids close to the potential transmembrane domain.

POSITIONAL CLONING OF *TSC2*

During 1992–3 linkage studies identified an approximately 1.5 Mb region of chromosome 16p as likely to contain the *TSC2* gene (Kandt et al. 1992, Kwiatkowski et al. 1993). At the same time, a family with both tuberous sclerosis and autosomal dominant polycystic kidney disease was found to segregate a translocation between chromosomes 16p and 22q. The mother and her daughter each carried a balanced translocation involving 16p13.3 (karyotypes 46,XX, t(16;22)(p13.3;q11.21)). They had signs of typical autosomal dominant polycystic kidney disease but no evidence of tuberous sclerosis. The son had severe learning disability, suffered with seizures, and exhibited repetitive autistic behaviours. He had inherited an unbalanced karyotype, 45, XY, -16,-22,+der(16)(16qter→16p13.3::22q11.21→22qter), and was therefore deleted for the chromosomal regions 16p13.3→16pter and 22q11.21 →22pter. Skin examination revealed facial angiofibromas and hypopigmented macules, and computed tomography of the brain revealed typical subependymal calcification, confirming the diagnosis of tuberous sclerosis. The translocation breakpoint on chromosome 16 in this family was shown to disrupt the previously unidentified *PKD1* gene (European Polycystic Kidney Disease Consortium 1994). It was reasoned that the son manifested tuberous sclerosis because of deletion of one copy of the *TSC2* gene, the implied location of which was telomeric to the translocation breakpoint on 16p13.3. The breakpoint was mapped by a combination of fluorescence in situ hybridization and pulsed field and conventional gel electrophoresis. It was defined as lying some 150 kb telomeric to 16AC2.5, the most centromeric flanking marker then identified for *TSC2*. The telomeric limit of the candidate region was greatly reduced by the position of a second breakpoint in a previously reported patient who had a *de novo* truncation of 16p (Wilkie et al. 1990), but no clinical or radiological evidence of tuberous sclerosis. The deletion in this patient effectively excluded approximately 1.1 Mb of the remaining 1.4 Mb *TSC2* candidate region.

A cosmid contig was constructed for the remaining 300 kb candidate region, and probes generated from it were used to analyse a panel of 255 unrelated TSC patients for rearrangements by pulsed field gel electrophoresis (PFGE) and Southern blotting. Five TSC patients were found to have genomic deletions between 30 kb and 100 kb in size, which involved the same 120 kb interval. cDNA clones were isolated corresponding to four genes in the interval, and one was found to be disrupted by all five deletions, making it a strong candidate for *TSC2*. Four smaller intragenic deletions were then identified in TSC patients, including a *de novo* deletion that was associated with a shortened *TSC2* transcript. These findings confirmed the identity of the *TSC2* gene. A previously unknown protein product of approximately 198 kDa was predicted from the sequence of the 5.5 kb transcript, and named tuberin (European Chromosome 16 Tuberous Sclerosis Consortium 1993) (Table 14.1).

Genomic Arrangement at the *TSC2* Locus

TSC2 has a complex genomic structure, comprising 41 coding exons and a noncoding leader exon (exon 1a, Kobayashi et al. 1997a) which are distributed over 44 kb of the genome. The sequence predicts a protein product of 1807 aminoacids (Maheshwar et al. 1996, Genbank accession numbers L48517–L48546). Immediately centromeric to *TSC2* is the *PKD1* gene which is mutated in autosomal dominant polycystic kidney disease. *TSC2* and *PKD1* are oriented 3′ to 3′ and their polyadenylation signals are separated by only 60bp (Harris et al. 1995). Immediately distal to *TSC2*, and oriented 5′ to 5′, is the *NTHL1* gene, originally designated *OCTS3* (European Chromosome 16 Tuberous Sclerosis Consortium 1993). *NTHL1* is a functional homologue of the *E. coli Nth* gene which encodes endonuclease III (Aspinwall et al. 1997), a major component of the base excision DNA repair pathway (Cunningham and Weiss 1985).

SEQUENCE ANALYSIS OF *TSC2*
Tuberin shows a region of homology with rap1GAP or GAP3, which extends over approximately 160 aminoacid residues encoded by exons 34 through 38 (Maheshwar et al. 1997). Over a stretch of 58 residues, the criteria for structural homology defined by Sander and Schneider (1991) are fulfilled. rap1GAP is a GTPase activating protein (GAP) which stimulates the hydrolysis of active GTP-bound rap1a and rap1b to their inactive GDP-bound forms (Rubinfeld et al. 1991). rap1a and b are members of the ras superfamily of small GTP-binding proteins whose functions include transduction of mitogenic signals from plasma membrane receptors to the nucleus (Yoshida et al. 1992, Lowy and Willumsen 1993, Ohtsuka et al. 1996, York et al. 1998). By catalysing the conversion of GTP-binding proteins to their inactive state, GAPs can function as negative regulators of cellular processes including proliferation.

INTER-SPECIES COMPARISONS OF *TSC2*
TSC2 orthologues have been characterized in the mouse (Kim et al. 1995, Olsson et al. 1996), the rat (Kobayashi et al. 1995a), the Japanese pufferfish, *Fugu rubripes* (Maheshwar et al. 1996), and *Drosophila* (Ito and Rubin 1999). The murine *TSC2* gene maps to mouse chromosome 17, in a conserved synteny group with human 16p13.3 (Olsson et al. 1995). The nucleotide identity of the human and mouse *TSC2* genes is approximately 85%, and deduced aminoacid identity of the products approximately 91%. The 58 aminoacid core of the rap1GAP homologous domain of tuberin shows only one conservative aminoacid change (Kim et al. 1995, Olsson et al. 1996). The rat *TSC2* gene shows a similar level of conservation (Kobayashi et al. 1995a). Its genomic structure has been determined, and all intron–exon boundaries are positioned as in the human gene. A comparative analysis of the *TSC2* gene in man and the Japanese pufferfish, species which have diverged over some 400 million years of evolution, has led to the identification of specific regions of sequence conservation (Maheshwar et al. 1996). Overall aminoacid identity with humans was 60% (similarity 79%), but four regions of the gene were more highly conserved. These included a region spanning the GAP-related domain, a hydrophobic N-terminal region, and two internal regions which did not show homology to other known proteins. These regions are likely to represent important functional domains.

Ito and Rubin (1999) recently showed that the *gigas* mutant in *Drosophila* results from mutation of the orthologue of the *TSC2* gene. The human and *Drosophila* predicted proteins are 26% identical (46% similar), with the highest level of homology (53% identity) spanning the GAP-related domain. Recent reports indicate the presence of conserved arginine fingers in GAP proteins which are important for their catalytic activity (Scheffzek et al. 1998). Although *TSC2/gigas* proteins have predicted arginine fingers, these do not resemble those of other known GAP subfamilies (Ito and Rubin 1999).

ALTERNATIVE SPLICING OF *TSC2*

Alternative splicing involving exon 25, the first 3bp of exon 26 and exon 31 has been documented in man (Xu et al. 1995, Maheshwar et al. 1996), mouse (Olsson et al. 1995, Xu et al. 1995), rat (Kobayashi et al. 1995a) and *Fugu* (Maheshwar et al. 1996). Other possible splice variants have been suggested by analysis of murine mRNA (Kim et al. 1995). Variation in expression of the different transcripts has been observed in different tissues and at different developmental stages. However, no clear pattern of developmentally regulated expression has been defined. Observation of the same alternative spliceforms in all organisms so far studied, particularly *Fugu*, points to the likelihood of functional significance. Many cell lines, including human lymphoblastoid and fibroblast lines, appear to exclusively express the isoform-lacking exon 25. Within this exon the residue Ser(946) is potentially a site for casein kinase phosphorylation, and Ser(970) and Ser(981) are potential protein kinase C phosphorylation sites. If these sites are variably phosphorylated, expression of the isoform-lacking exon 25 could be a mechanism for regulation of intermolecular signalling (Xu et al. 1995).

MUTATION ANALYSIS OF *TSC1* AND *TSC2*

In all, 591 cases with published TSC mutations (169 in *TSC1* and 422 in *TSC2*; Table 14.2) are reviewed here (European Chromosome 16 Tuberous Sclerosis Consortium 1993, Brook-Carter et al. 1994, Kumar et al. 1995a, 1995b, Verhoef et al. 1995, Vrtel et al. 1996, Wilson et al. 1996, Au et al. 1997, Jobert et al. 1997, Jones et al. 1997, Kumar et al. 1997, Maheshwar et al. 1997, Platten et al. 1997, Sampson et al. 1997, van Bakel et al. 1997a, 1997b, van Slegtenhorst et al. 1997, Yates et al. 1997, Ali et al. 1998, Au et al. 1998, Beauchamp et al. 1998, Dabora et al. 1998, Gilbert et al. 1998, Kwiatkowska et al. 1998, Wang et al. 1998, Young et al. 1998, Benit et al. 1999, Choy et al. 1999, Jones et al. 1999a, Mayer et al. 1999, Niida et al. 1999, Rose et al. 1999, Smith and Sperling 1999, van Slegtenhorst et al. 1999, Verhoef et al. 1999, Zhang et al. 1999a, Dabora et al. 2001).

In this chapter, we use the term 'mutation' to mean 'pathological change'. There is a total of 424 different reported mutations, 112 of *TSC1* and 312 of *TSC2*. Fifty-four mutations have been reported recurrently (21 of *TSC1* and 33 of *TSC2*),

TABLE 14.2
Summary of cases with published TSC mutations

Mutation	TSC1		TSC2	
Large deletions/ rearrangements	0	0%	69	16%
Insertions	29	17%	34	8%
Deletions	58	34%	97	23%
Nonsense	67	40%	86	20%
Point splicing	13	8%	52	12%
Missense	2	1%	84	20%
Total:	169		422	

accounting for 176 cases. Here we use a uniform +1 ATG for the numbering of the bases of both *TSC1* and *TSC2*, and include all alternatively spliced exons. We have used standard mutation nomenclature (Antonarakis et al. 1998). The GenBank reference sequences are AF013168 for *TSC1* and X75621 for *TSC2*. Complete listings of all *TSC1* and *TSC2* variations described here can be found on the TSC Variation Database site at http://expmed.bwh.harvard.edu/ts/

We classify missense mutations as pathogenic if they meet the following conditions: (1) they are present in a sporadic TSC patient or a founding family member; (2) they are not present in the unaffected parents of that patient; and (3) the TSC patient DNA sample had been completely screened for other changes in all exons of *TSC1* and *TSC2*. These criteria cannot, of course, be met in all circumstances. We therefore classified probable missense mutations ('mutation-p' in the online tables) as those for which these criteria were not met, but the sequence variation results in a significant alteration in the encoded aminoacid (a negative score in the aminoacid substitution matrix of Henikoff and Henikoff 1992). Other missense changes were not recorded here. Similar categories were applied to in-frame deletion mutations and splice mutations outside of the two invariant donor and acceptor bases. Changes listed in the TSC Variation Database as polymorphisms have been seen in one or more unaffected controls or in a patient with another clearly pathogenic mutation.

SINGLE-BASE SUBSTITUTIONS
In *TSC1*, 82 (48%) of the mutations are single-base substitutions, 82% of which are nonsense mutations (Table 14.2, Fig. 14.1). Most of the nonsense mutations are recurrent C to T transitions at 6 of the 7 CGA codons (encoding arginine, the only codon a single-base transition away from a nonsense codon and also containing a CpG). Deamination at CpG sites is a common mechanism of genetic change (Cooper and Youssoufian 1988) and is presumably the cause of these hotspots. The

only CGA codon without reported mutations was located near the 3' end of the gene where no mutations of any type have been identified. The six recurrent CpG mutation sites account for 55% of the nonsense mutations reported in *TSC1*. The other major category of single-base changes in *TSC1* is mutations affecting splicing (13 out of 82, 16%), only two of which have been reported recurrently (1029+1G>A and 211−1G>A). Two missense mutations have been reported in *TSC1*, but neither satisfied our criteria for proven pathogenicity.

Fifty-three per cent (222 out of 422) of *TSC2* mutations were point mutations (Table 14.2, Fig. 14.1). In contrast to *TSC1*, nonsense mutations in *TSC2* make up only 39% (86 out of 222) of this class. *TSC2* has seven CpG sites which can transition to nonsense codons. Mutations have been identified at five of these and comprise 36% of the nonsense mutations. *TSC2* missense mutations were also common and accounted for 38% (84 out of 222). *TSC2* has two CpG sites that appear to be mutational hotspots for missense mutations − 1831–2 (611R>W and 611R>Q) and 5024–5 (1675P>L). These two CpG sites contained 35 of the 84 (42%) verified or probable missense mutations. Other than the CpG sites, missense mutations were clustered in the region with rap1GAP homology (exons 34–38). Splice mutations make up the remaining 23% of point mutations in *TSC2*.

INSERTIONS AND DELETIONS

The *TSC1* mutation spectrum includes many insertions of less than 28bp (29 out of 169 mutations, 17%) and small deletions of less than 23bp (58 out of 169, 34%). Nearly all small insertions/deletions (indels) cause frameshifts in *TSC1*. Most small insertions (28 out of 29) arose from the duplication of an adjacent base or region. All recurrent insertions in *TSC1* are due to monomer adenosine runs, ranging in length from 2 to 7bp. Thirty-six of the 58 deletions (62%) removed an element of a tandem repeat (17 monomer, 11 dinucleotide, 7 tetranucleotide, and one other duplicated element). Both a deletion and an insertion were seen to affect the 23bp region between bases 1671 and 1693, which is flanked by 9bp repeats.

The indel mutation spectrum of *TSC2* comprised small insertions of up to 29bp (8%), small deletions of up to 34bp (23%), and large deletions and rearrangements (16%). Eighty-five per cent of the small insertion sequences were duplication events (29 out of 34). Of the small deletions, 54% were due to obvious repeated elements. Seven small deletions were seen recurrently and accounted for 30% of the deletions. One recurrent deletion, 5051–5068+16del34, removed one unit of a 34bp minisatellite-type element which is repeated for 2.3 units starting 18bp inside the splice acceptor site of exon 38 and continuing into the intron. One complex truncating change was also observed in *TSC2* consisting of both a deletion and an insertion. Unlike *TSC1*, a significant proportion of large deletions and rearrangements has been reported affecting *TSC2*. These include deletions ranging in size from ~1 kb to over 100 kb, as well as more complex rearrangements including

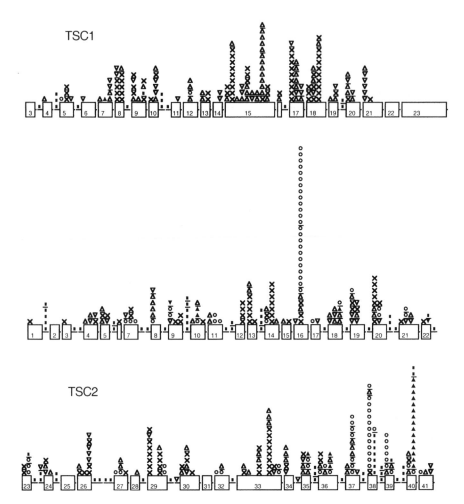

Fig. 14.1. Map of the sites of all published small mutations in *TSC1* and *TSC2*. Proportional drawings (boxes) of all of the exons of *TSC1* and *TSC2* are shown. Intron regions are not drawn to scale and are expanded only when a mutation is present. Mutation symbols are: × nonsense; □ splice site; Δ deletion; ▽ insertion; ○ missense; closed Δ in-frame deletion. A line separates mutations occurring at nearby but not identical nucleotide positions.

the translocation that led to the identification of *TSC2*. The deletion junctions have been sequenced in six cases, revealing a diversity of recombination mechanisms and joining sites (Dabora et al. 2000).

DETECTION METHODS

Comprehensive mutation analysis of the TSC genes has focused on coding exons 3–23 of *TSC1* and 1–41 of *TSC2*. The most common methods used have been SSCP and heteroduplex analysis (Wilson et al. 1996, Au et al. 1997, Jones et al. 1997, Ali et al. 1998, Au et al. 1998, Beauchamp et al. 1998, Gilbert et al. 1998, Kwiatkowska et al. 1998, Young et al. 1998, Jones et al. 1999a, Niida et al. 1999, van Slegtenhorst et al. 1999, Zhang et al. 1999a). The protein truncation test (PTT) (van Bakel et al. 1997a, Gilbert et al. 1998, Benit et al. 1999, Mayer et al. 1999), denaturing gradient gel electrophoresis (DGGE) (Dabora et al. 1998), and denaturing high performance liquid chromatography (DHPLC) (Choy et al. 1999, Jones et al. 1999b, 2000, Dabora et al. 2001) have also been used. Southern blot analysis of either normal or pulsed-field agarose gels has been the primary technique to assay for large deletions (European Chromosome 16 Tuberous Sclerosis Consortium 1993, Brook-Carter et al. 1994, Au et al. 1997, Jones et al. 1997, Sampson et al. 1997, Kwiatkowska et al. 1998, Young et al. 1998, Jones et al. 1999a, van Slegtenhorst et al. 1999). Recently, long-range PCR and quantitative PCR have also been used for the identification of large deletions (Jones et al. 1999a, Dabora et al. 2000, 2001).

Since small indels are the easiest types of mutation to identify using any strategy involving exon amplification and analysis, the true proportion of single-base substitution mutations and large deletions is likely to be underestimated for both *TSC1* and *TSC2*. Similarly, mutations that affect the internal regions of introns, 5′ and 3′ untranslated regions, and enhancer and promoter elements for each gene have not yet been looked for in detail by any laboratory. The expected frequency of both internal intronic and promoter/enhancer mutations in *TSC1* and *TSC2* is low (Jones et al. 1999a) and, to date, only four internal intronic mutations in *TSC2* (15, 15, 18, and 281bp from the exon border) have been reported following PTT screening (Mayer et al. 1999). Three of these changes were not present in the parental samples.

POLYMORPHISMS

In *TSC1,* 33 different polymorphisms have been identified. Ten (30%) occur in intronic sequence, 13 (39%) are silent, and 10 (30%) cause missense changes, four of which are nonconservative according to the BLOSUM62 matrix (Henikoff and Henikoff 1992). Four of the *TSC1* polymorphisms are relatively common, with rare allele frequency of 10% or greater. In *TSC2,* 81 different polymorphisms have been identified, consisting of one 3bp exonic deletion, two deletions in intronic sequences, 26 (32%) single-base changes in intronic regions, 19 (23%) missense changes of which six were nonconservative, and 33 (40%) silent changes in coding sequence. Five of these have rare allele frequency of more than 10%.

PERSPECTIVES ON MUTATION VARIATION AT THE TSC LOCI

Truncating mutations (nonsense, splicing, frameshift) make up 99% of the reported mutations in *TSC1* and 80% of those in *TSC2*. A similar high rate of truncating mutations is also observed in other tumour suppressor genes such as *RB1* (91% truncating, Lohmann 1999), *PTEN/MMAC1* (75% truncating, Ali et al. 1999), and *CDH1* (86% truncating in infiltrating lobular breast cancers, Berx et al. 1998). These genes also show heterogeneous mutation spectra, LOH in tumour cells and few exons escaping mutations. *RB1*, like *TSC1*, has a lack of CGA→TGA codon transitions at the 3′ end and concentration of nonsense mutations at CGA sites (Lohmann 1999).

No verified pathogenic missense mutations have been reported in *TSC1*, but there is no reason to think that this entire class of mutation would not occur. This prompts the question of how missense mutations might affect the function of hamartin and what might be the resultant clinical phenotype. Clearly some missense changes will have no effect on hamartin structure and function, including the 10 observed polymorphisms. However, we speculate that some *TSC1* missense mutations have dominant negative effects on the remaining normal hamartin allele, leading to an embryonic lethal or other severe phenotype, explaining why such mutations have not been identified in the TSC population.

CpG→TpG nonsense mutations are much more common in *TSC1* and *TSC2* than other types of nonsense mutation. They are 29 times more frequent in *TSC1* (32 observed occurrences in 59 CpGs that could create stops, compared to 8 occurrences in 375 non-CpG sites that could create stops) and 24 times more frequent in *TSC2*. This translates to nucleotide-specific mutation rates at the C of CpGs of 9.7- and 8-fold over the basal mutation rate, which is somewhat higher than the average increase in mutations at CpG sites of 5-fold over the basal mutation rate in a large series of human genetic disorders (Krawczak et al. 1998). Also similar to other series, deletion mutations in *TSC1* and *TSC2* occur about twice as often as insertion mutations. Nearly all deletion mutations were seen at short runs of simple sequence repeats (1–4 nucleotides), presumably occurring through slipped strand mispairing (Cooper and Krawczak 1991). Eighteen indel mutations have been seen recurrently in *TSC1* and *TSC2*, indicating the presence of hotspots for these mutations, the sequence basis for which is not evident.

The heterogeneous mutation spectra of *TSC1* and *TSC2* present a clear challenge in the design of a simple mutation identification strategy. The authors' research groups have independently explored the utility of DHPLC for mutational analysis in *TSC1* and *TSC2* (Choy et al. 1999, Jones et al. 2000, Dabora et al. 2001). The method was found to be more sensitive than both SSCP and heteroduplex analysis for detection of mutations in these genes. The limitations of the assay are the initial set-up cost and the necessity of maintaining the HPLC system, but it is otherwise robust and cost-effective for mutation screening. DHPLC scanning of all coding exons of *TSC1* and *TSC2* detects mutations in about 70% of cases with tuberous sclerosis (Jones et al. 2000, Dabora et al. 2001). Given that large deletions and rearrangements at the *TSC2* locus are present in a significant proportion of cases, and that such lesions will be missed using any exon-scanning technique, a combination of assays is necessary for truly comprehensive mutation testing in tuberous sclerosis.

In experienced centres the overall mutation detection rate in *TSC1* or *TSC2* for TSC patients remains in the range of 85–90% at best, even after the application of two or more mutation detection methods. Consequently, there remain 10–15% of TSC patients for whom no mutation can be identified. There are several possible explanations for this. First, all methods, including DHPLC and direct sequencing, have incomplete sensitivity. Second, intronic and promoter region mutations may contribute to the mutational load in both genes, and have not been extensively sought. Third, low-level mosaicism for a mutation in a TSC gene may cause a full TSC phenotype (Kwiatkowska et al. 1999) and may be very difficult to detect. Fourth, it is possible that there are additional genes, mutation of which causes a TSC syndrome. However, all reported large TSC families show linkage to either *TSC1* or *TSC2*, arguing against this last possibility.

TSC1 mutations have been identified in about 10–15% of sporadic TSC patients in several series, while *TSC2* mutations account for about 70%, with the causative gene as yet unidentified in the remainder (Kwiatkowska et al. 1998, Jones et al. 1999a, Niida et al. 1999). Several differences between the genes and their mutations may explain the apparent differences in mutation rate. First, missense mutations do not (or perhaps rarely) occur in *TSC1*, at least with a TSC phenotype. Second, a much higher rate of large rearrangements and deletions is seen in *TSC2*, probably reflecting differences in chromosomal location, genomic structural features, or the specific sequences present at the two loci. It is notable that the *TSC2* genomic region on 16p13.3 is characterized by many partial duplications likely to promote deletion and rearrangement. Third, the *TSC2* coding region is about 1.5 times longer than *TSC1*, and has approximately twice the number of splice sites, affording proportionally increased opportunity for all manner of small mutations.

GENOTYPE/PHENOTYPE CORRELATIONS
INCIDENCE OF SPORADIC VERSUS FAMILIAL *TSC1* AND *TSC2* MUTATIONS

Although *TSC2* mutations are about five times more common than *TSC1* mutations in sporadic TSC patients, the two genes appear to account for an equal proportion of mutations in large TSC families suitable for linkage analysis (Povey et al. 1994, Jones et al. 1997). Smaller TSC families with only 2 or 3 affected individuals are intermediate, in that *TSC1* mutation frequency is 15–50%, and *TSC2* accounts for the majority of the remainder (Niida et al. 1999, van Slegtenhorst et al. 1999, Dabora et al. 2001). These observations suggest that, on average, patients with *TSC1* mutations may be less severely affected than those with *TSC2* mutations, so that each new sporadic *TSC1* patient has a better chance of founding a family than a new *TSC2* patient. Comprehensive clinical evaluation of a large series of TSC patients with defined TSC mutations is required to evaluate this hypothesis, with consideration given to the age-dependent nature of the many manifestations of TSC, as well as the bias introduced by different methods of patient ascertainment.

INTELLECTUAL DISABILITY IN *TSC1* AND *TSC2*

Jones et al. (1997, 1999a) assessed the frequency of intellectual disability in sporadic cases as a reliable and important aspect of disease severity. Unlike many other components of the TSC phenotype which show age-dependent penetrance, intellectual disability is almost invariably present from early childhood, if it develops at all, and rarely escapes detection. Moderate to severe intellectual disability also clearly limits reproductive capacity. Intellectual disability was significantly more frequent among sporadic cases with *TSC2* mutations than among those with *TSC1* mutations (59 out of 88 cases versus 4 out of 13 cases, p = 0.0145, Jones et al. 1999a) (Table 14.1). However, other series have not replicated this finding (Kwiatkowska et al. 1998, Young et al. 1998, Niida et al. 1999, van Slegtenhorst et al. 1999).

CLINICAL SEVERITY OF *TSC1* AND *TSC2* MUTATIONS

In a recent analysis, a comprehensive clinical data instrument was applied to a cohort of 224 unselected TSC patients. Mutations were identified concurrently in 83%, including 22 sporadic cases with *TSC1* mutations and 129 sporadic cases with *TSC2* mutations. The study found that 8 out of 16 clinical features investigated occurred at a significantly higher frequency and/or with greater severity in *TSC2* than in *TSC1* sporadic cases (Table 14.3). These included: seizures (99% vs. 86%), moderate to severe learning disability (46% vs. 14%), mean number of subependymal nodules (6.7 vs. 1.7), tuber count (12.9 vs. 4.9), kidney angiomyolipomas (60% vs. 31%), mean grade of facial angiofibromas (1.5 vs. 0.9, on a severity scale of 0–3), forehead plaque (40% vs. 10%), and retinal hamartomas (27% vs. 0%). The observation that there is a lower frequency of sporadic TSC patients with *TSC1* mutations and a smaller number of cortical tubers and subependymal nodules in *TSC1* patients is consistent with the model that both germline and somatic mutations occur less frequently in *TSC1* than in *TSC2*. In this patient set, those patients without an identified mutation had clinical features that were on average significantly milder than those of *TSC2* patients and generally similar to those of *TSC1* patients, apart from kidney disease which was similar to the *TSC2* patient set. These observations suggest that a significant proportion of these patients have mosaicism for a *TSC2* mutation, causing a generally milder phenotype. Some of these patients might possibly have mutations in a third TSC gene, accounting for a small proportion of all cases.

TABLE 14.3
Comparison of clinical features in sporadic TSC patients with *TSC1* vs. *TSC2* mutations

	TSC1 Sporadic cases	*TSC2* Sporadic cases	P value *TSC1* vs. *TSC2*
Number of patients	22	129	
Age range (average age)	2–51 yrs (13.4)	1–44 yrs (11.2)	NS
Median age	9 yrs	10 yrs	
NEUROLOGIC			
Seizures	19/22 (86%)	127/128 (99%)	0.02
Learning disability (age >6)			
Mild + moderate + severe	7/14 (50%)	66/90 (73%)	NS
Moderate + severe	2/14 (14%)	41/90 (46%)	0.04
Mean LD grade (scale 0–3)	0.67	1.4	0.007
Subependymal nodules (SEN)	15/20 (75%)	127/136 (93%)	0.02
Mean SEN number	1.7	6.7	0.0002
SEGA	2/21 (9%)	13/118 (12%)	NS
Tubers (any)	13/15 (87%)	55/60 (92%)	NS
>10 tubers	1/9 (11%)	29/42 (69%)	0.002
Mean tuber number	4.4	12.9	0.002
RENAL			
Kidney cysts (grade 1–4)	3/19 (16%)	30/122 (25%)	NS
grade 2–4	0/19 (0%)	19/122 (16%)	NS (0.08)
grade 4	0/19 (0%)	5/122 (4%)	NS
Mean grade (scale 0–4)	0.16	0.52	NS (0.14)
Kidney AMLs	6/19 (31%)	72/121 (60%)	0.03
Mean grade (scale 0–3)	0.32	0.97	0.006
SKIN			
Hypomelanotic macules	20/21 (95%)	124/128 (97%)	NS
Facial angiofibromas (age >2)	13/22 (59%)	95/121 (78%)	NS
Mean grade (scale 0–3)	0.9	1.5	0.02
Shagreen patch	7/20 (35%)	68/130 (52%)	NS
Ungual fibroma	5/20 (25%)	26/128 (20%)	NS
Forehead plaque	2/20 (10%)	51/128 (40%)	0.01
OTHER			
Liver AMLs	0/15	9/117 (8%)	NS
Retinal hamartomas	0/16	32/117 (27%)	0.01
Cardiac rhabdomyoma	8/17 (47%)	58/117 (50%)	NS
LAM (females, age >16)	0/5	3/17 (18%)	NS

Notes:
Adapted from Dabora et al. 2001. SEGA = subependymal giant cell astrocytoma, AML = angiomyolipoma, LAM = lymphangioleiomyomatosis.
Learning disability was scored on a scale from 0 (none) to 3 (severe, no speech). Subependymal nodules were determined by high-resolution CT or MRI. Cortical tubers were determined by high-resolution MRI. Kidney cystic disease was graded on a scale from 0 (none) to 4 (severe). Facial angiofibromas and kidney AMLs were graded on a scale from 0 (none) to 3 (severe).

A Contiguous Gene Deletion Syndrome Involving *TSC2* and *PKD1*

Renal cysts are common in TSC patients, but only a small minority (approximately 2%) develop severe renal cystic disease similar to that classically defined as polycystic kidney disease (PKD). In these cases, the renal cystic disease is a serious complication accounting for significant morbidity and mortality, with frequent and early progression to renal failure (Sampson et al. 1997). Analysis of TSC patients with early-onset PKD has shown that contiguous deletions of *TSC2* and *PKD1* are present in the majority, while approximately 10% have other mutations at the *TSC2/PKD1* locus (Sampson et al. 1997).

Despite considerable evidence that *PKD1* plays a role in the aetiology of renal cystic disease in patients with tuberous sclerosis, there are significant clinical differences in these patients when compared to typical autosomal dominant polycystic kidney disease. First, renal cystic disease in patients with tuberous sclerosis often presents in childhood (Sedman et al. 1987, Sampson et al. 1997). In contrast, manifestation of autosomal dominant polycystic kidney is very unusual during childhood (Sedman et al. 1987). Second, the cystic epithelium in tuberous sclerosis comprises strongly eosinophilic, hypertrophic and hyperplastic cells which are considered unique (Bernstein 1993). The differences in natural history and pathology seem likely to reflect a significant difference in genetic pathogenesis in these two circumstances. Somatic inactivation of the second allele of *TSC2* occurs in hamartomas from *TSC2* patients, and inactivation of the second allele of *PKD1* has been demonstrated in cells that line the renal cysts of patients with *PKD1* mutations. In patients with deletions of *TSC2* and *PKD1*, genomic deletion of the second allele of both genes can occur in a single somatic event to ablate the growth suppressor activities of each gene in the same cell. A one-step double second-hit event may explain the unusual severity of the renal cystic disease in patients with *TSC2* and *PKD1* mutations.

Lymphangioleiomyomatosis and Pulmonary TSC

Lymphangioleiomyomatosis (LAM) is a disorder seen almost exclusively in females and is characterized by bronchiolar smooth muscle infiltration and cystic changes in the lung parenchyma. LAM patients often have angiomyolipoma of the kidneys and/or abdominal and hilar lymph nodes. Symptomatic LAM is estimated to occur in approximately one per million of the population without other evidence of TSC, but in up to 5% of females with TSC, implicating a role for the TSC genes in the aetiology of LAM. Loss of heterozygosity for markers in the *TSC2* region has been observed in renal angiomyolipomas and lymph nodes removed from women with LAM but without other signs of TSC (Smolarek et al. 1998). In addition, inactivating mutations affecting the retained *TSC2* allele have been demonstrated in affected tissues from five sporadic LAM patients, and these mutations are not present in unaffected tissues (Carsillo et al. 2000). These observations suggest that sporadic LAM is caused by first and second somatic hits of *TSC2* in individuals without TSC.

Thus far there is no evidence for involvement of the *TSC1* gene in sporadic LAM, but this may reflect the small number of patients studied to date.

Nine patients with TSC and LAM have now had their TSC gene mutations characterized (Jones et al. 1999a, Zhang et al. 1999b, Dabora et al. 2001). There were eight *TSC2* mutations of various kinds and one *TSC1* nonsense mutation. Thus, although the numbers are small, TSC patients with LAM have a variety of typical TSC mutations.

Recent studies have documented the occurrence of subclinical LAM in a high proportion of adult women with TSC, using high-resolution chest CT (Costello et al. 2000, Franz et al. 2001). Again, these women with subclinical LAM have a variety of mutations in *TSC1* and *TSC2* (Franz et al. 2001).

MOSAICISM

Mosaicism is the phenomenon in which two or more populations of cells with distinct genetic constitutions occur in an individual. Mosaicism occurs when mutation or chromosomal aberration (translocation, trisomy, or monosomy) occurs early during embryogenesis but after the fertilized egg undergoes one or more divisions. Both somatic (generalized) and germline (confined gonadal) mosaicism for *TSC1* and *TSC2* mutations have been described in many patients. These observations have important implications for gene testing and genetic counselling.

Mosaicism has been sought in several collections of patients who have been screened for mutations in the TSC genes. The highest level of mosaicism was reported in a series of patients with the contiguous gene syndrome due to deletion of both *TSC2* and *PKD1* (Sampson et al. 1997). In that series of 27 unrelated families, mosaicism was found in the first affected member in seven families (26%). This may reflect the dramatic renal involvement in these patients, making it easier to clinically detect disease in mosaic cases, and the nature of the assays used for detection of mosaicism (PFGE/Southern blotting and FISH). Patients with mosaicism were found to have less severe renal disease than those with full mutations, consistent with a dosage effect.

Verhoef et al. (1995, 1999) have presented evidence for mosaicism in founders of six TSC families (five somatic and one gonadal) in a series of 62 unrelated families with a mutation in either *TSC1* or *TSC2*. Somatic mosaicism for a *TSC1* mutation was recently identified in a severely affected patient with the deletion 2122delAC in only 30% of blood cells (Kwiatkowska et al. 1999). This patient had seizures, learning disability, multiple cortical tubers and subependymal nodules on brain imaging studies, and facial angiofibromas. Analysis of DNA samples obtained from urine, blood, buccal mucosa and hair indicated that the level of mosaicism varied from 0% in a buccal mucosa sample to 42% in a sample of urine cells.

At least ten sets of siblings affected by TSC but with apparently normal parents have been reported (Yates et al. 1997, Rose et al. 1999). In several instances, identical

TSC2 mutations have been found in DNA from affected siblings but not in blood-derived DNA from their parents. These observations strongly implicate gonadal mosaicism in a parent, although direct confirmation of this event through sampling of gonadal cells has not yet been performed. The incidence of this event is difficult to assess, as there is ascertainment bias in the identification and reporting of these patients (Rose et al. 1999). In our collective experience, the occurrence of two affected children with completely normal parents is observed in approximately 1% of sporadic TSC families.

FUNCTIONS OF THE TUBEROUS SCLEROSIS GENES
TUMOUR SUPPRESSOR PROPERTIES OF *TSC1* AND *TSC2*

Most individuals who have tuberous sclerosis, and certainly all those who have inherited the condition from an affected parent, carry a mutant tuberous sclerosis gene in each of their somatic cells. However, it is clear that a huge majority of these cells proliferate, differentiate and function normally, while, very occasionally, further localized events result in focal tumorigenesis. Knudson (1971) proposed that inherited predisposition to tumours might reflect the germline mutation of "tumour suppressor genes" and that tumour development might be the result of somatic "second-hit" mutations. Recent investigation of somatic mutations in a variety of tuberous sclerosis hamartomas supports classification of the TSC genes as tumour suppressor genes. Several groups have reported evidence for large somatic deletions of the wild-type *TSC1* or *TSC2* allele, manifested as "loss of heterozygosity" (Carbonara et al. 1994, Green et al. 1994a, 1994b). The observation of loss of heterozygosity implies clonality of hamartomas, and this has also been confirmed by demonstration of non-random X chromosome inactivation in hamartomas from female patients with tuberous sclerosis (Green et al. 1996). An intragenic somatic mutation together with the inherited germline mutation has also been documented in a renal cell carcinoma from a *TSC1* patient, supporting the tumour suppressor nature of the *TSC1* gene (van Slegtenhorst et al. 1997).

Although loss of heterozygosity has been documented in a wide variety of TSC hamartomas, and in more aggressive tumours including giant cell astrocytomas and renal cell carcinomas, it appears to be a more consistent finding in some types of lesion than in others. Henske et al. (1996) reported loss of heterozygosity in approximately half of angiomyolipomas and cardiac rhabdomyomas, but in none out of 14 cortical tubers and in only one out of 11 subependymal giant cell astrocytomas. The findings could reflect a different mutational spectrum in the different cell types, or even alternative mechanisms of tumorigenesis in the central nervous system (CNS). However, it is more likely that they reflect a mixture of normal and abnormal cells in lesions of the CNS.

Loss of heterozygosity has been documented infrequently at the *TSC1* locus, as compared to the *TSC2* locus (Table 14.1). In the largest study reported to date, loss was observed in hamartomas from 14 out of 25 patients informative for markers at the *TSC2* locus, but in only 1 out of 27 patients informative at the *TSC1* locus (Henske et al. 1996). Smaller studies have reported similar results (Carbonara et al. 1996, Sepp et al. 1996). The different rates of observed loss of heterozygosity at the *TSC1* and *TSC2* loci probably reflect unequal representation of *TSC1* and *TSC2* germline mutations among sporadic cases. It is also possible that the different relative frequencies of large genomic deletions (detectable by LOH analysis) versus more subtle mutations (small insertions or deletions, point mutations, genomic silencing) at the two loci, or differences in the growth characteristics of the resultant tumours (and hence the likelihood of their being excised), could contribute to these findings.

Chromosome 9 in general, and the 9q34 region in particular, is a frequent site of LOH in bladder carcinoma occurring in patients in the general population. One study has mapped the region of maximal LOH seen in bladder carcinoma to a small region containing the *TSC1* gene, and demonstrated the occurrence of inactivating mutation in the remaining normal allele of *TSC1* in 10% of carcinomas (Hornigold et al. 1999). This result is of borderline significance, and suggests that the *TSC1* gene may be a critical target for inactivation in bladder carcinogenesis, but more study is needed.

EXPRESSION OF *TSC1* AND *TSC2*

Northern blot analysis of *TSC1* expression indicates a major 8.6 kb transcript (with minor signals around 4 kb and 2.5 kb) that is widely expressed and particularly abundant in skeletal muscle (van Slegtenhorst et al. 1997). Northern blot analysis of *TSC2* expression shows a 5.5 kb transcript in a wide variety of human and rodent tissues (European Chromosome 16 Tuberous Sclerosis Consortium 1993, Geist and Gutmann 1995).

Detailed assessment of expression of both tuberin and hamartin in vivo by immunohistochemical analysis has been performed in several laboratories, with general agreement but some differences (Johnson et al. 1999, Plank et al. 1999, Fukuda et al. 2000, Gutmann et al. 2000, Mizuguchi et al. 2000a, Murthy et al. 2000). These differences seem likely to reflect the relatively low expression of both proteins in most cell types, the limitations of the antibodies available, and attempts by investigators to push microscopy techniques to their limit under these circumstances. Most reports indicate that the two proteins have similar expression patterns in all tissues examined. Some report that there are differences in expression in renal epithelial cells, astrocytes, or more generally (respectively Murthy et al. 2000, Gutmann et al. 2000, Fukuda et al. 2000).

In cultured cells, hamartin has been localized to the cytoplasm, with a punctate pattern of immunofluorescence (Plank et al. 1998), while tuberin has shown perinuclear staining (Wienecke et al. 1996). An association of tuberin with the cis-Medial Golgi was indicated by co-localization with mannosidase-II, and this was abolished in cells treated with brefeldin A, a drug which disrupts the Golgi apparatus.

SUBCELLULAR LOCALIZATION

Both hamartin and tuberin pellet from cytoplasmic extracts when centrifuged at $100,000 \times$ g for one hour (Plank et al. 1998, Nellist et al. 1999). Although this could be consistent with association of these proteins with cell membranes, it could also reflect the occurrence of these proteins in a large complex that pellets under these conditions without association with lipid. The failure of either protein to be solubilized from the pellet fraction when treated with anionic detergents suggests that lipid association does not explain this observation (Nellist et al. 1999).

CELLULAR ROLES OF HAMARTIN AND TUBERIN

HAMARTIN, EZRIN, AND THE ACTIN CYTOSKELETON

Lamb et al. (2000) provided evidence that hamartin binds to ezrin and to the other ERM family proteins, radixin and moesin, and participates in adhesion events and rho signalling. ERM proteins form crosslinks between cortical actin filaments and the plasma membrane. Using the yeast-based two-hybrid system, an N-terminal region of ezrin was identified that binds to aminoacids 881–1084 of hamartin, which consists of part of the coiled-coil region and some downstream sequence. This interaction was confirmed by co-immunoprecipitation of the two proteins from endothelial cells, but only 1% of cellular ezrin was bound to hamartin in this assay. A cortical distribution for hamartin in cultured endothelial cells was also shown, consistent with interaction with ezrin and actin, but conflicting with a high degree of association of hamartin with tuberin. Both micro-scale chromophore-assisted laser and antisense methods of inactivation of hamartin led to rapid endothelial cell retraction, accompanied by loss of focal adhesions, cell rounding and progressive detachment from the substrate (Lamb et al. 2000). Overexpression by transfection of both full-length and the N-terminal domain of hamartin (not containing the ERM binding domain) induced actin stress fibre formation through activation of the rho GTPase. These findings are intriguing, and may point to a critical function of hamartin. How they connect with the strong quantitative interaction between hamartin and tuberin is not clear.

GAP ACTIVITY OF TUBERIN

The GTPase activating properties of tuberin have been investigated biochemically. Modest GAP activity toward rap1a, but not rap2, ras, rho or rac, has been reported for native tuberin immunoprecipitated from K-562 cells (Wienecke et al. 1995). GST fusion proteins incorporating the GAP-containing C-terminal part of tuberin and expressed in *E. coli* and in Sf9 insect cells were reported to show similar activity, though at an even lower level (Wienecke et al. 1995). Recent evidence has pointed to mitogenic and oncogenic properties of rap1 and also a likely role in MAP kinase-mediated neuronal differentiation (York et al. 1998). Dysregulation of rap1 inactivation could potentially contribute to the abnormalities that characterize the TSC phenotype.

Similarly, tuberin has modest GAP activity for the GTPase Rab5, which serves a role in regulating endosome fusion (Xiao et al. 1997). Increased fluid-phase endocytosis as measured by horseradish peroxidase uptake has been reported in an Eker rat tumour-derived cell line deficient in tuberin, and re-expression of tuberin appeared to normalize this. The relevance of these observations to the aetiology of tuberous sclerosis remains speculative.

Role of Tuberin in Cell Cycle Control

A role for the TSC gene products in cell cycle control is implied by the abnormal proliferation of cells that results in hamartoma growth. Tuberin-deficient Eker rat-derived fibroblasts have been shown to have a faster transit through the cell cycle, with a reduced expression of one of the cyclin-dependent kinase inhibitors, p27KIP (Soucek et al. 1997, 1998a). However, the cytoplasmic localization of tuberin would appear to argue against a direct role for tuberin in the cell cycle events in the nucleus. Moreover, contrasting observations have been made in *Tsc2* null murine embryo-derived fibroblasts, in which growth is suppressed, and levels of p21CIP are elevated (Onda, Zhang and Kwiatkowski, unpublished observations). Overexpression of either tuberin or hamartin inhibits cell proliferation in many cell types, but the specificity and mechanism of this observation are uncertain (Miloloza et al. 2000).

Tuberin and Hamartin Interact Directly

Van Slegtenhorst et al. (1998) demonstrated an interaction between hamartin and tuberin in the yeast two-hybrid system, and a direct interaction between the two proteins has also been shown by co-immunoprecipation (Plank et al. 1998, van Slegtenhorst et al. 1998, Nellist et al. 1999). The association between tuberin and hamartin appears to be stoichiometric (Plank et al. 1998, Nellist et al. 1999), and gel filtration studies indicate that tuberin and hamartin are found in a complex of approximately 450 kDa (Nellist et al. 1999). The other components of this complex, if any, are yet to be defined. The existence of a tuberin-hamartin complex explains why complete deficiency of either protein (in hamartomas) has the same consequence – a deregulation of cell growth control. It is possible that tuberin has critical biochemical activities (e.g. GAP activity) that are modulated or localized through binding to hamartin.

ANIMAL MODELS FOR TUBEROUS SCLEROSIS

There is a naturally occurring rat mutation in *Tsc2*, and engineered mouse and *Drosophila* models for both *Tsc1* and *Tsc2* inactivation (Table 14.1).

The Eker Rat
Phenotype and histological analysis

The Eker rat was first described as an autosomal dominant, hereditary model of predisposition to renal adenoma and carcinoma in 1954 (Eker 1954). Kidney lesions vary in morphology and include pure cysts, cysts with papillary projections and solid adenomas (Eker et al. 1981), which can be seen as early as 4 months. A small minority of these tumours become malignant, with nuclear atypia, and expand to include the entire kidney, and metastasize to the lungs, pancreas and liver. Although there is some strain variability in the extent of kidney involvement and rapidity of tumour growth (Yeung et al. 1993), this has not been clearly quantitated. There is 100% penetrance of kidney involvement in Eker rats. The kidney tumours develop almost exclusively in the outer cortex and have variable staining characteristics even within a single cystadenoma (Eker et al. 1981). Histological studies have identified proximal tubular and collecting duct epithelial cells as the cells of origin of the Eker solid and cystic adenomas, respectively (Wolf et al. 1995). Three-dimensional reconstruction studies demonstrated that these lesions grow through the kidney by extending along the tubule of origin, with localized regions of cystic expansion with or without papillary growth (Eker et al. 1981).

Eker rats also develop pituitary adenomas (55% at 2 years), uterine leiomyomas and leiomyosarcomas (47–62% of females at 14 months to 2 years), and splenic hemangiomas (23–68% at 14 months to 2 years) (Everitt et al. 1992, Hino et al. 1994). They also develop a variety of brain lesions at low frequency, including lesions resembling human TSC subependymal nodules (Yeung et al. 1997) and cortical tubers (Mizuguchi et al. 2000b). Twenty-seven (63%) out of 43 Eker rats at 1.5 to 2 years had brain lesions (all <2 mm in diameter), consisting of mixtures of large and elongated cells that were found in both subependymal and subcortical regions (Yeung et al. 1997). Intralesional calcification was also seen, similar to human subependymal nodules. The large cells stained with GFAP and other glial and astrocytic markers. One out of six Eker rats examined in a second series had a cortical lesion similar to a cortical tuber (Mizuguchi et al. 2000b).

Mutation of the rat Tsc2 *homolog*

Genetic linkage studies localized the putative disease-causing gene in the Eker rat to a region of rat chromosome 10 that is syntenic to human chromosome 16p13 (Yeung et al. 1993). The identification of *TSC2* at 16p13 led to the analysis of the rat homolog (*Tsc2*) in Eker rats and to the identification of a mutation that resulted from insertion of a 6.3 kb intracisternal A particle (IAP) (Yeung et al. 1994, Kobayashi et al. 1995b) on one allele (*Tsc2Ek/+*). This disrupts codon 1272 of rat *Tsc2* and is predicted to have major effects on the mRNA and protein. Northern blot analysis of Eker tissues and tumours showed a series of faint mRNA bands that were larger in size than the normal *Tsc2* mRNA, representing hybrid species of *Tsc2*-IAP sequence (Yeung et al. 1994, Kobayashi et al. 1995b). A protein product derived from these novel mRNA species has not been identified.

Molecular analysis
Transfection of a plasmid encoding tuberin into Eker rat renal carcinoma cell lines suppressed growth and altered morphology (Orimoto et al. 1996), consistent with *Tsc2* being the gene responsible for the Eker phenotype. Kobayashi et al. (1997b) generated a transgenic Eker rat bearing an additional copy of the wild-type rat *Tsc2* gene and its upstream promoter element. The transgene completely compensated for the *Tsc2*Ek allele in a dosage-dependent manner, providing strong support for the two-hit model of *Tsc2* gene inactivation in the development of tumours in the Eker rat.

Loss of heterozygosity studies in Eker tumours have also provided strong evidence for the two-hit model of tumorigenesis and revealed organ-specific variation in the extent of LOH. Forty to 60% of renal tumours show LOH, compared to 0% of splenic hemangiomas, 36% of uterine leiomyomas, 35% of pituitary adenomas, and 0% of subependymal and subcortical hamartomas (Kubo et al. 1995a, Yeung et al. 1995, 1997). Since LOH analysis detects only large deletions, other mechanisms (e.g. point mutations or epigenetic modification) are likely to account for those tumours without LOH. Indeed, screening for intragenic mutations has shown that some renal tumours without LOH carry point mutations in the wild-type *Tsc2* allele (Kobayashi et al. 1997c). Renal tumours from Eker rats treated with chemical carcinogens, such as ENU, show a high frequency of point mutations but no LOH; such treatment greatly accelerates renal tumour formation (Hino et al. 1993).

Microdissection of cells from early tubular lesions revealed LOH very early during cystadenoma development, and it is probably the initiating molecular step in pathogenesis (Kubo et al. 1995b). Homozygous deletion of the *Ink4A* gene, an inhibitor of cyclin-dependent kinases, occurred in 14 out of 24 (58%) cell lines derived from Eker renal tumours. However, this finding was not seen in DNA from the corresponding tumours, suggesting that it occurred during the adaptation to tissue culture for establishment of these cell lines (Hino et al. 1995). p53 mutations have not been identified in Eker rat tumours (Horesovsky et al. 1995).

Tsc2 null rats
Rat embryos null for the *Tsc2* gene (*Tsc2*Ek/Ek) die at embryonic age 10–12 days, of uncertain causes. *Tsc2*Ek/Ek embryos in the Long–Evans strain display an abnormal head morphology with exencephaly in some cases and consistent overdevelopment of the forebrain neuroepithelium (Rennebeck et al. 1998). However, brain and skull development in *Tsc2*Ek/Ek embryos in the Fisher 344 strain is normal. Null embryos in each strain die at the same age, suggesting that other anatomic or physiologic processes are the cause of death.

Tsc1 AND *Tsc2* KNOCKOUT MICE

Two groups have engineered mice bearing targeted disruptions of the *Tsc1* (*Tsc1-*) and *Tsc2* (*Tsc2-*) genes (Kobayashi et al. 1999, Onda et al. 1999, Kobayashi et al. 2001, Kwiatkowski et al. 2002). All four result in early truncation of the protein product and were predicted to be inactivating.

Phenotype and histological analysis

The phenotypes of the *Tsc1* and *Tsc2* knockout mice are nearly identical and very similar to the Eker rat. *Tsc2+/-* mice develop renal lesions by 6 months, which appear to grow progressively throughout the life of the mouse (Kobayashi et al. 1999, Onda et al. 1999). Histologically, the lesions resemble cystadenomas, consisting of a spectrum of lesions including pure cysts, cysts with papillary projections and solid adenomas. Eight to 16 lesions were seen in analysis of five histologic sections from 12-month-old kidneys, suggesting that the total number per kidney was approximately 20–50 at that age. Renal carcinoma, characterized by nuclear atypia, massive growth and metastatic disease, developed in 5–10% of mice by 18 months, suggesting a very low rate of malignant progression for the cystadenomas (~1 in 1000), indicating that additional genetic or epigenetic events are required for transformation (Onda et al. 1999).

Other tumours are also seen in both the *Tsc1+/-* and *Tsc2+/-* mice (Kobayashi et al. 1999, Onda et al. 1999, Kobayashi et al. 2001, Kwiatkowski et al. 2002). Liver hemangiomas, characterized by endothelial and smooth muscle proliferation with large vascular spaces, are seen in about half of mice by 18 months. These lesions rupture with intraperitoneal haemorrhage and are the major cause of death in both *Tsc1+/-* and *Tsc2+/-* mice prior to age 18 months. Hemangiosarcomas develop on the tail, paws, or mouth region in about 7% of *Tsc2+/-* mice by 12 months. These lesions, consisting of proliferative spindle cells and aberrant vascular channels, do not metastasize, but are malignant by cytologic criteria and exhibit bone invasion. Brain lesions similar to those found in patients with tuberous sclerosis or in Eker rats have not been seen in *Tsc1+/-* or *Tsc2+/-* mice.

Strain-dependent differences in tumour development have been seen in both *Tsc1+/-* and *Tsc2+/-* mice (Onda et al. 1999, Kwiatkowski et al. 2002). Liver hemangiomas are more common in 129/SvJae mice, while kidney tumours predominate in all other mixed and pure strains (Kwiatkowski et al. 2002, Onda and Kwiatkowski, unpublished observations).

Histologic and immunohistochemical studies using a panel of cytoskeletal and membrane proteins expressed in limited segments of the normal mouse nephron identified the interstitial cell of the cortical collecting duct as the cell of origin of cystadenomas (Onda et al. 1999). The actin-binding protein gelsolin, which is normally expressed in interstitial cells of the kidney, was found to be overexpressed in all forms of cystadenoma, and may be used as a sensitive marker of early tumour development.

Molecular analysis
LOH was seen in 9 out of 37 (24%) renal cystadenomas and carcinomas, and in 7 out of 14 (50%) liver hemangiomas from *Tsc2+/-* mice, consistent with inactivation of the wild-type *Tsc2* allele. Immunohistochemical analysis also showed a consistent decrease in tuberin expression in the renal lesions in these mice (Onda et al. 1999).

Tsc2 *null mice*
Tsc2-/- embryos died at mid-gestation (E10.5–12.5) and were less developed than *Tsc2+/-* and wild-type littermates (Kobayashi et al. 1999, Onda et al. 1999). Consistent with the generalized developmental delay, a proportion of E8–E9 embryos had open neural tubes. *Tsc2-/-* embryos were paler, edematous and had pericardial effusions. Upon histologic analysis, liver hypoplasia was most striking and appeared to be the primary cause of fetal demise, with secondary growth retardation and circulatory failure from anaemia (Onda et al. 1999). *Tsc1-/-* embryos die with similar findings but survive on average about one day longer than *Tsc2-/-* embryos (Kwiatkowski et al. 2002)

The *Drosophila* Tsc2 Mutant, *Gigas*
Mutations in the *Drosophila* mutant, *gigas* (Ferrus and Garcia-Bellido 1976), have been found in the orthologue of *TSC2* (Ito and Rubin 1999). Homozygous *gigas* animals die during larval development. Using the FRT/FLP recombination system, it has been shown that homozygous *gigas* cells develop to an abnormally large size in the eye and wing. In the eye, all *gigas* cells are enlarged about 2–3 times in area, but the structure and organization are normal. Similarly, in the wing, *gigas* cells are larger but otherwise appear normal.

PERSPECTIVES ON ANIMAL MODELS
Although the phenotypes of the rodent models might seem extremely different from patients with tuberous sclerosis, there are similarities. In the human, rat and mouse, tumours develop at high frequency. Often these lesions exhibit loss of the wild-type allele, consistent with a pathogenic mechanism in which complete loss of functional tuberin leads to perturbed cell growth and differentiation. Although rodents and humans manifest different tumours, tumour progression is similar. The tumours have a low growth rate and quite possibly limited growth potential in the absence of additional genetic events. Malignancy is rare in both rodents and humans.

The absence of major brain manifestations in rodents is perhaps surprising given the marked brain pathology in human TSC. It is possible that the rarity of lesions in the rodent brain simply reflects its much smaller size and cell number compared to humans. However, it is also possible that the progenitor cells which give rise to human brain lesions have different mechanisms of tuberin-regulated cell growth and differentiation compared to the majority of rodent brain precursor cells.

The *Drosophila gigas* mutant is different from the mammalian models, in that the failure of cell growth control appears to occur only after completion of development and differentiation. It is notable that one hallmark feature of TSC cortical tubers is the presence of multinucleated giant cells, in which DNA replication has occurred in the absence of cell division, similar to the *gigas* cells. In addition, it is hoped that genetic approaches not possible in mammalian organisms will lead to the identification of genes and proteins that are involved in tuberin-related pathways of cell growth regulation in *Drosophila*.

CONCLUSIONS

The identification of the *TSC1* and *TSC2* genes has enabled the initiation of a wide range of experimental approaches to improve understanding of the pathogenesis of TSC. The products of the genes are novel proteins whose structures provide few immediate clues as to their likely cellular functions. However, biochemical analyses and use of animal models and their derived cells are likely to elucidate the pathways in which these genes and their encoded proteins participate.

Detailed study in multiple laboratories has provided considerable information on the nature and diversity of mutations that occur in *TSC1* and *TSC2*, causing TSC. Using this knowledge, gene-based diagnostic tests have been developed, and can aid genetic counselling by clarifying genetic status and enabling early prenatal diagnosis. Genotype-phenotype studies are revealing differences in overall disease severity between patients with *TSC1* and *TSC2* mutations. The immediate future should see technical developments that will increase the sensitivity of mutation detection, and the accrual of more accurate information on the risks of complications associated with *TSC1* and *TSC2* mutations.

NOTE ADDED IN PROOF

Major advances in our understanding of the function of tuberin and hamartin have recently been made. These are summarized here briefly, with apologies to those whose work is not cited due to space limitations.

Recent studies have used mutagenesis followed by a phenotypic screen in *Drosophila* to discover a connection between *Drosophila* homologs *Tsc1* and *Tsc2*, and the regulation of cell and organ size (Gao and Pan 2001, Potter et al. 2001, Tapon et al. 2001). Inactivation of *Tsc1* in the eye or wing leads to an increase in the size of the overall organ which is almost entirely due to an increase in cell size, similar to the effect of disruption of *Tsc2* (Ito and Rubin 1999). Increased expression of *Tsc1* and *Tsc2* (but not of either gene alone) in the eye leads to an opposite phenotype in which there are small eyes with fewer individual subunits (Gao and Pan 2001, Potter et al. 2001, Tapon et al. 2001). These observations suggest that *Tsc1/Tsc2* participate in the evolutionarily conserved PI3Kinase-Akt-S6Kinase pathway to regulate cell size. Genetic interaction studies in *Drosophila* then positioned *Tsc1/Tsc2* in this pathway at about the level of Tor (Target of rapamycin) (Gao and Pan 2001, Potter et al. 2001, Tapon et al. 2001, Gao et al. 2002, Potter et al. 2002). Furthermore, the *Drosophila Tsc2* protein was recognized to contain two to four Akt1 phosphorylation sites, and Akt1 phosphorylation of *Tsc2* was shown to cause disruption of the *Tsc1/Tsc2* complex.

Similar findings on the involvement of mammalian *Tsc1* and *Tsc2* in this pathway were made following the initial *Drosophila* studies and concurrent with the later work. In cultured mammalian cells lacking either *TSC1* or *TSC2*, there is constitutive high-level phosphorylation of S6K, 4E-BP1, and (in neuroepithelial cells) Stat3 (Goncharova et al. 2002, Kwiatkowski et al. 2002, Onda et al. 2002). In addition, these phosphorylations are rapidly reversed by treatment with the antibiotic rapamycin, consistent with activation of mTOR in the absence of *TSC1* or *TSC2* proteins. Activation of S6K in these cells leads to prominent phosphorylation of S6, a ribosomal protein component, and this molecular signature is relatively easily assessed in staining studies to show activation of this pathway both in cultured cell extracts and pathological samples from patients and mice (Goncharova et al. 2002, Kenerson et al. 2002, Kwiatkowski et al. 2002, El-Hashemite et al. 2003).

As in *Drosophila*, activated Akt phosphorylates *TSC2* at two to four different sites (Dan et al. 2002, Inoki et al. 2002, Manning et al. 2002), which appears to reduce its activity in inhibition of mTOR. High-level expression of *TSC1/TSC2* by transfection leads to inhibition of signalling pathways downstream of mTOR (Inoki et al. 2002).

Thus, in normal cells the *TSC1/TSC2* complex acts as an inhibitor of mTOR. When stimulated by growth factors or other agents, activation of Akt leads to phosphorylation of *TSC2* which leads to inactivation of the inhibitory activity of the *TSC1/TSC2* complex. In cells that are lacking either *TSC1* or *TSC2*, mTOR/S6Kinase activity is increased several-fold, and is no longer dependent upon several signals which normally regulate their activity including through the PI3Kinase pathway. Thus, this appears to be a fundamental biochemical defect in cells lacking *TSC1* or *TSC2*, which contributes to the growth of TSC hamartoma. It is a remarkably fortuitous circumstance that rapamycin, a clinically approved compound, has selective activity in the inhibition of mTOR. Thus, there is currently much guarded enthusiasm for the possibility that rapamycin will provide benefit for some of the clinical manifestations of TSC, and clinical trials are just beginning.

REFERENCES

Ali IU, Schriml L, Dean M (1999) Mutational spectra of *PTEN/MMAC1* gene: a tumour suppressor with lipid phosphatase activity. *JNCI* 91: 1922–32.

Ali JBM, Sepp T, Ward S, Green AJ, Yates JRW (1998) Mutations in the *TSC1* gene account for a minority of patients with tuberous sclerosis. *J Med Genet* 35: 969–72.

Antonarakis SE, and the Nomenclature Working Group (1998) Recommendations for a nomenclature system for human gene mutations. *Hum Mutat* 11: 1–3.

Aspinwall R, Rothwell DG, Roldan-Arjona T, Anselmino C, Ward CJ, Cheadle JP, Sampson JR,

Lindahl T, Harris PC, Hickson ID (1997) Cloning and characterisation of a functional homolog of *Escherichia coli* endonuclease III. *Proc Natl Acad Sci USA* 94: 109–14.

Au KS, Merrell J, Buckler A, Blanton SH, Northrup H (1996) Report of a critical recombination further narrowing the *TSC1* region. *J Med Genet* 33: 559–61.

Au KS, Rodriguez JA, Rodriguez E Jr, Dobyns WB, Delgado MR, Northrup H (1997) Mutations and polymorphisms in the tuberous sclerosis complex gene on chromosome 16. *Hum Mutat* 9: 23–9.

Au KS, Rodriguez JA, Finch JL, Volcik KA, Roach ES, Delgado MR, Rodriguez E Jr, Northrup H (1998) Germ-line mutational analysis of the *TSC2* gene in 90 tuberous-sclerosis patients. *Am J Hum Genet* 62: 286–94.

Beauchamp RL, Banwell A, McNamara P, Jacobsen M, Higgins E, Northrup H, Short P, Sims K, Ozelius L, Ramesh V (1998) Exon scanning of the entire *TSC2* gene for germline mutations in 40 unrelated patients with tuberous sclerosis. *Hum Mutat* 12: 408–16.

Benit P, Kara-Mostefa A, Hadj-Rabia S, Munnich A, Bonnefont JP (1999) Protein truncation test for screening hamartin gene mutations and report of new disease-causing mutations. *Hum Mutat* 14: 428–32.

Bernstein J (1993) Renal cystic disease in tuberous sclerosis complex. *Pediatr Nephrol* 7: 490–5.

Berx G, Becker KF, Hofler H, van Roy F (1998) Mutations of the human E-Cadherin (*CDH1*) gene. *Hum Mutat* 12: 226–37.

Boguski MS, McCormick F (1993) Proteins regulating ras and its relatives. *Nature* 366: 643–54.

Bourne HR, Sanders DA (1990) The GTPase superfamily – a conserved switch for diverse cell functions. *Nature* 348: 125–32.

Brook-Carter PT, Peral B, Ward CJ, Thompson P, Hughes J, Maheshwar MM, Nellist M, Gamble V, Harris PC, Sampson JR (1994) Deletion of the *TSC2* and *PKD1* genes associated with severe infantile polycystic kidney disease – a contiguous gene syndrome. *Nat Genet* 8: 328–32.

Carbonara C, Longa L, Grosso E, Borrone C, Garre MG, Brisigotti M, Migone M (1994) 9q34 loss of heterozygosity in a tuberous sclerosis astrocytoma suggests a growth suppressor-like activity also for the *TSC1* gene. *Hum Mol Genet* 3: 1829–32.

Carbonara C, Longa L, Grosso E, Mazzucco G, Borrone C, Garre ML, Brisigotti M, Filippi G, Scabar A, Giannotti A, Falzoni P, Monga G, Garini G, Gabrielli M, Riegler P, Dannesino C, Ruggieri M, Magro G, Migone N (1996) Apparent preferential loss of heterozygosity at *TSC2* over *TSC1* chromosomal regions in tuberous sclerosis hamartomas. *Genes Chromosom Cancer* 15: 18–25.

Carsillo T, Astrinidis A, Henske EP (2000) Mutations in the tuberous sclerosis complex gene *TSC2* are the cause of sporadic pulmonary lymphangioleiomyomatosis. *Proc Natl Acad Sci USA* 97: 6085–90.

Cheadle JP, Reeve MP, Sampson JR, Kwiatkowski DJ (2000) Molecular genetic advances in tuberous sclerosis. *Hum Genet* 107: 97–114.

Choy YS, Dabora SL, Hall F, Ramesh V, Niida Y, Franz D, Kasprzyk-Obara J, Reeve MP, Kwiatkowski DJ (1999) Superiority of Denaturing High Performance Liquid Chromatography over single-stranded conformation and conformation-sensitive gel electrophoresis for mutation detection in *TSC2*. *Ann Hum Genet* 63: 383–91.

Cooper DN, Krawczak M (1991) Mechanisms of insertional mutagenesis in human genes causing genetic disease. *Hum Genet* 87: 409–15.

Cooper DN, Youssoufian H (1988) The CpG dinucleotide and human genetic disease. *Hum Genet* 78: 151–5.

Costello LC, Hartman TE, Ryu JH (2000) High frequency of pulmonary lymphangi-oleiomyomatosis in women with tuberous sclerosis complex. *Mayo Clin Proc* 75: 591–4.

Cunningham RP, Weiss B (1985) Endonuclease III (*NTH*) mutants of *Escherichia coli*. *Proc Natl Acad Sci USA* 82: 474–8.

Dabora SL, Sigalas I, Hall F, Eng C, Vijg J, Kwiatkowski DJ (1998) Comprehensive mutation analysis of *TSC1* using two-dimensional DNA electrophoresis with DGGE. *Ann Hum Genet* 62: 491–504.

Dabora SL, Nieto A, Franz D, Jóźwiak S, van den Ouweland A, Kwiatkowski D (2000) Identification and characterization of 6 large (1.3kb–39kb) deletions in *TSC2* using long range PCR suggests diverse deletion mechanisms including Alu-mediated homologous recombination. *J Med Genet* 37: 877–82.

Dabora SL, Jóźwiak S, Franz DN, Roberts PS, Nieto AA, Chung J, Choy YS, Reeve MP, Thiele E, Egelhoff JC, Kasprzyk-Obara J, Domanska-Pakiela D, Kwiatkowski DJ (2001) Mutational analysis in a cohort of 224 tuberous sclerosis patients indicates increased severity of TSC2 compared with TSC1 disease in multiple organs. *Am J Hum Genet* 68(1): 64–80.

Dan HC, Sun M, Yang L, Feldman RI, Sui XM, Yeung RS, Halley DJ, Nicosia SV, Pledger WJ, Cheng, JQ (2002) PI3K/AKT pathway regulates TSC tumor suppressor complex by phosphorylation of tuberin. *J Biol Chem* 277: 35364–70.

Downward J (1990) The ras superfamily of small GTP-binding proteins. *Trends Biochem Sci* 15: 469–72.

Eker R (1954) Familial renal adenomas in Wistar rats. *Acta Path et Microbiol Scand* 34: 554–62.

Eker R, Mossige J, Johannessen JV, Aars H (1981) Hereditary renal adenomas and adenocar-cinomas in rats. *Diagn Histopathol* 4: 99–110.

El-Hashemite N, Zhang H, Henske EP, Kwiatkowski DJ (2003) Mutation in TSC2 and activation of mammalian target of rapamycin signaling pathway in renal angiomyolipoma. *Lancet* 361: 1348–9.

European Chromosome 16 Tuberous Sclerosis Consortium (1993) Identification and character-isation of the tuberous sclerosis gene on chromosome 16. *Cell* 75: 1305–15.

European Polycystic Kidney Disease Consortium (1994) The polycystic kidney disease 1 gene encodes a 14kb transcript and lies within a duplicated region on chromosome 16. *Cell* 77: 881–94.

Everitt JI, Goldsworthy TL, Wolf DC, Walker CL (1992) Hereditary renal cell carcinoma in the Eker rat: a rodent familial cancer syndrome. *J Urol* 148: 1932–6.

Ferrus A, Garcia-Bellido A (1976) Morphogenetic mutants detected in mitotic recombination clones. *Nature* 260: 425–6.

Franz DN, Brody A, Meyer C, Leonard J, Chuck G, Dabora S, Sethuraman G, Colby TV, Kwiatkowski DJ, McCormack FX (2001) Mutational and radiographic analysis of pulmonary disease consistent with lymphangioleiomyomatosis and micronodular pneumocyte hyperplasia in women with tuberous sclerosis. *Am J Respir Crit Care Med* 15; 164(4): 661–8.

Fryer AE, Chalmers A, Connor JM, Fraser I, Povey S, Yates AD, Yates JRW, Osborne JP (1987) Evidence that the gene for tuberous sclerosis is on chromosome 9. *Lancet* i: 659–61.

Fukuda T, Kobayashi T, Momose S, et al. (2000) Distribution of Tsc1 protein detected by immunohistochemistry in various normal rat tissues and the renal carcinomas of Eker rat: detection of limited colocalization with Tsc1 and Tsc2 gene products in vivo. *Lab Invest* 80: 1347–59.

Gao X, Pan D (2001) TSC1 and TSC2 tumor suppressors antagonize insulin signaling in cell growth. *Genes Dev* 15: 1383–92.

Gao X, Zhang Y, Arrazola P, Hino O, Kobayashi T, Yeung RS, Ru B, Pan D (2002) Tsc tumour suppressor proteins antagonize amino-acid TOR signalling. *Nat Cell Biol* 4: 699–704.

Geist RT, Gutmann DH (1995) The tuberous sclerosis 2 gene is expressed at high levels in the cerebellum and developing spinal cord. *Cell Growth Differ* 6: 1477–83.

Gilbert JR, Guy V, Kumar A, Wolpert C, Kandt R, Aylesworth A, Roses AD, Pericak-Vance MA (1998) Mutation and polymorphism analysis in the tuberous sclerosis 2 (*TSC2*) gene. *Neurogenetics* 1: 267–72.

Goncharova EA, Goncharov DA, Eszterhas A, Hunter DS, Glassberg MK, Yeung RS, Walker CL, Noonan D, Kwiatkowski DJ, Chou MM, Panettieri RA Jr, Krymskaya VP (2002) Tuberin regulates p70 S6 kinase activation and ribosomal protein S6 phosphorylation: a role for the TSC2 tumor suppressor gene in pulmonary lymphangioleiomyomatosis (LAM). *J Biol Chem* 277: 30958–67.

Green AJ, Johnson PH, Yates JRW (1994a) The tuberous sclerosis gene on chromosome 9q34 acts as a growth suppressor. *Hum Mol Genet* 3: 1833–4.

Green AJ, Smith M, Yates JRW (1994b) Loss of heterozygosity on chromosome 16p13.3 in hamartomas from tuberous sclerosis patients. *Nat Genet* 6: 193–6.

Green AJ, Sepp T, Yates JRW (1996) Clonality of tuberous sclerosis hamartomas shown by non-random X-chromosome inactivation. *Hum Genet* 97: 240–3.

Gutmann DH, Zhang Y, Hasbani MJ, et al. (2000) Expression of the tuberous sclerosis complex gene products, hamartin and tuberin, in central nervous system tissues. *Acta Neuropathol (Berl)* 99: 223–30.

Haines JL, Short MP, Kwiatkowski DJ, Jewell A, Andermann E, Bejjani B, Yang CH, Gusella JF, Amos JA (1991) Localisation of one gene for tuberous sclerosis within 9q32–9q34, and further evidence for heterogeneity. *Am J Hum Genet* 49: 764–72.

Harris PC, Ward CJ, Peral B, Hughes J (1995) Autosomal dominant polycystic kidney disease: molecular analysis. *Hum Mol Genet* 4: 1745–9.

Henikoff S, Henikoff J (1992) Amino acid substitution matrices from protein blocks. *Proc Natl Acad Sci USA* 89: 10915–19.

Henske EP, Scheithauer BW, Short MP, Wollmann R, Nahmias J, Hornigold N, van Slegtenhorst M, Welsh CT, Kwiatkowski DJ (1996) Allelic loss is frequent in tuberous sclerosis kidney lesions but rare in brain lesions. *Am J Hum Genet* 59: 400–6.

Hino O, Mitani H, Knudson AG (1993) Genetic predisposition to transplacentally induced renal cell carcinomas in the Eker rat. *Cancer Res* 53: 5856–8.

Hino O, Mitani H, Katsuyama H, Kubo Y (1994) A novel cancer predisposition syndrome in the Eker rat model. *Cancer Lett* 83: 117–21.

Hino O, Kobayashi E, Hirayama Y, Kobayashi T, Kubo Y, Tsuchiya H, Kikuchi Y, Mitani H (1995) Molecular genetic basis of renal carcinogenesis in the Eker rat model of tuberous sclerosis (*Tsc2*). *Mol Carcinog* 14: 23–7.

Horesovsky G, Recio L, Everitt J, Goldsworthy T, Wolf DC, Walker C (1995) p53 status in spontaneous and dimethylnitrosamine-induced renal cell tumours from rats. *Mol Carcinog* 12: 236–40.

Hornigold N, van Slegtenhorst M, Nahmias J, Ekong R, Rousseaux S, Hermans C, Halley D, Povey S, Wolfe J (1997) A 1.7-megabase sequence-ready cosmid contig covering the *TSC1* candidate region in 9q34. *Genomics* 41: 385–9.

Hornigold N, Devlin J, Davies AM, Aveyard JS, Habuchi T, Knowles MA (1999) Mutation of the 9q34 gene TSC1 in sporadic bladder cancer. *Oncogene* 18: 2657–61.

Inoki K, Li Y, Zhu T, Wu J, Guan KL (2002) TSC2 is phosphorylated and inhibited by Akt and suppresses mTOR signalling. *Nat Cell Biol* 4: 648–57.

Ito N, Rubin G (1999) *Gigas*, a *Drosophila* homolog of tuberous sclerosis gene product-2, regulates the cell cycle. *Cell* 96: 529–39.

Janssen LAJ, Sandkuyl LA, Merkens EC, Maat-Kievit JA, Sampson JR, Fleury P, Hennekan RCM, Grosveld GC, Lindhout D, Halley DJ (1990) Genetic heterogeneity in tuberous sclerosis. *Genomics* 8: 237–42.

Janssen B, Sampson JR, van der Est M, Deelen W, Verhoef S, Daniels I, Hesseling A, Brook-Carter P, Nellist M, Lindhout D, Sandkuijl L, Halley D (1994) Refined localisation of *TSC1* by combined analysis of 9q34 and 16p13 data in 14 tuberous sclerosis families. *Hum Genet* 94: 437–40.

Jobert S, Bragado-Nilsson E, Samolyk D, Pedespan JM, Marchal C, Reichert S, Mallet J, Pitiot G (1997) Deletion of 11 amino acids in tuberin associated with severe tuberous sclerosis phenotypes: evidence for a new essential domain in the first third of the protein. *Eur J Hum Genet* 5: 280–7.

Johnson MW, Emelin JK, Park SH, Vinters HV (1999) Co-localization of *TSC1* and *TSC2* gene products in tubers of patients with tuberous sclerosis. *Brain Pathol* 9: 45–54.

Jones AC, Daniells CE, Snell RG, Tachataki M, Idziaszczyk SA, Krawczak M, Sampson JR, Cheadle JP (1997) Molecular genetic and phenotypic analysis reveals differences between *TSC1* and *TSC2* associated familial and sporadic tuberous sclerosis. *Hum Mol Genet* 6: 2155–61.

Jones AC, Shyamsundar MM, Thomas MW, Maynard J, Idziaszczyk S, Tomkins S, Sampson JR, Cheadle JP (1999a) Comprehensive mutation analysis of *TSC1* and *TSC2* and phenotypic correlations in 150 families with tuberous sclerosis. *Am J Hum Genet* 64: 1305–15.

Jones AC, Austin J, Hansen N, Hoogendoorn B, Oefner PJ, Cheadle JP, O'Donovan MC (1999b) Optimal temperature selection for mutation detection by denaturing HPLC and comparison to single-stranded conformation polymorphism and heteroduplex analysis. *Clin Chem* 45: 1133–40.

Jones AC, Sampson JR, Hoogendoorn B, Cohen D, Cheadle JP (2000) Application and evaluation of denaturing HPLC for molecular genetic analysis in tuberous sclerosis. *Hum Genet* 106(6): 663–8.

Kandt RS, Haines JL, Smith M, Northrup H, Gardner RJM, Short MP, Dumars K, Roach ES, Steingold S, Wall S, Blanton SH, Flodman P, Kwiatkowski DJ, Jewell A, Weber JL, Roses AD, Pericak-Vance MA (1992) Linkage of an important gene locus for tuberous sclerosis to a chromosome 16 marker for polycystic kidney disease. *Nat Genet* 2: 37–41.

Kenerson HL, Aicher LD, True LD, Yeung RS (2002) Activated mammalian target of rapamycin pathway in the pathogenesis of tuberous sclerosis complex renal tumors. *Cancer Res* 62: 5645–50.

Kim KK, Pajak L, Wang H, Field LJ (1995) Cloning, developmental expression, and evidence for alternative splicing of the murine tuberous sclerosis (*Tsc2*) gene product. *Cell Mol Biol Res* 41: 515–26.

Knudson AG (1971) Mutation and cancer: statistical study of retinoblastoma. *Proc Natl Acad Sci USA* 68: 820–3.

Kobayashi T, Nishizawa M, Hirayama Y, Kobayashi E, Hino O (1995a) cDNA structure, alternative splicing and exon-intron organisation of the predisposing tuberous sclerosis (*Tsc2*) gene of the Eker rat model. *Nucleic Acids Res* 23: 2608–13.

Kobayashi T, Hirayama Y, Kobayashi E, Kubo Y, Hino O (1995b) A germline insertion in the tuberous sclerosis (*Tsc2*) gene gives rise to the Eker rat model of dominantly inherited cancer. *Nat Genet* 9: 70–4.

Kobayashi T, Urakami S, Cheadle JP, Aspinwall R, Harris P, Sampson JR, Hino O (1997a)

Identification of a leader exon and a core promoter for the rat tuberous sclerosis 2 (*Tsc2*) gene and structural comparison with the human homolog. *Mammalian Genome* 8: 554–8.

Kobayashi T, Mitani H, Takahashi R, Hirabayashi M, Ueda M, Tamura H, Hino O (1997b) Transgenic rescue from embryonic lethality and renal carcinogenesis in the Eker rat model by introduction of a wild-type *Tsc2* gene. *Proc Natl Acad Sci USA* 94: 3990–3.

Kobayashi T, Urakami S, Hirayama Y, Yamamoto T, Nishizawa M, Takahara T, Kubo Y, Hino O (1997c) Intragenic *Tsc2* somatic mutations as Knudson's second hit in spontaneous and chemically induced renal carcinomas in the Eker rat model. *Jpn J Cancer Res* 88: 254–61.

Kobayashi T, Minowa O, Kuno J, Mitani H, Hino O, Noda T (1999) Renal carcinogenesis, hepatic hemangiomatosis, and embryonic lethality caused by a germ-line *Tsc2* mutation in mice. *Cancer Res* 59: 1206–11.

Kobayashi T, Minowa O, Sugitani Y, Takai S, Mitani H, Kobayashi E, Noda T, Hino O (2001) A germ-line Tsc1 mutation causes tumor development and embryonic lethality that are similar, but not identical, to those caused by Tsc2 mutation in mice. *Proc Natl Acad Sci USA* 98: 8762–7.

Krawczak M, Ball E, Cooper D (1998) Neighboring-nucleotide effects on the rates of germ-line single-base-pair substitution in human genes. *Am J Hum Genet* 63: 474–88.

Kubo Y, Kikuchi Y, Mitani H, Kobayashi E, Kobayashi T, Hino O (1995a) Allelic loss at the tuberous sclerosis (*Tsc2*) gene locus in spontaneous uterine leiomyosarcomas and pituitary adenomas in the Eker rat model. *Jpn J Cancer Res* 86: 828–32.

Kubo Y, Klimek F, Kikuchi Y, Bannasch P, Hino O (1995b) Early detection of Knudson's two-hits in preneoplastic renal cells of the Eker rat model by the laser microdissection procedure. *Cancer Res* 55: 989–90.

Kumar A, Kandt RS, Wolpert C, Roses AD, Pericak-Vance MA, Gilbert JR (1995a) Mutation analysis of the *TSC2* gene in an African-American family. *Hum Mol Genet* 4: 2295–8.

Kumar A, Wolpert C, Kandt RS, Segal J, Pufky J, Roses AD, Pericak-Vance MA, Gilbert JR (1995b) A *de novo* frame-shift mutation in the tuberin gene. *Hum Mol Genet* 4: 1471–2.

Kumar A, Kandt RS, Wolpert C, Roses AD, Pericak-Vance MA, Gilbert JR (1997) A novel splice site mutation (156+1G>A) in the *TSC2* gene. *Hum Mutat* 9: 64–5.

Kwiatkowska J, Jóźwiak S, Hall F, Henske E, Haines J, McNamara P, Braiser J, Wigowska-Sowinska J, Kasprzyk-Obara J, Short MP, Kwiatkowski DJ (1998) Comprehensive analysis of the *TSC1* gene: observations on frequency of mutation, associated features, and nonpenetrance. *Ann Hum Genet* 62: 277–85.

Kwiatkowska J, Wigowska-Sowinska J, Napierala D, Slomski R, Kwiatkowski DJ (1999) Mosaicism in tuberous sclerosis as a potential cause of the failure of molecular diagnosis. *New Engl J Med* 340: 703–7.

Kwiatkowski DJ, Armour J, Bale AE, Fountain JW, Goudie D, Haines JL, Knowles MA, Pilz A, Slaugenhaupt S, Povey S (1993) Report on the second international workshop on human chromosome 9. *Cytogenet Cell Genet* 64: 94–106.

Kwiatkowski DJ, Zhang H, Bandura JL, Heiberger KM, Glogauer M, El-Hashemite N, Onda H (2002) A mouse model of TSC1 reveals sex-dependent lethality from liver hemangiomas, and up-regulation of p70S6 kinase activity in Tsc1 null cells. *Hum Mol Genet* 11: 525–34.

Lamb RF, Roy C, Diefenbach TJ, Vinters HV, Johnson MW, Jay DG, Hall A (2000) The *TSC1* tumour suppressor hamartin regulates cell adhesion through ERM proteins and the GTPase Rho. *Nat Cell Biol* 2: 281–7.

Lohmann DR (1999) *RB1* gene mutations in retinoblastoma. *Hum Mutat* 14: 283–8.

Lowy DR, Willumsen BM (1993) Function and regulation of ras. *Ann Rev Biochem* 62: 851–91.

Maheshwar MM, Sandford R, Nellist M, Cheadle JP, Sgotto B, Vaudin M, Sampson JR (1996) Comparative analysis and genomic structure of the tuberous sclerosis 2 (*TSC2*) gene in human and pufferfish. *Hum Mol Genet* 5: 131–7.

Maheshwar MM, Cheadle JP, Jones AC, Myring J, Fryer AE, Harris PC, Sampson JR (1997) The GAP-related domain of tuberin, the product of the *TSC2* gene, is a target for missense mutations in tuberous sclerosis. *Hum Mol Genet* 6: 1991–6.

Manning BD, Tee AR, Logsdon MN, Blenis J, Cantley LC (2002) Identification of the tuberous sclerosis complex-2 tumor suppressor gene product tuberin as a target of the phosphoinositide 3-kinase/akt pathway. *Mol Cell* 10: 151–62.

Mayer K, Ballhausen W, Rott H-D (1999) Mutation screening of the entire coding regions of the *TSC1* and the *TSC2* gene with the protein truncation test (PTT) identifies frequent splicing defects. *Hum Mutat* 14: 401–11.

Miloloza A, Rosner M, Nellist M, Halley D, Bernaschek G, Hengstschlager M (2000) The TSC1 gene product, hamartin, negatively regulates cell proliferation. *Hum Mol Genet* 9: 1721–7.

Mizuguchi M, Ikeda K, Takashima S (2000a) Simultaneous loss of hamartin and tuberin from the cerebrum, kidney and heart with tuberous sclerosis. *Acta Neuropathol (Berl)* 99: 503–10.

Mizuguchi M, Takashima S, Yamanouchi H, et al. (2000b) Novel cerebral lesions in the Eker rat model of tuberous sclerosis: cortical tuber and anaplastic ganglioglioma. *J Neuropathol Exp Neurol* 59: 188–96.

Murthy V, Haddad LA, Smith N, Pinney D, Tyszkowski R, Brown D, Ramesh V (2000) Similarities and differences in the subcellular localization of hamartin and tuberin in the kidney. *Am J Physiol Renal Physiol* 278: F737–F746.

Nellist M, Brook-Carter PT, Connor JM, Kwiatkowski DJ, Johnson P, Sampson JR (1993) Identification of markers flanking the tuberous sclerosis locus on chromosome 9 (*TSC1*). *J Med Genet* 30: 224–7.

Nellist M, van Slegtenhorst MA, Goedbloed M, van den Ouweland AMW, Halley DJ, van der Sluijs P (1999) Characterization of the cytosolic tuberin-hamartin complex: tuberin is a cytosolic chaperone for hamartin. *J Biol Chem* 274: 35647–52.

Niida Y, Lawrence-Smith N, Banwell A, Hammer E, Lewis J, Beauchamp R, Sims K, Ramesh V, Ozelius L (1999) Analysis of both *TSC1* and *TSC2* for germline mutations in 126 unrelated patients with tuberous sclerosis. *Hum Mutat* 14: 412–22.

Northrup H, Beaudet AL, O'Brien WE, Herman GE, Lewis RA, Pollack MS (1987) Linkage of tuberous sclerosis to ABO blood-group. *Lancet* 2: 804–5.

Northrup H, Kwiatkowski DJ, Roach ES, Dobyns WB, Lewis RA, Herman GE, Rodriguez E, Daiger SP, Blanton SH (1992) Evidence for genetic heterogeneity in tuberous sclerosis: one locus on chromosome 9 and at least one locus elsewhere. *Am J Hum Genet* 51: 709–20.

Ohtsuka T, Shimuzu K, Yamamori B, Kuroda S, Takai Y (1996) Activation of brain B-raf protein kinase by rap1B small GTP-binding protein. *J Biol Chem* 271: 1258–61.

Olsson PG, Sutherland HF, Nowicka U, Korn B, Poutska A, Frischauf AM (1995) The mouse homolog of the tuberin gene (*Tsc2*) maps to a conserved synteny group between mouse chromosome-17 and human 16p13.3. *Genomics* 25: 339–40.

Olsson PG, Schofield JN, Edwards YH, Frischauf AM (1996) Expression and differential splicing of the mouse *Tsc2* homolog. *Mammalian Genome* 7: 212–15.

Onda H, Lueck A, Marks PW, Warren HB, Kwiatkowski DJ (1999) *Tsc2*(+/-) mice develop tumours in multiple sites that express gelsolin and are influenced by genetic background. *J Clin Invest* 104: 687–95.

Onda H, Crino PB, Zhang H, Murphey RD, Rastelli L, Rothberg BEG, Kwiatkowski DJ (2002) Tsc2 null murine neuroepithelial cells are a model for human tuber giant cells, and show activation of an mTOR pathway. *Mol Cell Neurosc* 21: 561–74.

Orimoto K, Tsuchiya H, Kobayashi T, Matsuda T, Hino O (1996) Suppression of the neoplastic phenotype by replacement of the *Tsc2* gene in Eker rat renal carcinoma cells. *Biochem Biophys Res Commun* 219: 70–5.

Osborne JP, Fryer A, Webb D (1991) Epidemiology of tuberous sclerosis. *Ann NY Acad Sci* 615: 125–7.

Plank TL, Yeung RS, Henske EP (1998) Hamartin, the product of the tuberous sclerosis 1 (*TSC1*) gene, interacts with tuberin and appears to be localised to cytoplasmic vesicles. *Cancer Res* 58: 4766–70.

Plank TL, Logginidou H, Klein-Szanto A, Henske EP (1999) The expression of hamartin, the product of the *TSC1* gene, in normal human tissues and in TSC1- and TSC2-linked angiomyolipomas. *Mod Pathol* 12: 539–45.

Platten M, Meyer-Puttlitz B, Blumcke I, Waha A, Wolf HK, Nothen MM, Louis DN, Sampson JR, von Deimling A (1997) A novel splice site associated polymorphism in the tuberous sclerosis 2 (*TSC2*) gene may predispose to the development of sporadic gangliogliomas. *J Neuropathol Exp* 56: 806–10.

Potter CJ, Huang H, Xu T (2001) Drosophila Tsc1 functions with Tsc2 to antagonize insulin signaling in regulating cell growth, cell proliferation, and organ size. *Cell* 105: 357–68.

Potter CJ, Pedraza LG, Xu T (2002) Akt regulates growth by directly phosphorylating Tsc2. *Nat Cell Biol* 4: 658–65.

Povey S, Burley MW, Attwood J, Benham F, Hunt D, Jeremiah SJ, Franklin D, Gillett G, Malas S, Robson EB, Tippett P, Edwards JH, Kwiatkowski DJ, Super M, Mueller R, Fryer A, Clarke A, Webb D, Osborne J (1994) Two loci for tuberous sclerosis: one on 9q34 and one on 16p13. *Ann Hum Genet* 58: 107–27.

Rennebeck G, Kleymenova EV, Anderson R, Yeung RS, Artzt K, Walker CL (1998) Loss of function of the tuberous sclerosis 2 tumour suppressor gene results in embryonic lethality characterised by disrupted neuroepithelial growth and development. *Proc Natl Acad Sci USA* 95: 15629–34.

Rose VM, Au KS, Pollom G, Roach ES, Prashner HR, Northrup H (1999) Germ-line mosaicism in tuberous sclerosis: how common? *Am J Hum Genet* 64: 986–92.

Rubinfeld B, Munemitsu S, Clark R, Conroy L, Watt K, Crosier WJ, McCormick F, Polakis P (1991) Molecular cloning of a GTPase activating protein specific for the Krev-1 protein p21rap1. *Cell* 65: 1033–42.

Sampson JR, Scahill SJ, Stephenson JBP, Mann L, Connor JM (1989a) Genetic aspects of tuberous sclerosis in the West of Scotland. *J Med Genet* 26: 28–31.

Sampson JR, Yates JRW, Pirrit LA, Fleury P, Winship I, Beighton P, Connor JM (1989b) Evidence for genetic heterogeneity in tuberous sclerosis. *J Med Genet* 26: 511–16.

Sampson JR, Janssen LAJ, Sandkuijl LA, and the Tuberous Sclerosis Collaborative Group (1992) Linkage investigation of three putative tuberous sclerosis determining loci on chromosome 9q, 11q, and 12q. *J Med Genet* 29: 861–6.

Sampson JR, Maheshwar MM, Aspinwall R, Thompson P, Cheadle JP, Ravine D, Roy S, Haan E, Bernstein J, Harris PC (1997) Renal cystic disease in tuberous sclerosis: role of the polycystic kidney disease 1 gene. *Am J Hum Genet* 61: 843–51.

Sander C, Schneider R (1991) Database of homology-derived protein structures and the structural meaning of sequence alignment. *Proteins* 9: 56–68.

Satake N, Kobayashi T, Kobayashi E, Izumi K, Hino O (1999) Isolation and characterisation of a rat homologue of the human tuberous sclerosis 1 gene (*Tsc1*) and analysis of its mutations in rat renal carcinomas. *Cancer Res* 59: 849–55.

Scheffzek K, Ahmadian MR, Whittinghofer A (1998) GTPase-activating proteins: helping hands to complement an active site. *Trends in Biochem Sciences* 23: 257–62.

Sedman A, Bell P, Manco-Johnson M, Schrier R, Warady BA, Heard EO, Butler-Simon N, Gabow P (1987) Autosomal dominant polycystic kidney disease in childhood: a longitudinal study. *Kidney Int* 31: 1000–5.

Sepp T, Green AJ, Yates JRW (1996) Loss of heterozygosity in tuberous sclerosis hamartomas. *J Med Genet* 33: 962–4.

Smith M, Sperling D (1999) Novel 23-base-pair duplication mutation in *TSC1* exon 15 in an infant presenting with cardiac rhabdomyomas. *Am J Med Genet* 84: 346–9.

Smolarek TA, Wessner LL, McCormack FX, Mylet JC, Menon AG, Henske EP (1998) Evidence that lymphangiomyomatosis is caused by *TSC2* mutations: chromosome 16p13 loss of heterozygosity in angiomyolipomas and lymph nodes from women with lymphangiomyomatosis. *Am J Hum Genet* 62: 810–15.

Soucek T, Pusch O, Wienecke R, DeClue JE, Hengstschlager M (1997) Role of the tuberous sclerosis gene-2 product in cell cycle control. *J Biol Chem* 272: 29301–8.

Soucek, T, Yeung RS, Hengstschlager M (1998a) Inactivation of the cyclin-dependent kinase inhibitor p27 upon loss of the tuberous sclerosis complex gene-2. *Proc Natl Acad Sci USA* 95: 15653–8.

Tapon N, Ito N, Dickson BJ, Treisman JE, Hariharan IK (2001) The drosophila tuberous sclerosis complex gene homologs restrict cell growth and cell proliferation. *Cell* 105: 345–55.

van Bakel I, Sepp T, Ward S, Yates JRW, Green AJ (1997a) Mutations in the *TSC2* gene: analysis of the complete coding sequence using the protein truncation test (PTT). *Hum Mol Genet* 6: 1409–14.

van Bakel I, Sepp T, Yates JR, Green AJ (1997b) An EcoRV polymorphism in exon 40 of the tuberous sclerosis 2 (*TSC2*) gene. *Mol Cell Probes* 11: 75–6.

van Slegtenhorst M, Janssen B, Nellist M, Ramlakhan S, Hermans C, Hesseling A, van den Ouweland A, Kwiatkowski DJ, Eussen B, Sampson JR, de Jong P, Halley D (1995) Cosmid contigs from the tuberous sclerosis candidate region on chromosome 9q34. *Eur J Hum Genet* 3: 78–86.

van Slegtenhorst M, deHoogt R, Hermans C, Nellist M, Janssen B, Verhoef S, Lindhout D, van den Ouweland A, Halley D, Young J, Burley M, Jeremiah S, Woodward K, Nahmias J, Fox M, Ekong R, Osborne J, Wolfe J, Povey S, Snell RG, Cheadle JP, Jones AC, Tachataki M, Ravine D, Sampson JR, Reeve MP, Richardson P, Wilmer F, Munro C, Hawkins TL, Sepp T, Ali JBM, Ward S, Green AJ, Yates JRW, Kwiatkowska J, Henske EP, Short MP, Haines JH, Jóźwiak S, Kwiatkowski DJ (1997) Identification of the tuberous sclerosis gene *TSC1* on chromosome 9q34. *Science* 77: 805–8.

van Slegtenhorst M, Nellist M, Nagelkerken B, Cheadle J, Snell R, van den Ouweland A, Reuser A, Sampson J, Halley D, van der Sluijs P (1998) Interaction between hamartin and tuberin, the *TSC1* and *TSC2* gene products. *Hum Mol Genet* 7: 1053–7.

van Slegtenhorst M, Verhoef S, Tempelaars A, Bakker L, Wang Q, Wessels M, Bakker R, Nellist M, Lindhout D, Halley D, van den Ouweland A (1999) Mutational spectrum of the *TSC1* gene in a cohort of 225 tuberous sclerosis complex patients: no evidence for genotype-phenotype correlation. *J Med Genet* 36: 285–9.

Verhoef S, Vrtel R, van Essen TV, Bakker L, Sikkens E, Halley D, Lindhout D, van den

Ouweland A (1995) Somatic mosaicism and clinical variation in tuberous sclerosis complex. *Lancet* 345: 202.

Verhoef S, Bakker L, Tempelaars AMP, Hesseling-Janssen ALW, Mazurczak T, Jóźwiak S, Fois A, Bartalini G, Zonnenberg BA, van Essen AJ, Lindhout D, Halley DJJ, van den Ouweland AMW (1999) High rate of mosaicism in tuberous sclerosis complex. *Am J Hum Genet* 64: 1632–7.

Vrtel R, Verhoef S, Bouman K, Maheshwar MM, Nellist M, van Essen AJ, Bakker PL, Hermans CJ, Bink-Boelkens MT, van Elburg RM, Hoff M, Lindhout D, Sampson J, Halley DJ, van den Ouweland AM (1996) Identification of a nonsense mutation at the 5' end of the *TSC2* gene in a family with a presumptive diagnosis of tuberous sclerosis complex. *J Med Genet* 33: 47–51.

Wang Q, Verhoef S, Tempelaars AM, Bakker PL, Vrtel R, Hesseling-Janssen AL, Nellist M, Oranje AP, Stroink H, Lindhout D, Halley DJ, van den Ouweland AM (1998) Identification of a large insertion and two novel point mutations (3671del8 and S1221X) in tuberous sclerosis complex (TSC) patients. *Hum Mutat* 11: 331–2.

Wienecke R, Konig A, DeClue JE (1995) Identification of tuberin, the tuberous sclerosis-2 product – tuberin possesses specific rap1GAP activity. *J Biol Chem* 270: 16409–14.

Wienecke R, Maize JC, Shoarinejad F, Vass WC, Reed J, Bonifacino JS, Resau JH, de Gunzburg J, Yeung RS, DeClue JE (1996) Co-localization of the *TSC2* product tuberin with its target rap1 in the Golgi apparatus. *Oncogene* 13: 913–23.

Wienecke R, Maize JC, Reed JA, de Gunzburg J, Yeung RS, DeClue JE (1997) Expression of the *TSC2* product tuberin and its target rap1 in normal human tissues. *Am J Path* 150: 43–50.

Wilkie AOM, Buckle VJ, Harris PC, Lamb J, Barton NJ, Reeders ST, Lindenbaum RH, Nicholls RD, Barrow M, Bethlenfalvay NC, Hutz MH, Tolmie JL, Wetherall DJ, Higgs DR (1990) Clinical features and molecular analysis of the (-thalassemia/mental retardation syndromes. I. Cases due to deletions involving chromosome band 16p13.3. *Am J Hum Genet* 46: 1112–26.

Wilson PJ, Ramesh V, Kristiansen A, Bove C, Jóźwiak S, Kwiatkowski DJ, Short MP, Haines JL (1996) Novel mutations detected in the *TSC2* gene from both sporadic and familial TSC patients. *Hum Mol Genet* 5: 249–56.

Wolf DC, Whiteley HE, Everitt JI (1995) Preneoplastic and neoplastic lesions of rat hereditary renal cell tumours express markers of proximal and distal nephron. *Vet Pathol* 32: 379–86.

Xiao G-H, Shoarinejad F, Jin F, Golemis EA, Yeung RS (1997) The tuberous sclerosis 2 gene product, tuberin, functions as a rab5 GTPase activating protein (GAP) in modulating endocytosis. *J Biol Chem* 272: 6097–100.

Xu L, Sterner C, Maheshwar MM, Wilson PJ, Nellist M, Short PM, Haines JL, Sampson JR, Ramesh V (1995) Alternative splicing of the tuberous sclerosis 2 (*TSC2*) gene in human and mouse tissues. *Genomics* 27: 475–80.

Yates JR, van Bakel I, Sepp T, Payne SJ, Webb DW, Nevin NC, Green AJ (1997) Female germline mosaicism in tuberous sclerosis confirmed by molecular genetic analysis. *Hum Mol Genet* 6: 2265–9.

Yeung RS, Buetow KH, Testa JR, Knudson AG Jr (1993) Susceptibility to renal carcinoma in the Eker rat involves a tumour suppressor gene on chromosome 10. *Proc Natl Acad Sci USA* 90: 8038–42.

Yeung RS, Xiao GH, Jin F, Lee WC, Testa JR, Knudson AG (1994) Predisposition to renal carcinoma in the Eker rat is determined by germ-line mutation of the tuberous sclerosis 2 (*Tsc2*) gene. *Proc Natl Acad Sci USA* 91: 11413–16.

Yeung RS, Xiao GH, Everitt JI, Jin F, Walker CL (1995) Allelic loss at the tuberous sclerosis 2 locus in spontaneous tumours in the Eker rat. *Mol Carcinog* 14: 28–36.

Yeung RS, Katsetos CD, Klein-Szanto A (1997) Subependymal astrocytic hamartomas in the Eker rat model of tuberous sclerosis. *Am J Pathol* 151: 1477–86.

York RD, Yao H, Dillon T, Ellig CL, Eckert SP, McCleskey EW, Stork PJS (1998) rap1 mediates sustained MAP-kinase activation induced by nerve growth factor. *Nature* 392: 622–6.

Yoshida Y, Kawata M, Miura Y, Musha T, Sasaki T, Kikuchi A, Takai Y (1992) Microinjection of smg/rap1/Krev-1 p21 into Swiss 3T3 cells induces DNA synthesis and morphological changes. *Mol Cell Biol* 12: 3407–14.

Young JM, Burley MW, Jeremiah SJ, Jeganathan D, Ekong R, Osborne JP, Povey S (1998) A mutation screen of the *TSC1* gene reveals 26 protein truncating mutations and 1 splice site mutation in a panel of 79 tuberous sclerosis patients. *Ann Hum Genet* 62: 203–13.

Zhang H, Namba E, Yamamoto T, Ninomiya H, Ohno K, Mizuguchi M, Takeshita K (1999a) Mutational analysis of *TSC1* and *TSC2* genes in Japanese patients with tuberous sclerosis complex. *J Hum Genet* 44: 391–6.

Zhang H, Yamamoto T, Nanba E, Kitamura Y, Terada T, Akaboshi S, Yuasa I, Ohtani K, Nakamoto S, Takeshita K, Ohno K (1999b) Novel *TSC2* mutation in a patient with pulmonary tuberous sclerosis: lack of loss of heterozygosity in a lung cyst. *Am J Med Genet* 82: 368–70.

15
NEUROPATHOLOGY

Masashi Mizuguchi and Okio Hino

The pathology of tuberous sclerosis complex (TSC) is characterized by the development of hamartias and hamartomas in various organs, such as the brain, kidneys and heart. In the brain, there are three types of nodular lesions: cortical tubers, heterotopic nodules in the white matter, and subependymal nodules. The first two are static lesions (hamartias) closely related to epilepsy, learning disability and other neuropsychiatric symptoms of many TSC patients, whereas subependymal nodules often behave as a benign tumour (hamartoma), causing progressive hydrocephalus in a minority of cases. In the kidneys and heart, the most common hamartomas are angiomyolipomas and rhabdomyomas, respectively (Bender and Yunis 1982, Gomez 1987, Richardson 1991).

TSC is an autosomal dominant disorder manifested with variable phenotypes. Linkage studies have shown genetic heterogeneity of TSC, with the responsible genes on chromosome 9q34 (*TSC1*) and 16p13.3 (*TSC2*) (Fryer et al. 1987, Kandt et al. 1992), although there is little clinico-pathological distinction between these two. Compatible with their role as tumour suppressor genes, loss of heterozygosity (LOH) for alleles in 9q34 and 16p13.3 has been observed in the TSC-associated hamartomas (Carbonara et al. 1994, Green et al. 1994a, 1994b).

MORPHOLOGY OF CEREBRAL LESIONS

When brains of TSC patients are examined at surgery or necropsy, cortical tubers appear as a focal enlargement of the gyri, and are firm to palpation. They often protrude slightly above their neighbouring gyri, and occasionally have a central dimple (umbilication). Their number varies from zero to double digits, and their size ranges from a few millimetres to several centimetres (Bender and Yunis 1982, Gomez 1987, Richardson 1991).

Tubers can be found in the fetal cerebrum as early as 20 weeks gestation (Chow and Chow 1989, Park et al. 1997). On sectioning, tubers appear as undefined, pale nodules. Histologically, normal cortical lamination and the boundary between the grey and white matter are blurred (Fig. 15.1). There is usually a decrease in the number of neurons, as well as astrogliosis. Amyloid bodies are often found in excessive number. In the subpial layer, astrogliosis and aggregates of small round cells, which probably represent a remnant of the subpial germinal matrix layer, may be found. The major feature of tubers is the presence of abnormal giant cells, which

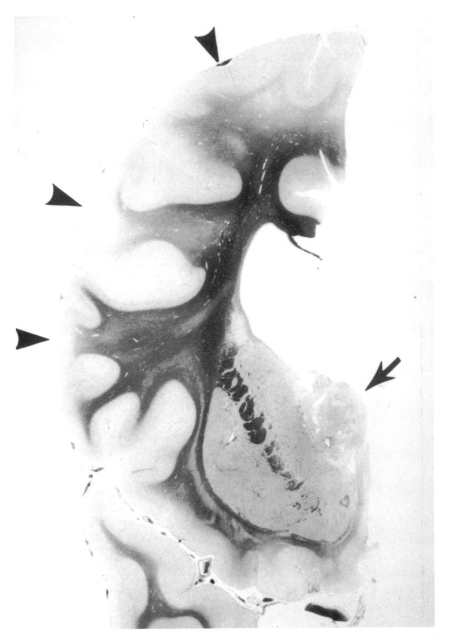

Fig. 15.1. Coronal section of the brain of a patient with tuberous sclerosis, stained with luxol fast blue and cresyl violet. There are cortical tubers (arrowheads) and a subependymal giant cell astrocytoma (arrow).

are 5 to 10 times larger than common neurons and astrocytes. These cells randomly show either a neuron-like or astrocyte-like appearance, or both (Fig. 15.2A and B). They may be scattered in a disorganized manner, or appear in clusters (Bender and Yunis 1982, Gomez 1987, Richardson 1991).

The white matter heterotopic nodules occur most frequently in the subcortical region underlying a cortical tuber. They show pathologic features similar to those of cortical tubers, such as the presence of giant cells (Fig. 15.2C), astrogliosis (especially around the blood vessels), and an excess of amyloid bodies. Several additional features, such as hypomyelination, loss of axons, and the presence of ectopic neurons with satellitosis, are also noted (Bender and Yunis 1982, Gomez 1987, Richardson 1991).

Subependymal nodules arise from the brain tissue surrounding the lateral ventricles, and protrude into the lumen (Fig. 15.1). In most cases the lesions are multiple, and vary in size from a few millimetres to several centimetres. They are often located along the thalamostriatus sulcus, assuming a "candle-guttering" appearance. Histologically, they are composed of round giant cells and spindle-shaped cells, both of which resemble astrocytes (Fig. 15.2D). The central part shows calcification.

During childhood and adolescence, subependymal nodules in some patients show a propensity to grow slowly. Occasionally the enlarged nodules obstruct the

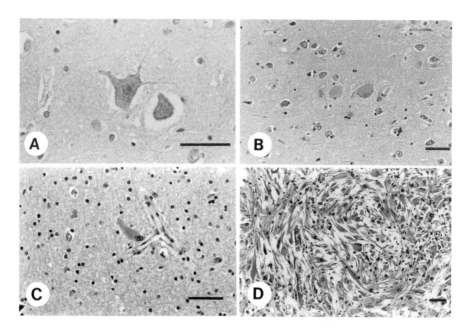

Fig. 15.2. Abnormal giant cells in a cortical tuber (A and B), a subcortical white matter heterotopic nodule (C), and a subependymal giant cell astrocytoma (D), showing neuron-like (A), astrocyte-like (B and D), or intermediate (C) features. Hematoxylin and eosin. Bars: 50 mm.

foramen of Monro, causing progressive hydrocephalus. Such behaviour simulates that of a benign tumour, and the constituent cells resemble gemistocytic (giant) astrocytes, hence the term "subependymal giant cell astrocytoma (SEGA)". However, from the cytological point of view, there is no essential difference between subependymal nodules and SEGAs. The tumours are well vasculized, and do not undergo malignant transformation (Bender and Yunis 1982, Gomez 1987, Richardson 1991).

CHARACTERISTICS OF ABNORMAL GIANT CELLS

Abnormal giant cells are the pathological hallmark of the TSC cerebral lesions. The histogenesis of these cells remains still ambiguous.

Under electron microscopic observation (Arseni et al. 1975, De Chadarevian and Hollenberg 1979, Bender and Yunis 1980, 1982, Trombey and Mirra 1988, Hirose et al. 1995), some giant cells show distinct neuronal features, whereas others resemble gemistocytic astrocytes. Cells with intermediate features are also seen (Fig. 15.2). Immunohistochemically, some giant cells are positive for neuronal markers, and others for astrocytic antigens (Hirose et al. 1995, Lopes et al. 1996). Occasionally, a single giant cell expresses both the neuronal and astrocytic features, either cytologically or immunohistochemically (Table 15.1). These findings indicate abnormal differentiation of these giant cells.

In addition, some abnormal giant cells express nestin (Yamanouchi et al. 1997) (Fig. 15.3) and other intermediate filament proteins specific for immature CNS cells (Table 15.1). The overdue expression of these markers in immature CNS cells represents another aspect of their abnormal differentiation.

EXPRESSION AND FUNCTION OF THE *TSC* GENE PRODUCTS

The two genes responsible for TSC, *TSC1* and *TSC2*, were cloned in 1997 and 1993, respectively (European Chromosome 16 Tuberous Sclerosis Consortium 1993, van Slegtenhorst et al. 1997). The product of *TSC1*, hamartin, is a protein with molecular weight of about 130 kilodalton, which is widely expressed in the brain, kidney, heart and many other organs (Plank et al. 1999, Gutmann et al. 2000, Mizuguchi et al. 2000a). Although much remains to be clarified about its function, hamartin interacts with the ezrin-radixin-moiesin family of actin-binding proteins, thereby activating the small GTP-binding protein Rho. The resultant assembly of actin fibres promotes cell adhesion to their substrate (Lamb et al. 2000). Thus, hamartin may suppress tumorigenesis via a Rho-mediated signalling pathway regulating cellular adhesion.

The *TSC2* gene product, tuberin, is a protein of about 180 kilodalton. Like hamartin, tuberin is widely expressed in most organs (Geist and Gutmann 1995, Kerfoot et al. 1996, Mizuguchi et al. 1997, Wienecke et al. 1997). Tuberin has a region homologous to guanosine triphosphatase (GTPase)-activating proteins (GAPs) near its carboxy terminus, and indeed possesses GAP activities for Rap1, a member

TABLE 15.1
Cytological and immunohistochemical characteristics of abnormal giant cells

	Neuronal features	Astrocytic features
Light microscopic	Large, centrally placed nucleus with a prominent nucleolus Nissl bodies Neurofibrils	Convoluted or multiple nuclei without prominent nucleoli
Electron microscopic	Lamellar stacks of rough endoplastic reticulum Microtubules Synapses Dense-core granules	Glial filaments Numerous lysosomes
Immunohistochemical	Neurofilament proteins Class IIIb-tubulin Microtubule-associated protein 2 Calbindin D-28k Neuron-specific enolase Chromogranin A Somatostatin Met-enkephalin 5-Hydroxytryptamine Neuropeptide Y	Glial fibrillary acidic protein S-100 protein ß-Crystallin *Immature features* Nestin Vimentin Microtubule-associated protein 1B

of the Ras superfamily that may function as a positive mitogenic signalling molecule (Wienecke et al. 1995), and for Rab5, a modulator of fluid-phase endocytosis (Xiao et al. 1997). Tuberin plays a role in cell cycle control by inhibiting the transition from G0/G1 to S phase (Soucek et al. 1997). A *Drosophila* homolog of *TSC2*, *gigas*, also regulates the cell cycle by blocking DNA replication or promoting mitosis (Ito and Rubin 1999). On the other hand, much remains to be elucidated about the possible role of tuberin in cellular differentiation. It has recently been shown that in neuroblastoma cell lines, tuberin expression is upregulated upon induction of neuronal differentiation (Soucek et al. 1998).

Although hamartin and tuberin have no structural homology mutually, they bind and interact with each other in vitro, mediated by their coiled-coil domains (Plank et al. 1998, van Slegtenhorst et al. 1998). Tuberin may act as a chaperone which prevents hamartin from self-aggregation (Nellist et al. 1999). These interactions may account for the similarities of phenotypes between *TSC1* and *TSC2* mutations.

Hamartin and tuberin also show a similar pattern of distribution in vivo. From an immunohistochemical point of view, both the proteins are localized in the

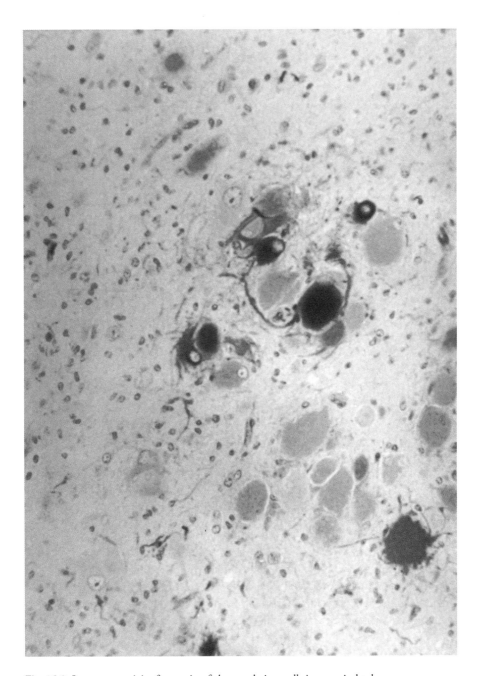

Fig. 15.3. Immunoreactivity for nestin of abnormal giant cells in a cortical tuber.

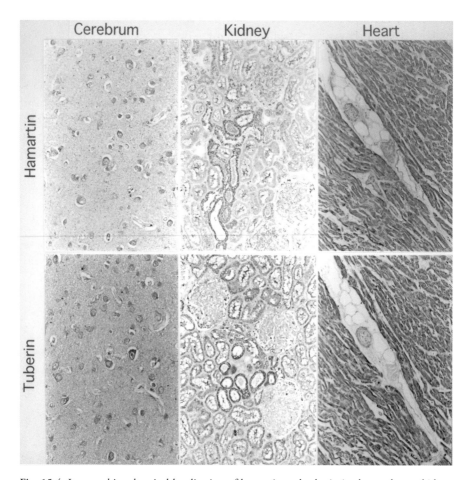

Fig. 15.4. Immunohistochemical localization of hamartin and tuberin in the cerebrum, kidney and heart of control patients, showing nearly identical distribution of the two proteins.

uriniferous and collecting tubules in the kidneys, and in the myocardium in the heart (Plank et al. 1999, Mizuguchi et al. 2000a) (Fig. 15.4). In the brain, positive immunoreactivities are present in the cytoplasm of neurons and astrocytes (Gutmann et al. 2000, Mizuguchi et al. 2000a) (Fig. 15.4). However, the two proteins do not always co-localize; some differences in their distribution have recently been demonstrated (Gutmann et al. 2000, Murthy et al. 2000).

ALTERATION OF THE *TSC* GENE PRODUCTS IN TSC LESIONS
Studies on the expression of hamartin and tuberin have disclosed a variable degree of their loss in TSC lesions, confirming their critical role in the pathogenesis of TSC. However, there is a considerable discrepancy among these studies, making interpretation of their findings difficult.

In the kidney and heart, hamartomas (renal angiomyolipomas and cardiac rhabdomyomas) show a focal reduction of immunoreactivity for hamartin and/or tuberin (Mizuguchi et al. 1997, Plank et al. 1999, Mizuguchi et al. 2000a), nicely fitting with the two-hit model of tumorigenesis (Knudson 1971). A recent study found the loss of either hamartin or tuberin in *TSC1-* and *TSC2*-linked angiomyolipomas, respectively. These findings may enable distinction between *TSC1* and *TSC2* mutations by immunohistochemical means (Plank et al. 1999). By contrast, our recent study demonstrated simultaneous loss of both proteins (Mizuguchi et al. 2000a) (Fig. 15.5). This finding appears to agree with the putative interactions

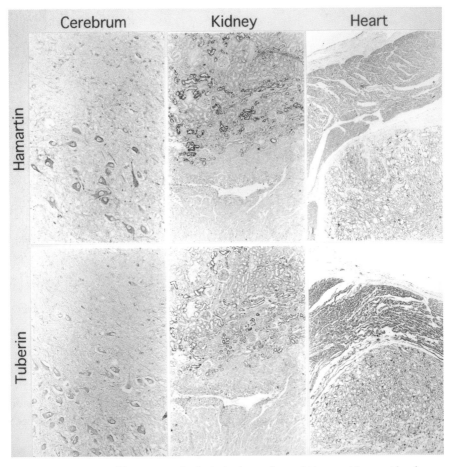

Fig. 15.5. Expression of hamartin and tuberin in the cerebrum, kidney and heart with tuberous sclerosis. The staining patterns of the two proteins are similar. In the cerebrum, the overall labelling intensity is decreased, although abnormal giant cells of a tuber (bottom) show positive labelling. In a renal angiomyolipoma and a cardiac rhabdomyoma (lower half of each panel), there is loss of immunoreactivity for both hamartin and tuberin.

described above, and may well account for the phenotypic similarity between *TSC1* and *TSC2* mutations.

With regard to the cerebrum, the situation is even more confusing. Based on the results of immunohistochemical studies, many investigators agree that SEGAs show loss of hamartin and/or tuberin (Henske et al. 1997, Kimura et al. 1997, Arai et al. 1998). This finding is further supported by our Western blotting data which demonstrated semi-quantitatively their reduction in three SEGAs (Mizuguchi et al. 1996, 2000a). What is problematic is their expression in cortical tubers. The results of our Western blotting studies revealed the reduction of both hamartin and tuberin in a tuber of one patient with a *TSC2* mutation (Fig. 15.6). However, immunostaining using the same tissue materials disclosed positive labelling of abnormal giant cells, the intensity of which is by no means negligible (Mizuguchi et al. 1996, 2000a) (Fig. 15.7). Other investigators have observed that the TSC gene expression, either at mRNA or protein levels, is normal or even enhanced in giant cells (Kerfoot et al. 1996, Menchine et al. 1996, Arai et al. 1998, Jones et al. 1999). This apparently contradicts the two-hit model of their developmental origin.

Genetic studies have so far failed to clarify this issue (Henske et al. 1996). When DNA extracted from frozen tissue materials of cortical tubers is used, it is difficult

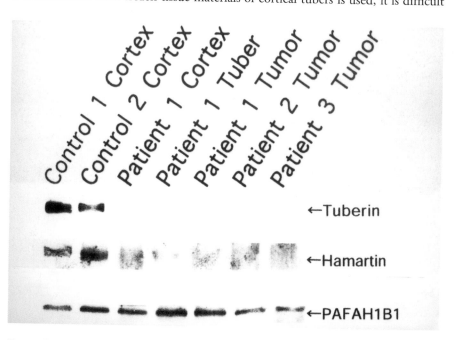

Fig. 15.6. Western blotting for hamartin and tuberin of cerebral tissues from control patients (left two lanes) and from those with tuberous sclerosis (right five lanes). Both the proteins are abundant in control cortices, but decreased in all the TSC tissues. The amount of a control protein, PAFAH1B1, is unaltered. Tumour denotes subependymal giant cell astrocytoma.

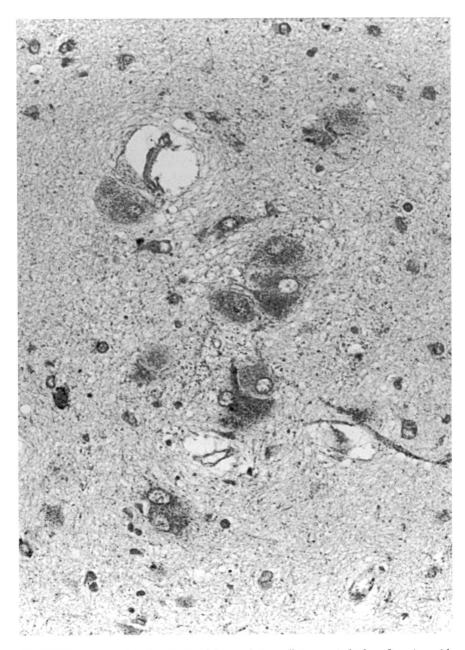

Fig. 15.7. Immunoreactivity for tuberin of abnormal giant cells in a cortical tuber of a patient with TSC (Patient 1 of Fig. 15.6) carrying a *TSC2* mutation.

to detect LOH in abnormal giant cells. To further elucidate their cytogenesis, DNA analyses of single cells should provide useful information (Crino et al. 1996).

CEREBRAL LESIONS OF THE EKER RAT MODEL

Pathologic studies on human material are often hampered by several obstacles. First, the opportunity to obtain cerebral tissues, especially from mild cases, is limited. Second, the DNA diagnosis of TSC is not only laborious, but also fails to reveal the causative mutation in about a third of cases (Jones et al. 1999, Zhang et al. 1999, Yamashita et al. 2000). It is often impossible to determine the genotype of old necropsy cases because neither blood samples nor frozen tissues are available. Third, human TSC is genetically heterogeneous. Different types of mutations may result in inconsistent findings in immunohistochemical studies. The phenotypes are highly variable even in a single family, which also complicates analyses.

These problems can be overcome by the use of animal models of TSC. The Eker rat is an autosomal dominant trait caused by a germline insertion mutation in the rat *Tsc2* gene (Kobayashi et al. 1995). Carriers of the mutation always develop multiple renal cell carcinomas (Everitt et al. 1992, Hino et al. 1993). Although no clinical signs of neurological dysfunction have been described so far, we and other investigators have recently found the following CNS lesions:

Cortical tuber. This lesion shows features similar to those of human tubers, such as the loss of normal cortical lamination, decrease in neuronal density and astrogliosis. There are many abnormal giant cells (cytomegalic neurons), showing intense immunoreactivity for non-phosphorylated neurofilament protein (NF), a marker for mature neurons (Mizuguchi et al. 2000b).

Subcortical hamartoma. This lesion shows hypomyelination and focal calcification, and consists of abnormal large cells intermingled with elongated cell processes. Some of these cells are positive for glial fibrillary acidic protein (GFAP), a marker for astrocytes. Others are immunoreactive for NF (Yeung et al. 1997, Mizuguchi et al. 2000b).

Subependymal hamartoma. This occurs most frequently in the basal ganglia. Its histologic and immunohistochemical features are similar to those of subcortical hamartomas (Yeung et al. 1997, Mizuguchi et al. 2000b).

Anaplastic ganglioglioma. This malignant neoplasm consists of densely packed tumour cells exhibiting pleomorphism, nuclear atypism and a high mitotic index. Immunohistochemically, some tumour cells are positive for synaptophysin, NF and other neuronal markers, whereas others are immunoreactive for GFAP, vimentin and other glial markers (Mizuguchi et al. 2000b).

Each of the first three lesions above has its counterpart in human TSC (Table 15.2). By contrast, anaplastic ganglioglioma is absent from the brains of TSC patients, where occurrence of a malignant brain tumour is exceedingly rare (Padmaltha et al. 1980). In general, the incidence of malignancies, such as renal cell

TABLE 15.2
Human TSC and Eker rat cerebral lesions

Human TSC	Eker rat
Cortical tuber	Cortical tuber
Heterotopic nodule in the white matter	Subcortical hamartoma
Subependymal nodule (giant cell astrocytoma)	Subependymal hamartoma
	Anaplastic ganglioglioma

carcinomas and splenic hemangiosarcomas, is much higher in Eker rats than in human TSC patients (Hino et al. 1994).

In all the Eker rat cerebral lesions, there is loss of tuberin immunoreactivity (Mizuguchi et al. 2000b). The molecular mechanism by which this occurs is currently under investigation. From the standpoint of clinical neuroscience, studies on the rat cortical tuber are the most important. This is because we currently know too little about the pathogenetic mechanism of tubers, which cause most of the distressing neurological symptoms in human TSC patients.

ACKNOWLEDGEMENTS
We thank Professors Sachio Takashima (National Institute of Neuroscience), Hideo Yamanouchi (Dept of Pediatrics, Dokkyo University School of Medicine) and Yoichi Nakazato (Dept of Pathology, Gunma University School of Medicine) for their helpful comments. This research was supported in part by a Grant-in-Aid for Scientific Research (10670753) from the Ministry of Education, Science and Culture, Japan, Grants for Research on Neurocutaneous Diseases (3310) from the Ministry of Health and Welfare, Japan, and a Grant for Pharmaceutical Safety and Research, Japan.

REFERENCES
Arai Y, Ackerley CA, Becker LE (1998) Loss of the *TSC2* product tuberin in subependymal giant-cell tumors. *Acta Neuropathol* 98: 233–9.

Arseni C, Alexianu M, Horvat L, Alexianu D (1975) Fine structure of atypical cells in tuberous sclerosis. *Acta Neuropathol* 21: 185–93.

Bender BL, Yunis EJ (1980) Central nervous system pathology of tuberous sclerosis in children. *Ultrastruct Pathol* 1: 287–99.

Bender BL, Yunis EJ (1982) The pathology of tuberous sclerosis. *Pathol Annu* 17: 339–82.

Carbonara C, Longa L, Grosso E, Borrone C, Garre MG, Brisigotti M, Migone N (1994) 9q34 loss of heterozygosity in a tuberous sclerosis astrocytoma suggests a growth suppressor-like activity also for the TSC1 gene. *Hum Mol Genet* 3: 1829–32.

Chow TM, Chow SM (1989) Tuberous sclerosis in the premature infant: a report of a case with immunohistochemistry on the CNS. *Clin Neuropathol* 8: 45–52.

Crino PB, Trojanowski JQ, Dichter MA, Eberwine J (1996) Embryonic neural markers in tuberous sclerosis: single-cell molecular pathology. *Proc Natl Acad Sci USA* 93: 14152–7.

De Chadarevian J-P, Hollenberg RD (1979) Subependymal giant-cell tumor of tuberous sclerosis: a light and ultrastructural study. *J Neuropathol Exp Neurol* 38: 419–33.

European Chromosome 16 Tuberous Sclerosis Consortium (1993) Identification and characterization of the tuberous sclerosis gene on chromosome 16. *Cell* 75: 1305–15.

Everitt JI, Goldworthy TL, Wolf DC, Walker CL (1992) Hereditary renal cell carcinoma in the Eker rat: a rodent familial cancer syndrome. *J Urol* 148: 1932–6.

Fryer AE, Chalmers A, Connor JM, Fraser I, Povey S, Yates AD, Yates JRW, Osborne JP (1987) Evidence that the gene for tuberous sclerosis is on chromosome 9. *Lancet* 1: 659–61.

Geist RT, Gutmann DH (1995) The tuberous sclerosis 2 gene is expressed at high levels in the cerebellum and developing spinal cord. *Cell Growth Differ* 6: 1477–83.

Gomez MR (1987) Tuberous sclerosis. In: Gomez MR, Adams RD (eds) *Neurocutaneous Diseases. A Practical Approach*, Boston: Butterworths, pp 30–52.

Green AJ, Johnson PH, Yates JR (1994a) The tuberous sclerosis gene on chromosome 9q34 acts as a growth suppressor. *Hum Mol Genet* 3: 1833–4.

Green AJ, Smith M, Yates JR (1994b) Loss of heterozygosity on chromosome 16p13.3 in hamartomas from tuberous sclerosis patients. *Nat Genet* 6: 193–6.

Gutmann DH, Zhang Y, Hasbani MJ, Goldberg MP, Plank TL, Henske EP (2000) Expression of the tuberous sclerosis complex gene products, hamartin and tuberin, in central nervous system tissues. *Acta Neuropathol* 99: 223–30.

Henske EP, Scheithauer BW, Short MP, Wollmann R, Nahmias J, Hornigold N, van Slegtenhorst M, Welsh CT, Kwiatkowski DJ (1996) Allelic loss is frequent in tuberous sclerosis kidney lesions but rare in brain lesions. *Am J Hum Genet* 59: 400–6.

Henske EP, Wessner LL, Golden J, Scheithauer BW, Vortmeyer AO, Zhuang Z, Klein-Szanto AJP, Kwiatkowski DJ, Yeung RS (1997) Loss of tuberin in both subependymal giant cell astrocytomas and angiomyolipomas supports a two-hit model for the pathogenesis of tuberous sclerosis tumors. *Am J Pathol* 151: 1639–47.

Hino O, Klein-Szanto AJP, Freed JJ, Testa JR, Brown DQ, Vilensky M, Yeung RS, Tartof KD, Knudson AG (1993) Spontaneous and radiation-induced renal tumors in the Eker rat model of inherited cancer. *Proc Natl Acad Sci USA* 90: 327–31.

Hino O, Mitani H, Katsuyama H, Kubo Y (1994) A novel cancer predisposition syndrome in the Eker rat model. *Cancer Lett* 83: 117–21.

Hirose T, Scheithauer BW, Lopes MBS, Gerber HA, Altermatt HJ, Hukee MJ, VandenBerg SR, Charlesworth JC (1995) Tuber and subependymal giant cell astrocytoma associated with tuberous sclerosis: an immunohistochemical, ultrastructural, and immunoelectron microscopic study. *Acta Neuropathol* 90: 387–99.

Ito N, Rubin GM (1999) *Gigas*, a *Drosophila* homolog of tuberous sclerosis gene product-2, regulates the cell cycle. *Cell* 96: 529–39.

Johnson MW, Emelin JK, Park S-H, Vinters HV (1999) Co-localization of TSC1 and TSC2 gene products in tubers of patients with tuberous sclerosis. *Brain Pathol* 9: 45–54.

Jones AC, Shyamsunder MM, Thomas MW, Maynard J, Idziaszczyk S, Tomkins S, Sampson JR, Cheadle JP (1999) Comprehensive mutation analysis of *TSC1* and *TSC2* and phenotypic correlations in 150 families with tuberous sclerosis. *Am J Hum Genet* 64: 1305–15.

Kandt RS, Haines JL, Smith M, Northrup H, Gardner RJM, Short MP, Dumars K, Roach ES, Steingold S, Wall S, Blanton SH, Flodman P, Kwiatkowski DJ, Jewell A, Weber JL, Roses AD, Piricak-Vance MA (1992) Linkage of an important gene locus for tuberous sclerosis to a chromosome 16 marker for polycystic kidney disease. *Nat Genet* 2: 37–41.

Kerfoot C, Wienecke R, Menchine M, Emelin J, Maize JC Jr, Welsh CT, Norman MG, DeClue JE, Vinters HV (1996) Localization of tuberous sclerosis 2 mRNA and its protein product tuberin in normal human brain and in cerebral lesions of patients with tuberous sclerosis. *Brain Pathol* 6: 367–77.

Kimura N, Watanabe M, Date F, Kitamoto T, Kimura I, Horii A, Nagura H (1997) HMB-45 and tuberin in hamartomas associated with tuberous sclerosis. *Mod Pathol* 10: 952–9.

Knudson AGJ (1971) Mutation and cancer: statistical study of retinoblastoma. *Proc Natl Acad Sci USA* 68: 820–3.

Kobayashi T, Hirayama Y, Kobayashi E, Kubo Y, Hino O (1995) A germline insertion in the tuberous sclerosis (*Tsc2*) gene gives rise to the Eker rat model of dominantly inherited cancer. *Nat Genet* 9: 70–4.

Lamb RF, Roy C, Diefenbach TJ, Vinters HV, Johnson DG, Hall A (2000) The *TSC1* tumor suppressor hamartin regulates cell adhesion through ERM proteins and the GTPase Rho. *Nat Cell Biol* 2: 281–7.

Lopes MB, Altermatt HJ, Scheithauer BW, Shepherd CW, VandenBerg SR (1996) Immuno-histochemical characterization of subependymal giant cell astrocytomas. *Acta Neuropathol* 91: 368–75.

Menchine M, Emelin JK, Mischel PS, Haag TA, Norman MG, Pepkowitz SH, Welsh CT, Townsend JT, Vinters HV (1996) Tissue and cell-type specific expression of the tuberous sclerosis gene, *TSC2*, in human tissues. *Mod Pathol* 9: 1071–80.

Mizuguchi M, Kato M, Yamanouchi H, Ikeda K, Takashima S (1996) Loss of tuberin from cerebral tissues with tuberous sclerosis and astrocytoma. *Ann Neurol* 40: 941–4.

Mizuguchi M, Kato M, Yamanouchi H, Ikeda K, Takashima S (1997) Tuberin immuno-histochemistry in brain, kidneys and heart with or without tuberous sclerosis. *Acta Neuropathol* 94: 525–31.

Mizuguchi M, Ikeda K, Takashima S (2000a) Simultaneous loss of hamartin and tuberin from the cerebrum, kidney and heart with tuberous sclerosis. *Acta Neuropathol* 99: 503–10.

Mizuguchi M, Takashima S, Yamanouchi H, Nakazato Y, Mitani H, Hino O (2000b) Novel cerebral lesions in the Eker rat model of tuberous sclerosis: cortical tuber and anaplastic ganglioglioma. *J Neuropathol Exp Neurol* 59: 188–96.

Murthy V, Haddad LA, Smith N, Pinney D, Tyskowski R, Brown D, Ramesh V (2000) Similarities and differences in the subcellular localization of hamartin and tuberin in the kidney. *Am J Physiol Renal Physiol* 278: F737–46.

Nellist M, van Slegtenhorst MA, Goedbloed M, van den Ouweland AMW, Halley DJJ, van der Sluijs P (1999) Characterization of the cytosolic tuberin-hamartin complex. Tuberin is a cytosolic chaperone for hamartin. *J Biol Chem* 274: 35647–52.

Padmaltha C, Harruff RC, Ganick D, Hafez GB (1980) Glioblastoma multiforme with tuberous sclerosis. Report of a case. *Arch Pathol Lab Med* 104: 649–50.

Park SH, Pepkowitz SH, Kefoot C, de Rosa MJ, Poukens V, Wienecke R, DeClue JE, Vinters HV (1997) Tuberous sclerosis in a 20-week gestation fetus: immunohistochemical study. *Acta Neuropathol* 94: 180–6.

Plank TL, Yeung RS, Henske EP (1998) Hamartin, the product of the tuberous sclerosis 1 (*TSC1*) gene, interacts with tuberin and appears to be localized to cytoplasmic vesicles. *Cancer Res* 58: 4766–70.

Plank TL, Loggindou H, Klein-Szanto A, Henske EP (1999) The expression of hamartin, the product of the *TSC1* gene, in normal human tissues and in *TSC1*- and *TSC2*-linked angiomyolipomas. *Mod Pathol* 12: 539–45.

Richardson EP Jr (1991) Pathology of tuberous sclerosis. Neuropathologic aspects. *Ann NY Acad Sci* 615: 128–39.

Soucek T, Pusch O, Wienecke R, DeClue JE, Hengstschlager M (1997) Role of the tuberous sclerosis gene-2 product in cell cycle control. Loss of the tuberous sclerosis gene-2 induces quiescent cells to enter S phase. *J Biol Chem* 272: 29301–8.

Soucek T, Holzl G, Bernaschek G, Hengstschlager M (1998) A role of the tuberous sclerosis gene-2 product during neuronal differentiation. *Oncogene* 16: 2197–204.

Trombey IK, Mirra SS (1988) Ultrastructure of tuberous sclerosis: cortical tuber and subependymal tumor. *Ann Neurol* 9: 174–81.

van Slegtenhorst M, de Hoogt R, Hermans C, Nellist M, Janssen B, Verhoef S, Lindhout D, van den Ouweland A, Halley D, Young J, Burley M, Jeremiah S, Woodward K, Nahmias J, Fox M, Ekong R, Osborne J, Wolfe J, Povey S, Snell RG, Cheadle JP, Jones AC, Tachataki M, Ravine D, Sampson JR, Reeve MP, Richardson P, Wilmer F, Munro C, Hawkins TL, Sepp T, Ali JBM, Ward S, Green AJ, Yates JRW, Kwiatkowska J, Henske EP, Short MP, Haines JH, Jóźwiak S, Kwiatkowski DJ (1997) Identification of the tuberous sclerosis gene *TSC1* on chromosome 9q34. *Science* 277: 805–8.

van Slegtenhorst M, Nellist M, Nagelkerken B, Cheadle J, Snell R, van den Ouweland A, Reuser A, Sampson J, Halley D, van der Sluijs P (1998) Interaction between hamartin and tuberin, the TSC1 and TSC2 gene products. *Hum Mol Genet* 7: 1053–7.

Wienecke R, Konig A, DeClue JE (1995) Identification of tuberin, the tuberous sclerosis-2 product. Tuberin possesses specific Rap1GAP activity. *J Biol Chem* 170: 16409–14.

Wienecke RW, Maize JC Jr, Reed JA, de Gunzburg J, Yeung RS, DeClue JE (1997) Expression of the *TSC2* product tuberin and its target Rap1 in normal human tissues. *Am J Pathol* 150: 43–50.

Xiao GH, Shoarinejad F, Jin F, Golemis EA, Yeung RS (1997) The tuberous sclerosis 2 gene product, tuberin, functions as a Rab5 GTPase activating protein (GAP) in modulating endocytosis. *J Biol Chem* 272: 6097–100.

Yamanouchi H, Jay V, Rutka JT, Takashima S, Becker LE (1997) Evidence of abnormal differentiation in giant cells of tuberous sclerosis. *Pediatr Neurol* 17: 49–53.

Yamashita Y, Ono J, Okada S, Wataya-Kaneda M, Yoshikawa K, Nishizawa M, Hirayama Y, Kobayashi E, Seyama K, Hino O (2000) Analysis of all exons of *TSC1* and *TSC2* genes for germline mutation in Japanese patients with tuberous sclerosis: report of 10 mutations. *Am J Med Genet* 90: 123–6.

Yeung RS, Katsetos CD, Klein-Szanto A (1997) Subependymal astrocytic hamartoma in the Eker rat model of tuberous sclerosis. *Am J Pathol* 151: 1477–86.

Zhang H, Nanba E, Yamamoto T, Ninomiya H, Ohno K, Mizuguchi M, Takeshita K (1999) Mutational analysis of *TSC1* and *TSC2* genes in Japanese patients with tuberous sclerosis complex. *J Hum Genet* 44: 391–6.

16
MOLECULAR NEUROBIOLOGY

Peter B Crino

The tuberous sclerosis complex (TSC) is an autosomal disorder resulting from mutations in one of two genes, *TSC1* or *TSC2* (for review, see Short et al. 1995, Crino and Henske 1999). Epilepsy occurs in 70 to 80% of TSC patients (Shepherd 1999). The CNS lesions of TSC include tubers in the cerebral cortex, and subependymal nodules (SENs) and subependymal giant cell astrocytomas (SEGAs) in the ventricular system (Richardson 1991, Hirose et al. 1995). Recently, the clinical diagnostic criteria for TSC were revised into major and minor features which provide the latest approach to accurate diagnosis of TSC (Roach et al. 1998). Tubers, SENs and SEGAs are considered major criteria for TSC (Roach et al. 1998).

Tubers are developmental abnormalities of cerebral cortical cytoarchitecture identified in TSC patients, characterized histologically by disorganized cortical lamination and cells with aberrant morphologies (Richardson 1991). These characteristic brain lesions with a potato- or root-like (hence tuber) consistency were first described by Bourneville in 1880. It is likely that tubers result from aberrant neuronal migration during corticogenesis. Tubers are directly related to the more common neurological manifestations of TSC including epilepsy, learning disability (LD) and autism. These symptoms are highly variable in age of onset and severity in patients with TSC.

Tubers exhibit abnormal metabolism on FDG-PET imaging, and correlative EEG/MRI analysis has revealed that tubers are epileptogenic (Tamaki et al. 1990, Chugani et al. 1998, Guerreiro et al. 1998). Seizures in TSC patients are often refractory to medical management despite anticonvulsant polytherapy. Surgical resection of tubers may be necessary to achieve adequate seizure control (Bebin et al. 1993, Guerreiro et al. 1998).

In contrast, SENs are nodular lesions which extend into the ventricles and are typically asymptomatic. SENs which enlarge can cause hydrocephalus and are referred to as SEGAs. This chapter will address the neuropathologic features of tubers, SENs and SEGAs, and specifically evaluate the molecular pathogenesis of these lesions as it relates to the genetic mutations responsible for TSC.

NEUROPATHOLOGY OF TSC LESIONS
The neuropathologic hallmarks of TSC, including tubers, SENs and SEGAs, have been comprehensively reviewed (Richardson 1991, Scheithauer and Reagan 1999).

Of these TSC lesions, tubers are most closely associated with epilepsy, LD and autism. SENs are largely asymptomatic and seem to be unrelated to neurological symptoms. However, SENs that continue to grow are designated as SEGAs, and these lesions can cause compression and obstructive hydrocephalus. In severe cases, SEGAs can lead to patient death. Additional though more infrequent CNS manifestations of TSC include regions of focal cortical dysplasia that are radiographically and histologically distinct from tubers, white matter migration lines, cerebellar foliar atrophy, Purkinje cell loss, and tuber-like hamartomas in the cerebellum. The spinal cord and peripheral nerves are surprisingly unaffected in TSC.

Tubers are found most commonly in the fronto-parietal cortical regions (but may be found in any cortical region) and are present in over 80% of TSC patients (Richardson 1991, Wiestler et al. 1997). Tubers may be detected radiographically in the neonatal period, and have been identified histologically in fetal life as earlier as 20 weeks gestation (Sonigo et al. 1996, Park et al. 1997). On gross pathologic examination, tubers are firm, well-circumscribed nodules which span flattened gyri and sulci. On microscopic examination, the normal hexalaminar structure of neocortex is lost within the tuber and the grey-white junction is blurred (Fig. 16.1). Interestingly, the cytoarchitecture of cerebral cortex surrounding tubers is typically

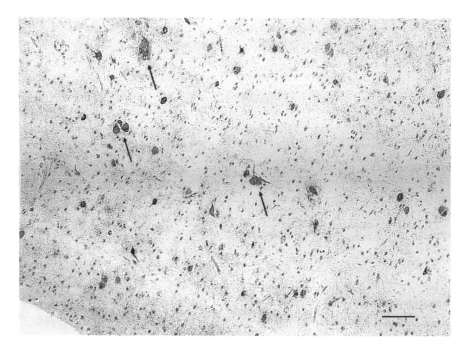

Fig. 16.1. Section of a cortical tuber resected during epilepsy surgery immunolabelled with nestin antibodies. Note heterogeneous population of cell types including giant cells and dysmorphic neurons.

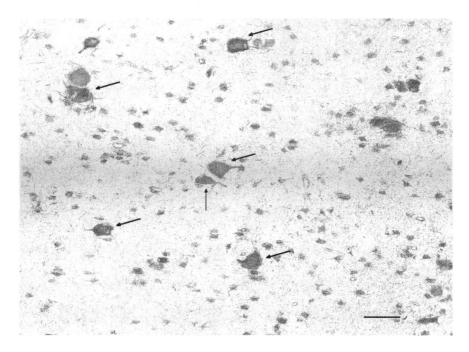

Fig. 16.2. Section of tuber immunolabelled with NeuN antibodies. Note GCs expressing this neuronal marker (large arrows) that are adjacent to DNs (short arrow).

normal, suggesting that tubers result from a developmental defect affecting a restricted population of neuronal precursor cells during corticogenesis. The most prominent abnormal cell types in tubers are large dysplastic neurons (DNs) and giant cells (GCs, see below), as well as bizarrely shaped astrocytes (Fig. 16.2). DNs exhibit disrupted radial orientation in cortex and abnormal dendritic arborization. Heterotopic neurons scattered in the deep white matter are also a frequent finding. Restricted foci of gliosis and cortical dysplasia may also be identified in patients with other manifestations of TSC which are histologically distinct from tubers.

Subependymal nodules are well-circumscribed lesions found along the surface of the lateral ventricles and rarely within the aqueduct and fourth ventricle (Richardson 1991, Wiestler et al. 1997, Scheithauer and Reagan 1999). They occur in approximately 80% of TSC patients and may be present in the neonatal period. SENs may extend into the surrounding white matter and abut the basal ganglia. SENs do not undergo neoplastic transformation, but a subpopulation of SENs may exhibit exuberant cell growth and are then classified as SEGAs which are WHO grade I tumours. SEGAs typically develop within the first two decades of life, but may be detected in infancy (Tien et al. 1990). Many of the cellular constituents of features of SENs and SEGAs, such as GCs, are similar to those of tubers (see below). However, the cellular packing density in SENs/SEGAs is greater than in tubers, and these lesions have the cytopathologic appearance of a tumour. For example, in SEGAs, multinucleated cells may be seen with rare mitotic figures and cellular pleomorphism. In addition to GCs, a heterogeneous array of astrocytic, polygonal, epithelioid, and spindle-cell populations may also be seen. Vascular endothelial proliferation and necrosis may be observed, yet SEGAs exhibit a low mitotic index, as evidenced by MIB-1 immunolabelling, which reinforces the benign nature of these lesions (Gyure and Prayson 1997, Scheithauer and Reagan 1999). Despite the histologic similarities between SENs and SEGAs, the molecular events that govern ongoing cellular proliferation within SENs and a transition into SEGAs remain to be defined.

GCs are the hallmark histologic cell type within tubers, SENs and SEGAs which is unique to TSC (Fig. 16.3). They are large (80–150 microns in diameter), polygonal or ovoid eosinophilic cells which extend short, thickened processes of unclear identity (i.e. axons or dendrites). GCs are distributed from the pial surface to the

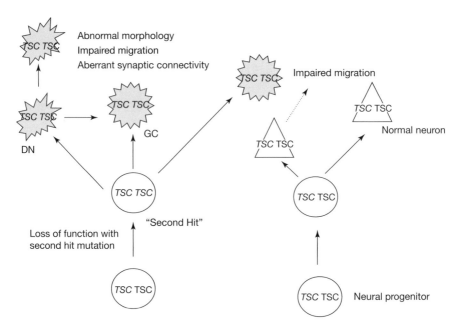

Fig. 16.3. Schematic of giant cell formation by second-hit mechanism. A neural progenitor cell has one normal TSC allele and one existing TSC mutation (italics and bold). A second-hit mutation occurs and there is inactivation of the normal allele so that the cells contain two mutated TSC genes. The progenitor cell with two mutations can give rise to a giant cell (GC) only or to a mixed population of GCs and dysplastic neurons (DNs). These cells exhibit abnormal morphology, make aberrant synaptic connections, and migrate to inappropriate laminae. In addition, GCs (or DNs) may block the migratory pathways of adjacent "normal" neurons containing only one mutated TSC gene, and further disrupt the formation of appropriate synaptic connections during brain development.

subcortical white matter without clear radial or laminar orientation and they may appear in clusters. They do not exhibit preference for superficial or deeper parts of cortex.

The cell lineage and phenotype of GCs have been a matter of some debate, since GCs have been shown to express both glial and astrocytic markers. Indeed, a fundamental question regarding the pathogenesis of CNS lesions in TSC is which cell precursors, i.e. glial or neuronal, give rise to GCs in tubers, SENs and SEGAs during early brain development. Early evidence argued independently for neuronal or glial lineage of giant cells, based on identification of neuronal or glial structural features using electron microscopy (Trombley and Mirra 1981, Yamanouchi et al. 1997). For example, the identification of rough endoplasmic reticulum, intermediate filaments extending into processes of ambiguous morphology, prominent paranu-clear Golgi zones, and dense-core granules (suggestive of secretory vesicles) in giant cells suggested neuronal features. In contrast, a subpopulation of GCs in SENs and SEGAs are immunoreactive for GFAP, vimentin or S-100, which suggests a glial phenotype. The predominant cellular phenotype of the subependymal nodules in the Eker rat model of TSC (see below) is astrocytic (Yeung et al. 1997).

Recent immunohistochemical and molecular analyses have identified neuronal mRNAs and proteins such as neuron-specific enolase, tubulin, microtubule-associated proteins (MAPs), and intermediate filaments in giant cells within tubers (Hirose et al. 1995, Crino et al. 1996, Lopes et al. 1996). In addition, a small proportion of giant cells in SEGAs express met-enkephalin, b-endorphin, serotonin and neuropeptide Y, suggesting a neural lineage (Hirose et al. 1995). CD44, a cell adhesion molecule, which mediates cell–cell and cell–matrix interactions, is expressed near GCs in both tubers and SEGAs (Arai et al. 2000b). CD44 is expressed in astrocytic processes, predominantly in white matter and subpial regions, suggesting its involvement in the maintenance of a stable CNS cytoarchitecture. Tuber sections probed with antibodies recognizing the neural marker NeuN, a DNA binding protein present in mature neurons, exhibit a heterogeneous staining pattern (Fig. 16.3; Crino, unpublished results).

Some of the GCs and most of the DNs are labelled, but a small proportion are unlabelled, suggesting either a mixed neuroglial phenotype or that these cell types are phenotypically immature. Dysmorphic neurons express a variety of neuronal markers, e.g. cytoskeletal elements, neurotransmitter receptor subunits, which suggest that they are indeed of neuronal phenotype. These neural markers have been identified within a subpopulation of GCs in SEGAs and SENs, suggesting that GCs in tubers are more closely akin to neurons whereas those in SENs/SEGAs may reflect a more mixed population. Synaptophysin immunoreactivity has been reported along the cell membrane of GCs (Lippa et al. 1993), and single cell mRNA analysis from microdissected GCs has shown that these cells express NMDA, GluR and GABA$_A$ receptor subunit mRNAs (White et al. 2001), suggesting the possibility of synaptic connectivity between GCs and surrounding neurons. One compelling question is whether GCs are capable of synaptic transmission and, if so, whether they potentiate excitatory or inhibitory activity. To date, there has been no direct electrophysiological analysis or characterization of DNs or GCs in acute slice preparations from tubers. However, electron microscopic analyses have also identified desmosomal or gap junction-like connections between GCs and surrounding neurons (Huttenlocher and Heydemann 1984), and GCs express the gap junction mRNA connexin 26 (Crino et al. 1996). Electronic cellular interactions via gap junctions may contribute to the epileptogenicity of tubers, as has been suggested for temporal neocortex of epilepsy patients (Naus et al. 1991).

GCs in tubers express mRNA and proteins that are typically found in immature neurons and neuroepithelial precursor cells such as nestin (Crino et al. 1996), MAP2C (Yamanouchi et al. 1997) and the NMDA 2D receptor subunit (White et al. 2001). Recent evidence suggests that these cell types express doublecortin and collapsing response mediator protein-4 (Crino, unpublished observations) which are expressed in recently generated cell types. One possible explanation is that these markers may indicate that GCs have failed to terminally differentiate prior to migration into cortex, or that they have retained an immature phenotype within the tubers.

MOLECULAR NEUROBIOLOGY OF TSC

The identification of the *TSC1* and *TSC2* genes has aided in understanding the molecular events that lead to tuber, SEN and SEGA formation. Recent work has suggested that hamartin and tuberin are components of a pathway that modulates cellular proliferation and cell cycle passage, perhaps via a direct protein–protein interaction between the two molecules. The *TSC1* encoded protein hamartin has virtually no homology to known vertebrate genes. Hamartin mRNA and protein are widely expressed in normal tissues including the brain, liver, adrenal cortex, cardiac muscle, skin and kidney. Hamartin is highly expressed in G(0)-arrested cells as well as throughout the ongoing cell cycle, and an encoded coiled-coil domain may permit functional interaction with tuberin throughout the cell cycle. In fact, identification of an encoded coiled-coil domain in the carboxy region of hamartin (van Slegtenhorst et al. 1998) raised the possibility of a functional protein–protein interaction with tuberin (and other proteins) which has recently been demonstrated in *Drosophila* (Potter et al. 2001).

It is likely that hamartin interacts directly with tuberin and may be localized to cytoplasmic vesicles (Plank et al. 1998). Recent studies suggest that hamartin interacts with the ezrin-radixin-moesin (ERM) family of actin-binding proteins and thus may play an important role in mediating cell–cell interactions, cell adhesion, and potentially cell migration (Lamb et al. 2000). Interaction of endogenous hamartin with ERM-family proteins is required for activation of the intracellular signalling protein, Rho. Inhibition of hamartin function in vitro disrupts the formation and maintenance of focal adhesions and results in loss of attachment to the cell substrate. In contrast, hamartin overexpression in vitro in cells lacking focal adhesions results in activation of the small GTP-binding protein Rho, assembly of actin stress fibres, and formation of focal adhesions. Loss of functional hamartin in *TSC1*-associated TSC cases leads to altered adhesion to extracellular matrix proteins or adjacent cells, and thus, in developing cortex, loss of effective cell–cell communication may initiate the development of tubers via a compromise of cell migration and loss of cell adhesion cues. Furthermore, ongoing cellular proliferation in SEGAs may result from failed Rho-mediated cell–cell contact cues, and, thus, a Rho-mediated signalling pathway regulating cell adhesion may constitute a rate-limiting step in formation of these lesions.

Tuberin mRNA and protein are widely expressed in normal tissues including the brain, liver, adrenal cortex, cardiac muscle, skin and kidney (Geist et al. 1996). Tuberin mRNA and protein have been detected throughout the developing and adult brain, e.g. cortical and hippocampal pyramidal neurons, cerebellar Purkinje cells, brainstem motor nuclei, choroid plexus epithelium, and spinal cord (Geist and Gutmann 1995, Geist et al. 1996). In the mouse, tuberin expression is greatest during embryogenesis and in non-neuronal tissues, e.g. lymphocytes and epithelia, which undergo high mitotic turnover, suggesting a role in cell division. In TSC patients, alterations in tuberin mRNA or protein expression have been reported in tubers and SEGAs (Kerfoot et al. 1996, Mizuguchi et al. 1996). Tuberin immunore-activity was moderate to strong in neurons and reactive astrocytes of control brains, but was reduced in brains with tuberous sclerosis. A surprising finding in some TSC patients is the detection of intense tuberin immunoreactivity in GCs within tubers and SEGAs. Staining intensity of abnormal giant cells varied from negative to moderate in cortical tubers, subependymal nodules and subependymal giant cell astrocytomas.

Tuberin contains a hydrophobic N-terminal domain and a conserved 163 aminoacid carboxy terminal region which exhibits sequence homology to the catalytic domain of a GTPase activating protein (GAP) for Rap1. As a member of the superfamily of Ras-related protein, it is likely that Rap1 functions in the regulation of DNA synthesis and cell cycle transition. Tuberin displays GAP activity for Rap1, but not Rap2, Ha-Ras, Rac, or Rho (Wienecke et al. 1997), and co-localizes with Rap1 in the Golgi apparatus in several cell lines (Wienecke et al. 1996). The GAP activity of functional tuberin may modulate the effects of Rap1 on G- to S-phase transition during cell division. Thus, *TSC2* mutations might result in constitutive activation of Rap1. If tuberin functions as a tumour or growth suppressor (see below), activation of Rap1 pathways may lead to enhanced cell proliferation or incomplete cellular differentiation. For example, antisense inhibition of tuberin expression in cultured fibroblasts induced quiescent G0 arrested cells to re-enter the cell cycle and shortened the time in G1 of actively dividing cells (Soucek et al. 1997). In neuroblastoma cell lines, antisense inhibition of tuberin expression inhibited neuronal differentiation (Soucek et al. 1998). Using the yeast two-hybrid system, tuberin interaction with rabaptin-5, an effecter of Rab5, has been reported (Xiao et al. 1997). Tuberin exhibits GAP activity for Rab5, which is believed to be a critical component of the docking and fusion component of the endocytic pathway. These findings suggest that tuberin may be Golgi-localized in order to perform a functional role as a negative regulator of endocytosis via Rab5. Consistent with this model, the rate of fluid-phase endocytosis was increased in Eker rat cells lacking tuberin (Xiao et al. 1997). Finally, recent evidence suggests that tuberin can bind and selectively modulate gene transcription mediated by members of the steroid receptor super-family of genes (Henry et al. 1998).

Recent studies in *Drosophila* suggest that hamartin and tuberin form a func-tional heteromeric complex that is an important component of a pathway that modulates insulin receptor or insulin-like growth factor mediated signalling (Potter et al. 2001, Gao and Pan 2001). This pathway functions downstream of the cell signalling molecule Akt to regulate cell growth and potentially cell size. Thus, loss of hamartin or tuberin function following *TSC1* or *TSC2* mutations may result in enhanced proliferation of neural and astrocytic precursor cells and increased cell size characteristic of dysplastic neurons and giant cells commonly found in tubers of TSC. Of course, enhanced cell size may compromise neuronal migration and account for the loss of lamination within tubers. Alternatively, loss of hamartin or tuberin function may independently compromise neural migration via an interac-tion with ERM or actin-binding proteins. Recently it has been shown that hamartin and tuberin interact with the G2/M cyclin-dependent kinase CDK1 and its regulatory cyclins A and B (Catania et al. 2001). Abnormalities of radial glia have also been implicated in the pathogenesis of TSC (Park et al. 1997).

A rat strain (the Eker rat) serves as a model system to study the pathology of TSC (Yeung et al. 1994). A spontaneous germline mutation in the rat homologue of the human *TSC2* gene (*Tsc2*) results in a truncated isoform of tuberin lacking its C-terminal GAP element (see below). The Eker strain is predisposed to multiple neoplasias involving the kidneys, spleen and uterus. It was recently demonstrated that subependymal and subcortical hamartomas (tubers) identified in Eker rats are histologically similar to human subependymal nodules and tubers (Yeung et al. 1997).

Several lines of evidence indicate that both TSC genes are tumour suppressor genes. For example, germline *TSC1* and *TSC2* mutations appear to be inactivating, and restoration of normal tuberin function in cells cultured from the Eker rat results in a suppression of tumorigenicity (Jin et al. 1996). Loss of allelic heterozygosity (LOH) occurs in renal angiomyolipomas and cardiac rhabdomyomas, and supports a "two-hit" model for these lesions in TSC (Henske et al. 1996). In a given tumour,

LOH occurs at either *TSC1* or *TSC2*, but not at both loci. In SEGAs, *TSC1* or *TSC2* LOH has been detected in both the epithelioid and the spindle-cell populations, indicating that these two cells arose from a single precursor cell (Carbonara et al. 1994, Henske et al. 1996, 1997).

DEVELOPMENTAL PATHOGENESIS OF TUBERS, SENs AND SEGAs

It is likely that tubers result from the effects of *TSC1* or *TSC2* mutations on one of several steps during cortical development, including cell proliferation, differentiation or migration. The cellular effects of the TSC gene mutations in developing cortex occur at least as early as mid- to late corticogenesis since nascent cortical tubers have been identified in embryonic brains as early as 20 weeks gestation (Park et al. 1997). Similarly, SENs may be formed during embryogenesis, or, like SEGAs, may appear in childhood or adulthood. The link between altered function of tuberin and hamartin and the genesis of tubers, SENs and SEGAs, however, remains to be defined. It is likely that tubers derive from early progenitor cells in the ventricular zone (VZ), while SENs and SEGAs may derive from neuroepithelial cell precursors in the subventricular zone (SVZ) or VZ. Current data suggest that these proteins regulate cellular proliferation and potentially cellular movement, and thus the morphologic appearance of tubers and SEGAs suggests alterations in these cellular domains. For example, antisense inhibition of tuberin expression in cultured cells fosters cell proliferation (Soucek et al. 1997), and it is likely that hamartin contributes to the formation of focal adhesions necessary for cellular migration (Lamb et al. 2000). Further understanding of the downstream cellular events resulting from *TSC1* or *TSC2* mutations may highlight specific cellular pathways or select cell types that account for the histologic manifestations of these lesions. Indeed, it remains to be shown that the same processes are altered in tubers, SENs and SEGAs.

There have been several theories proposed to explain how tubers, SENs and SEGAs may form during cortical development (Fig. 16.3). For example, it is believed that all neuroepithelial progenitor cells carry a single allelic TSC gene mutation. In view of the focal nature of these lesions, one hypothesis is that a "second-hit" mutation in the existing normal TSC allele occurs within a single neuroepithelial cell in the VZ or SVZ as a result of inherent susceptibility or random mutation. As a consequence of the two mutations within this precursor cell, there is loss of hamartin or tuberin function and the ensuing downstream events may alter one of several steps involved in cellular proliferation or differentiation. This model suggests that all the cells within a tuber, SEN or SEGA derive from the initial cell sustaining a "second-hit" TSC mutation.

A problem with this hypothesis is that while LOH may account for SEN and SEGA formation and has indeed been demonstrated in SEGAs, LOH occurs rarely, if ever, in tubers (Henske et al. 1996, Niida et al. 2001). In fact, it is difficult to account for the overt cellular heterogeneity observed in tubers if all cells are derived from a common precursor cell. One possibility is that the precursor cell sustaining the "second hit" can yield progeny of disparate cell phenotypes via intrinsic programs or stochastic events. Similarly, LOH at either *TSC1* or *TSC2* loci was not identified in glioneuronal malformations with cellular morphology that was similar to tubers (*forme fruste* TSC; Normann et al. 1997). The failure to detect LOH in tubers suggests either an experimental artifact that disrupts the LOH, or that tubers form by a mechanism that is distinct from that of other lesions in TSC. One experimental contaminant is the presence of normal neurons (containing only the germline TSC mutation), which could migrate into tubers by non-radial migration routes (Reid et al. 1995), as well as astrocytes and oligodendrocytes. If only one in five neurons were to migrate into a tuber by non-radial pathways, then the LOH assay may not be reliable. A second possibility is that only certain cell types in tubers, e.g. giant cells, reflect progeny of neuroepithelial precursor cells that sustained a second-hit mutation. If so, then LOH would not be identified in whole tubers but instead would be confined to a select cell population in tubers. This model has important implications since all cells in tubers would not derive as a downstream effect of the TSC mutation, and in fact some would be innocent bystander cells, e.g. dysplastic neurons. A third possibility is that tubers may form by an alternative mechanism such as haploinsufficiency. If haploinsufficiency is an important mechanism in TSC, the focal nature of tubers suggests that additional somatic events may be involved, and the formation of tubers during cortical development may result from stochastic events superimposed on the setting of haploinsufficiency. In this hypothetical scenario, additional non-mutational events, such as regional localization, hypoxic injury, viral illness, or random DNA mutational events, could lead to the development of abnormal cell types. Indeed, these effects may not be confined to single cells but rather may affect a small subpopulation of cell types. A final possibility is that second-hit mutations may occur in several precursor cell types at once or in close anatomic and temporal proximity, and thus tubers might derive from a series of mutational events occurring during early corticogenesis. There is no clear explanation as to why multiple neural precursor cells would be affected in such close anatomic proximity or at distinct developmental epochs.

Regardless of mechanism, two critical questions regarding the formation of tubers and SEGAs derive from the observed cellular heterogeneity of these lesions. First, do mutational events such as a "second-hit" TSC gene mutation occur in the same subpopulations of neuroepithelial precursor cells in all TSC patients; and second, do these events occur at the same developmental epoch in all TSC patients? These questions are relevant to tuber and SEGA formation since variable mutational events occurring in disparate precursor cell populations or at different developmental time-points could result in cells populating tubers or SEGAs with remarkably distinct phenotypes. For example, one possibility is that any single neuronal precursor cell subtype might yield both GCs and DNs in all tubers in all TSC patients. If this were the case, then the observed cellular heterogeneity within tubers would reflect mutational events in an early neuroepithelial precursor that then differentiates into multiple cell types, some with similar phenotypes and others with distinct phenotypes. Thus, cellular heterogeneity in tubers and SEGAs may also reflect TSC mutations occurring at distinct time-points. If a mutation were to occur in an early progenitor cell, then the progeny of that cell may be more diverse than if such a mutation were to occur in a more mature precursor cell where the progeny would be a more restricted phenotype. Recent studies using retroviral tagging strategies have demonstrated that clonally derived cells may give rise to quite diverse cell populations, including pyramidal and multipolar cells and even astrocytes (Reid et al. 1995).

An alternative possible explanation for the observed heterogeneity of protein expression and cell morphology of DNs and GCs may be that in some cases a second-hit mutation occurs in a cell destined to become a pyramidal cell, while in others it occurs within a cell destined to become an astrocyte. These disparities may explain why GCs have been reported to express a variety of often conflicting neural and glial protein lineage markers. In contrast, only specific precursor cells may be capable of becoming a GC or a DN and, hence, a requirement might be that second-hit mutations occur in specific precursor cells. Thus, the phenotypic pathologic variability reported in tubers and SEGAs may suggest that, in some patients, GCs in tubers are largely derived from an astrocytic precursor cell, whereas in other patients, tubers are populated by GCs that derive from neuronal precursors. In fact, these differences might be observed within the same patient, so that a proportion of tubers may be neuronal and a portion astrocytic. These possibilities have important theoretical functional ramifications: for example, tubers derived from neural precursors might be more epileptogenic than those derived from astrocytes, which would explain why, in some TSC patients, only one of several tubers is epileptogenic.

An important additional issue is whether all the cellular constituents of tubers or SEGAs directly result from TSC gene mutations. In other words, do all cells within these lesions necessarily reflect downstream effects of TSC gene mutations, or are some cell types, e.g. astrocytes or DNs, merely "innocent bystanders" whose functional attributes, such as locating the appropriate laminar destination, have been altered by the presence of aberrant GCs? On this view, the GCs would be the "two-hit" cells that migrate, albeit abnormally, into the cortical plate and which disrupt migration of adjacent "single-hit" neurons. The cortical dysplasia observed in tubers would reflect a secondary or bystander effect in which "normal" (single mutation) neurons fail to migrate appropriately due to the disruption of migratory pathways by GCs.

Conversely, DNs may reflect the "two-hit" cells that cannot migrate correctly and that induce cytomegaly in GCs through the effects of a released growth factor. Indeed, the mutational status of other cells within tubers or SEGAs, i.e. endothelial cells or macrophages, remains unknown. These considerations are vital towards understanding the pathogenesis of tubers and SEGAs and especially how tuberin or hamartin dysfunction results in abnormal cytoarchitecture and potentially epileptogenesis. In contrast, in the latter scenario, the effects of altered tuberin or hamartin function would be evident in both neurons and giant cells, and thus *TSC1* and *TSC2* may serve as epilepsy susceptibility genes.

THE NEUROBIOLOGICAL BASIS OF EPILEPTOGENESIS IN TUBERS

Like other forms of cortical dysplasia, tubers are often identified as epileptic foci in TSC patients. In view of the cellular heterogeneity of these lesions, an important question is which cell types in tubers contribute to epileptogenesis? For example, if GCs in tubers express neuronal markers, then it is logical to hypothesize that these cells are somehow related to the epileptogenicity of tubers in cortex. In contrast, the synaptic connectivity of GCs remains to be defined and, thus, adjacent DNs may be responsible for aberrant hyperexcitability and seizure onset.

To date, the molecular pathogenesis of seizure initiation within tubers has not been characterized, and the pharmacologic features of DNs and GCs in tubers have not been fully defined. For example, the electrophysiologic, e.g. excitatory or inhibitory, firing properties of DNs and GCs have not been investigated. Variable GAD65 and NR 1 receptor immunoreactivity has been reported in "tuberous sclerosis-like lesions" (Wolf et al. 1995), and mRNA encoding the GABA A α2, 3 and 5 subunits was detected in GCs (Crino et al. 1996). A recent study using immunohistochemical techniques has demonstrated GluR subunit 2 and 3 expression in tubers and SEGAs (Arai et al. 2000a). PET imaging has demonstrated that epileptogenic tubers exhibit increased uptake of a-[^{11}C]-methyl-L-tryptophan which is metabolized to quinolinic acid, a potent agonist at NMDA sites (Chugani et al. 1998). In contrast, reduced iomezenil binding to benzodiazepine sites has been reported by PET in tubers (Fujita et al. 1997). These data suggest that an imbalance between excitatory and inhibitory synaptic transmission may be linked with seizure initiation in tubers.

A recent study has addressed the contribution of altered transcription of genes encoding glutamatergic and GABAergic receptors and uptake sites to seizure initiation in tubers (White et al. 2001). cDNA arrays containing GABA A (GABAAR), GluR, NMDA (NR) receptor subunits, GAD65, the vesicular GABA transporter (VGAT) and the neuronal (EAAC1) glutamate transporter cDNAs were probed with amplified poly (A) mRNA (aRNA) from tubers or normal neocortex to identify changes in gene expression. Increased levels of EAAC1, NR2B and 2D subunit mRNAs and diminished levels of GAD65, VGAT, GluR1 and GABAAR α1 and α2 were observed in tubers. Ligand binding experiments in frozen tuber homogenates demonstrated an increase in functional NR2B-containing receptors and a decrease in NR2A-containing sites. GCs and DNs are immunoreactive for the neuronal glutamate transporter, EAAC1 mRNA and protein (White et al. 2001). EAAC1 is expressed largely by excitatory neurons such as cortical pyramidal neurons. It is likely that reduced GAD65 and VGAT mRNA levels detected in tuber sections compared with control sections reflected diminished numbers of GABAergic neurons within tubers. If GCs and most DNs are in fact excitatory, then the physiologic effects of enhanced NR or GluR-mediated excitation and diminished GABAAR-mediated inhibition on these cells could be more pronounced. In this same study, cDNA arrays were then probed with aRNA from single, microdissected DNs, GCs or normal neurons. Enhanced expression of GluR 3, 4 and 6 and NR2B and 2C subunit mRNAs was noted in the DNs, whereas only the NR2D mRNA was upregulated in GCs. GABAAR α1 and α2 mRNA levels were reduced in both DNs and GCs compared to control neurons. Differential expression of GluR, NR, and GABAAR mRNAs in tubers reflected cell-specific changes in gene transcription, which argued for a distinct molecular phenotype of DNs and GCs, and suggested that DNs and GCs may make differential contributions to epileptogenesis in TSC. Since genotype analysis of just one TSC case was available in these studies, the authors concluded that either: (a) uniform alterations in neurotransmitter receptor subunit gene transcription may be a downstream effect of mutations in either the *TSC1* or *TSC2* locus; or (b) that the cases analysed in fact resulted from mutations in the *TSC2* gene. Indeed, further studies to establish the relationship between specific mutations in the *TSC1* or *TSC2* gene and changes in neurotransmitter receptor subunit mRNA expression may prove crucial in understanding epilepto-genesis in TSC. Without question, a critical and necessary future study will be to define the electrophysiological properties of select cell types in tubers.

SUMMARY

As the functions of the *TSC1* and *TSC2* gene products are defined, a clearer understanding of how these genes regulate normal cortical development will be generated. Several important questions remain that are under intense investigation. For example, understanding the relationship between tuberin and hamartin function and neuroglial proliferation and the role that mutations in these genes may play in aberrant neural migration will provide critical insights into the pathogenesis of tuber and SEGA formation. The electrophysiological properties of GCs and DNs in tubers can be defined so that new antiepileptic drugs can be designed specifically to treat seizures in TSC. Identification of the genes and proteins that modulate tran-sition from SEN to SEGA may provide important target molecules to regulate the growth of SEGAs and obviate the need for neurosurgical intervention. Finally, the relationship between tubers and epilepsy, learning disability and autism remains to be defined.

ACKNOWLEDGEMENTS

The author wishes to thank the Tuberous Sclerosis Alliance (TSA), the Center Without Walls, the Esther A. and Joseph Klingenstein Fund, and NIMH K0801658 for financial support.

REFERENCES

Arai Y, Takashima S, Becker LE (2000a) Downregulation of glutamate receptor subunit 2(3) in subependymal giant cell tumor. *Pediatr Neurol* 23(1): 37–41.

Arai Y, Takashima S, Becker LE (2000b) CD44 expression in tuberous sclerosis. *Pathobiology* 68: 87–92.

Bebin EM, Kelly PJ, Gomez MR (1993) Surgical treatment for epilepsy in cerebral tuberous sclerosis. *Epilepsia* 34: 651–7.

Bourneville DM (1880) Contributions a l'étude de l'idiotie. III. Sclérose tubéreuse des circonvolutions cérébrales. *Arch Internat Neurol* 1: 81–91.

Carbonara C, Longa L, Grosso E, et al. (1994) 9q34 loss of heterozygosity in a tuberous sclerosis astrocytoma suggests a growth suppressor-like activity also for the TSC1 gene. *Hum Mol Genet* 3: 1829–32.

Catania MG, Mischel PS, Vinters HV (2001) Hamartin and tuberin interaction with the G2/M cyclin-dependent kinase CDK1 and its regulatory cyclins A and B. *J Neuropathol Exp Neurol* 60(7): 711–23.

Chugani DC, Chugani HT, Muzik O, Shah JR, Shah AK, Canady A, Mangner TJ, Chakraborty PK (1998) Imaging epileptogenic tubers in children with tuberous sclerosis complex using alpha-[11C]methyl-L-tryptophan positron emission tomography. *Ann Neurol* 44: 858–66.

Consortium ECTS (1993) Identification and characterization of the tuberous sclerosis gene on chromosome 16. *Cell* 75: 1305–15.

Crino PB, Henske EP (1999) New development in neurobiology of tuberous sclerosis complex. *Neurology* 53: 1384–90.

Crino PB, Dichter MA, Trojanowski JQ, Eberwine JH (1996) Embryonic neuronal markers in tuberous sclerosis: single cell molecular pathology. *Proc Nat Acad Sci (USA)* 93: 14152–7.

Fujita M, Hashikawa K, Nagai T, Kodaka R, Uehara T, Nishimura T (1997) Decrease of the central type benzodiazepine receptor in cortical tubers in a patient with tuberous sclerosis. *Clin Nucl Med* 22: 130–1.

Gao X, Pan D (2001) TSC1 and TSC2 tumor suppressors antagonize insulin signaling in cell growth. *Genes Dev* 15: 1383–92.

Geist RT, Gutmann DH (1995) The tuberous sclerosis 2 gene is expressed at high levels in the cerebellum and developing spinal cord. *Cell Growth Diff* 6: 1477–83.

Geist RT, Reddy AJ, Zhang J, Gutmann DH (1996) Expression of the tuberous sclerosis 2 gene product, tuberin, in adult and developing nervous system tissues. *Neurobiol Disease* 3: 111–20.

Gomez MR (1988) *Tuberous Sclerosis*. New York: Raven Press.

Guerreiro MM, Andermann F, Andermann E, Palmini A, Hwang P, Hoffman HJ, Otsubo H, Bastos A, Dubeau F, Snipes GJ, Olivier A, Rasmussen T (1998) Surgical treatment of epilepsy in tuberous sclerosis: strategies and results in 18 patients. *Neurology* 51: 1263–9.

Gyure KA, Prayson RA (1997) Subependymal giant cell astrocytoma: a clinicopathologic study with HMB45 and MIB-1 immunohistochemical analysis. *Mod Pathol* 10: 313–17.

Henry KW, Yuan X, Koszewski NJ, Onda H, Kwiatkowski DJ, Noonan DJ (1998) Tuberous sclerosis gene 2 product modulates transcription mediated by steroid hormone receptor family members. *J Biol Chem* 273: 20535–9.

Henske E, Neumann H, Scheithauer B, Herbst E, Short M, Kwiatkowski D (1995) Loss of heterozygosity in the tuberous sclerosis (TSC2) region of chromosome band 16p13 occurs in sporadic as well as TSC-associated renal angiomyolipomas. *Genes Chrom Cancer* 13: 295–8.

Henske E, Scheithauer B, Short M, et al. (1996) Allelic loss is frequent in tuberous sclerosis kidney lesions but rare in brain lesions. *Am J Hum Genet* 59: 400–6.

Henske E, Wessner L, Golden J, et al. (1997) Loss of tuberin in both subependymal giant cell astrocytomas and angiomyolipomas supports a two-hit model for the pathogenesis of tuberous sclerosis tumors. *Am J Path* 151: 1639–47.

Hirose Y, Scheithauer BW, Lopes MBS, et al. (1995) Tuber and subependymal giant cell astrocytoma associated with tuberous sclerosis: an immunohistochemical, ultrastructural, and immunoelectron microscopic study. *Acta Neuropathol* 90: 387–99.

Huttenlocher PR, Heydemann PT (1984) Fine structure of cortical tubers in tuberous sclerosis. *Ann Neurol* 16: 595–602.

Jin F, Wieneke R, Xiao G-H, Maize J, DeClue J, Yeung R (1996) Suppression of tumorigenicity by the wild type tuberous sclerosis 2 (Tsc2) gene and its C-terminal region. *Proc Nat Acad Sci (USA)* 93: 9154–9.

Johnson MW, Emelin JK, Park SH, Vinters H (1999) Co-localization of TSC1 and TSC2 gene products in tubers of patients with tuberous sclerosis. *Brain Pathol* 9(1): 45–54.

Kerfoot C, Wienecke R, Menchine M, et al. (1996) Localization of tuberous sclerosis 2 mRNA and its protein product tuberin in normal human brain and in cerebral lesion of patients with tuberous sclerosis. *Brain Pathol* 6: 367–77.

Lamb RF, Roy C, Diefenbach TJ, Vinters HV, Johnson MW, Jay DG, Hall A (2000) The TSC1 tumour suppressor hamartin regulates cell adhesion through ERM proteins and the GTPase Rho. *Nat Cell Biol* 2(5): 281–7.

Lippa CF, Pearson D, Smith TW (1993) Cortical tubers demonstrate reduced immunoreactivity for synapsin I. *Acta Neuropathol* 85: 449–51.

Lopes MBS, Altermatt HJ, Scheitauer BW, Shepard CW, VandenBerg SR (1996) Immuno-histochemical characterization of subependymal giant cell astrocytomas. *Acta Neuropathol* 91: 368–75.

Mizuguchi M, Kato M, Yamanouchi H, Ikeda K, Takashima S (1996) Loss of tuberin from cerebral tissues with tuberous sclerosis and astrocytoma. *Ann Neurol* 40: 941–4.

Mizuguchi M, Kato M, Yamanouchi H, Ikeda K, Takashima S (1997) Tuberin immuno-histochemistry in brain, kidneys and heart with or without tuberous sclerosis. *Acta Neuropathol (Berl)* 94(6): 525–31.

Naus CC, Bechberger JF, Paul DL (1991) Gap junction gene expression in human seizure disorder. *Exp Neurol* 111: 198–203.

Niida Y, Stemmer-Rachamimov AO, Logrip M, Tapon D, Perez R, Kwiatkowski DJ, Sims K, MacCollin M, Louis DN, Ramesh V (2001) Survey of somatic mutations in tuberous sclerosis complex (TSC) hamartomas suggests different genetic mechanisms for pathogenesis of TSC lesions. *Am J Hum Genet* 69(3): 493–503.

Normann S, Green AJ, van Bakel I, et al. (1997) Tuberous sclerosis-like lesions in epileptogenic human neocortex lack allelic loss at the TSC1 and TSC2 regions. *Acta Neuropathol (Berl)* 93: 93–6.

O'Callaghan FJ, Shiell AW, Osborne JP, Martyn CN (1998) Prevalence of tuberous sclerosis estimated by capture-recapture analysis. *Lancet* 351: 149.

Padmalatha C, Harruff R, Ganick D, Hafez G (1980) Glioblastoma multiforme with tuberous sclerosis. Report of a case. *Arch Pathol Lab Med* 104: 649–50.

Park SH, Pepkowitz SH, Kerfoot C, et al. (1997) Tuberous sclerosis in a 20-week gestation fetus: immunohistochemical study. *Acta Neuropathol (Berl)* 94: 180–6.

Plank TL, Yeung RS, Henske EP (1998) Hamartin, the product of the tuberous sclerosis 1 (TSC1) gene, interacts with tuberin and appears to be localized to cytoplasmic vesicles. *Cancer Res* 58(21): 4766–70.

Potter CJ, Huang H, Xu T (2001) Drosophila Tsc1 functions with Tsc2 to antagonize insulin signaling in regulating cell growth, cell proliferation, and organ size. *Cell* 105: 357–68.

Povey S, Burley M, Attwood J, et al. (1994) Two loci for tuberous sclerosis: one on 9q34 and one on 16p13. *Ann Hum Genet* 58: 107–27.

Reid CB, Liang I, Walsh C (1995) Systematic widespread clonal organization in cerebral cortex. *Neuron* 15: 299–310.

Richardson EP (1991) Pathology of tuberous sclerosis. *Ann NY Acad Sci* 615: 128–39.

Roach ES, Gomez MR, Northrup H (1998) Tuberous sclerosis complex consensus conference: revised clinical diagnostic criteria. *J Child Neurol* 13(12): 624–8.

Scheithauer BW, Reagan TJ (1999) Neuropathology in the tuberous sclerosis complex. In: Gomez MR, Sampson JR, Whittemore VH (eds) *Tuberous Sclerosis Complex, 3rd edn.* New York: Oxford University Press, pp 101–21.

Shepherd CW (1999) The epidemiology of the tuberous sclerosis complex. In: Gomez MR, Sampson JR, Whittemore VH (eds) *Tuberous Sclerosis Complex, 3rd edn.* New York: Oxford University Press, pp. 101–21.

Short MP, Richardson EP, Haines J, Kwiatkowski DJ (1995) Clinical, neuropathological, and genetic aspects of the tuberous sclerosis complex. *Brain Path* 5: 173–9.

Sonigo P, Elmaleh A, Fermott L, Delezoide AL, Mirlesse V, Brunelole F (1996) Prenatal MRI diagnosis of fetal cerebral tuberous sclerosis. *Pediatr Radiol* 26: 1–4.

Soucek T, Pusch O, Wienecke R, DeClue J, Hengstschlager M (1997) Role of the tuberous sclerosis gene-2 product in cell cycle control. *J Biol Chem* 272: 29301–8.

Soucek T, Holzl G, Bernaschek G, Hengstschlager M (1998) A role of the tuberous sclerosis gene-2 product during neuronal differentiation. *Oncogene* 16: 2197–204.

Tamaki K, Okuno T, Ito M, Asato R, Konishi J, Mikawa H (1990) Magnetic resonance imaging in relation to EEG epileptic foci in tuberous sclerosis. *Brain Dev* 12: 316–20.

Tien RD, Hesselink JR, Duberg A (1990) Rare subependymal giant cell astrocytoma in a neonate with tuberous sclerosis. *Am J Neuroradiol* 11: 1251–2.

Trombley IK, Mirra SS (1981) Ultrastructure of tuberous sclerosis: cortical tuber and subependymal tumor. *Ann Neurol* 9: 174–81.

van Bakel I, Sepp T, Ward S, Yates J, Green A (1997) Mutations in the TSC2 gene: analysis of the complete coding sequence using the protein truncation test (PTT). *Hum Mol Genet* 6: 1409–14.

van Slegtenhorst M, de Hoogt R, Hermans C, Nellist M, Janssen B, et al. (1997) Identification of the tuberous sclerosis gene TSC1 on chromosome 9q34. *Science* 277: 805–8.

van Slegtenhorst M, Nellist M, Nagelkerken B, et al. (1998) Interaction between hamartin and tuberin, the TSC1 and TSC2 gene products. *Hum Mol Genet* 7: 1053–7.

von Recklinghausen, FD (1863) Ein Herz von einen Neurogeborenen. *Verb Berl Ges Geburt* 15: 73.

White R, Hua Y, Lynch DR, Henske E, Crino P (2001) Differential transcription of neuro-transmitter receptor subunits and uptake sites in giant cells and dysplastic neurons in cortical tubers. *Ann Neurol* 49: 67–78.

Wienecke R, Konig A, DeClue J (1995) Identification of tuberin, the tuberous sclerosis-2 product. *J Biol Chem* 270: 16409–14.

Wienecke R, Maize J, Shoarinejad F, et al. (1996) Co-localization of the TSC2 product tuberin with its target Rap1 in the Golgi apparatus. *Oncogene* 13: 913–23.

Wienecke R, Maize J, Reed J, deGunzburg J, Yeung R, DeClue J (1997) Expression of the TSC2 product tuberin and its target Rap1 in normal human tissues. *Am J Pathol* 150: 43–50.

Wiestler O, Lopez B, Crino PB (1997) Tuberous sclerosis complex and subependymal astro-cytoma. In: Kleihues P, Cavenee WK (eds) *Pathology and Genetics: Tumors of the Nervous System*. Lyon: International Agency for Research on Cancer, pp 182–5.

Wolf HK, Birkholz T, Wellmer J, Blumcke I, Pietsch T, Wiestler OD (1995) Neurochemical profile of glioneuronal lesions from patients with pharmacoresistant focal epilepsies. *J Neuropathol Exp Neurol* 54: 689–97.

Xiao G, Shoarinejad F, Jin F, Golemis E, Yeung R (1997) The tuberous sclerosis-2 gene product, tuberin, functions as a Rab5 GAP in modulating endocytosis. *J Bio Chem* 272: 6097–100.

Yamanouchi H, Jay V, Rutka JT, Takashima S, Becker LE (1997) Evidence of abnormal differentiation in giant cells of tuberous sclerosis. *Pediatr Neurol* 17: 49–53.

Yeung RS, Xiao GH, Jin F, Lee WC, Testa JR, Knudson AG (1994) Predisposition to renal carcinoma in the Eker rat is determined by germ-line mutation of the tuberous sclerosis 2 (TSC2) gene. *Proc Nat Acad Sci (USA)* 91: 11413–16.

Yeung RS, Katsetos CD, Klein-Szanto A (1997) Subependymal astrocytic hamartomas in the Eker rat model of tuberous sclerosis. *Am J Pathol* 151: 1477–86.

17
FUTURE DIRECTIONS

Paolo Curatolo and Nunzio Bottini

Despite the great achievements of the last years and rapid advances in our knowledge about tuberous sclerosis complex (TSC), many questions remain unanswered and will constitute the basis for further research in the field. In the future TSC will also provide an important model to investigate relationships between strategically located morphological abnormalities and mechanisms of cognition and behaviour.

Furthermore, TSC will continue to be a very exciting area of research in the field of pediatric neuroscience for all those interested in cell migration, differentiation and proliferation, oncogenesis, epileptogenesis, and molecular genetic programming of brain development.

It is not possible to discuss in detail all these important issues, but we will try to focus on future directions in some areas of research, where we hope that important achievements will shortly be obtained.

FUNCTIONS OF THE TSC GENES
According to the new classification of CNS malformations, which provides for the integration of both morphological and molecular genetic criteria, TSC lesions are classified as primary disorders of cellular lineage, involving both hamartomatous tissue architecture and cytological dysplasia with mixed neuronal and glial protein expression in the same cell. The mechanisms by which loss of tuberin and hamartin expression produces the TSC lesions are still unclear, but modern molecular biology seems to hold the greatest promise for unravelling these mechanisms in the near future and identifying the physiological functions of tuberin and hamartin in human tissues.

The dissection of the role of the TSC complex in specific signal transduction pathways regulating cell growth and proliferation is currently being carried out by several research groups, and many exciting new findings have been reported during the last few years. In the insulin signalling system, genetic studies in *Drosophila* were the first to position tuberin upstream or parallel to the cell growth regulator mTOR and upstream to the S6 kinase (S6K) (Potter et al. 2001). Negative regulation of S6K activation by tuberin has recently been reported by different groups (Goncharova et al. 2002, Inoki et al. 2002, Tee et al. 2002), and it is likely to play an important role in tuberin tumour suppressor activity.

Recent studies have also shown that tuberin and hamartin share with other signal transduction molecules the ability to be reversibly phosphorylated on tyrosine and serine/threonine residues during signalling (Aicher et al. 2001, Manning et al. 2002, Potter et al. 2002). The physiological relevance of tuberin phosphorylation on tyrosine is not completely clear yet, but it seems to regulate its interaction with hamartin (Aicher et al. 2001, Nellist et al. 2001) and apparently affects tuberin cellular location (Lou et al. 2001). Tuberin is one of the main targets of serine/threonine kinases located downstream of PI3K in several signalling systems, including insulin, PDGF and IGF-1. During insulin signal transduction, phosphorylation of tuberin on S939/T1462 by AKT is able to suppress its inhibitory activity on S6K activation, apparently without affecting the tuberin–hamartin interaction (Dan et al. 2002, Inoki et al. 2002, Manning et al. 2002).

Some future trends in TSC molecular research are relatively easy to predict. The relationship between tuberin/hamartin and mTOR in the regulation of cell growth and proliferation and the role of tuberin in pathways downstream of PI3K in several signalling systems warrant further investigation. Several results on tuberin/hamartin phosphorylation are available, but more biochemical efforts are needed in order to clarify phosphorylation sites, responsible kinases and the physiological role of phosphorylation of TSC molecules. Future research will also undoubtedly address possible changes in localization, and/or expression of TSC molecules during signalling, and their possible interaction with scaffolding and signalling molecules. Two-hybrid studies with both tuberin and hamartin have been completed or are in progress; for example, using this procedure, recently the 14–3-3 molecule has been identified as an interactor of the tuberin/hamartin complex (Nellist et al. 2002). The analysis of molecules interacting with tuberin and hamartin will also help in understanding TSC clinical variability (which may be extensive even between affected siblings), which is most probably influenced by the interactions of *TSC1* and *TSC2* with other genes in the various target organs, such as the brain, kidneys and heart. Therefore, it is possible that such interacting molecules will turn out to be 'phenotype modifier' genes: it is likely that studies aimed at characterizing such genes will require an international collaboration of patients, clinicians and geneticists worldwide.

Finally, molecular biology studies will, it is hoped, lead to the identification of the factors that drive the development of SEGAs from SENs and provide new pharmacological targets to control the growth of SEGAs, preventing the need for neurosurgery. The same targets could be useful in preventing tuber formation during fetal brain development.

PATHOPHYSIOLOGICAL MECHANISMS

There is no doubt that different parts of the TSC genes have different functions, and it is likely that we will soon learn the distinctive role of different mutations. It is possible that different mutations have different physiological effects and they may contribute differently to lowering the epileptogenic threshold. Many questions are still unanswered. What role do the TSC genes play in determining the presence of sporadic epilepsy in some patients and early-onset intractable seizures in others? Since tubers are present from the gestational age, what is the epileptogenic trigger and when does it start working? In the future we should learn more about how the mutant gene is responsible for abnormal firing and consequent epilepsy. Furthermore, what do the mutant cells do to the brain? Is the onset of epilepsy related to different exon mutations? Several laboratories are presently intensively studying mutation characterization in order to address this important issue. The increased sensitivity of mutation detection due to technical development of gene-based diagnostic tests will provide more accurate information on the risk of complications associated with different *TSC1* and *TSC2* mutations. This will open an avenue for child neurologists for the study of new correlations between the genotype and the phenotypes.

In families with a known TSC mutation, gene mutation carriers can be followed up even before birth in order to determine the natural course of TSC. Close monitoring in the first months of life is important for early detection of seizures and particularly of infantile spasms (Curatolo et al. 2002). Immediate treatment of infantile spasms should be attempted, as there is evidence that this increases the chance of successful seizure control, and potentially reduces the risk or the severity of learning disability.

Efforts are on their way to improve the image quality of MRI and to extract more information from the anatomical data than is apparent on standard tomographic visualization. Advanced MRI analysis methods and quantitative analysis may better characterize the tuber. Functional imaging may offer the best hope for future neuroimaging advances in epilepsy. The newest aspects of PET for epilepsy imaging are the development of tracers that can image neurotransmitters and neurotransmitter receptor systems to study abnormal brain tissue responsible for seizures, and mechanisms of intrinsic epileptogenicity, showing excess of excitatory NMDA-mediated transmission with impaired GABA-mediated transmission in localized cortical zones (Di Michele et al. 2003). In addition, the advent of more powerful magnets will enhance the role of magnetic resonance spectroscopy to measure both aminoacids and energy-related metabolite. Defining the cellular, and molecular, characteristics of the neural network in tubers is important for developing new, more effective pharmacological treatments able to reach the specific tuber cell types responsible for the initiation and the propagation of the epileptic discharge.

There will also be great interest in using imaging to assess therapeutic effects. Both MRS and flumazenil PET imaging of GABA changes in the epileptic zone are promising in this regard. There is no doubt that integration of morphological and functional data will further improve, explaining enhanced epileptogenicity in some areas.

In TSC, epilepsy arises from interaction among multiple areas, all of which have increased excitability. Evaluation of refractory epilepsy should employ strategies that define specific firing patterns able to activate specific neurotransmitter receptors. The hunt for the epileptogenic focus will be launched by new source localization techniques approaches, and mainly by magnetic source imaging, which will show us where the seizures really begin and the neural networks of generalizations. We will be looking for early detection of epileptogenic cortical tubers even before seizure onset.

NEUROBIOLOGY OF BEHAVIOURAL PHENOTYPES

Recent evidence suggests that generalized epilepsy during early development, and functional deficits in the temporal lobes of the brain, may be associated with autism. The presence of tubers in the temporal lobes seems a necessary but not sufficient risk factor for the development of an autistic spectrum disorder (Bolton et al. 2002). There is a critical early stage of brain maturation during which temporal lobe epileptiform discharges on EEG perturb the development of brain systems that underpin social intelligence and possibly other cognitive skills, thereby inducing an autistic spectrum disorder. The links between brain structure and behaviour are under study.

Autistic spectrum disorders may also reflect a direct effect of the abnormal genetic program. Exciting new developments in molecular genetics of autism are in progress. Autism is more frequently associated with *TSC2* mutations. Recent evidence suggests that a potential susceptibility gene located on chromosome 16p13 exists (Lucarelli et al. 2003). Positional cloning of susceptibility genes in autism may provide important clues in the understanding of autistic behaviour associated with TSC. The genetic dissection of the short arm of chromosome 16 in autism will help to more precisely localize a susceptibility gene, and clarify its position with respect to the *TSC2* locus.

There is evidence for a widespread cortical disorganization and structural abnormalities throughout the brain, not just associated with tubers and nodules. It is possible that some of the cognitive deficits in TSC relate to the function of the *TSC1* and *TSC2* gene on neuronal maturation. Vulnerability in systems associated with regulation of attention, as well as with planning and organization, is a neuro-cognitive pattern frequently found even in the most able individual with the disorder, reminding us of the importance of finding the crucial interface between the cognitive-behavioural endophenotype and the genotypes

EARLY RATIONAL TREATMENT FOR EPILEPSY

New clinical research is also under way that will lead to better treatment of the TSC manifestations. Presently, the treatment of epilepsy remains a major challenge, and many patients with TSC continue to have intractable seizures. A more science-based, rational drug choice for individual patients will replace the largely empirical approach to the pharmacological management of epilepsy we still have today. Advances in drug therapy have opened up research into appropriate polytherapy, since children with TSC often have several different seizure types. Good effective practice has been researched into, looking at the best polytherapy for different seizures, using only two medications. New drugs delivery systems for freeing small quantities of specific antiepileptic drug directly to targeted brain zones could be a future option.

New neuroprotective strategies should allow the development of seizure prevention strategies to minimize the effect of recurrent seizures on immature brains. We will probably understand much more about pre-ictal changes, and when a tuber is becoming epileptogenic, which will enable us to anticipate diagnosis of seizures and to initiate early treatment. Furthermore, prevention of generalized and catastrophic epilepsies, such as epileptic spasms and Lennox–Gastaut syndrome, will be possible. We will see a lot of development in this area in the next decade. Evidence suggests that we can now predict medical intractability, and we can now easily and not invasively identify TSC patients who are highly likely to become seizure-free following surgical treatment.

In future there will be an increasing role for epileptic surgery programs. Multicentre assessment prospective studies using standardized selection criteria, surgical protocols to evaluate seizure outcomes, and quality of life following epilepsy surgery will provide more information on the long-term prognosis. Prognostic factors for epilepsy surgery outcome should help child neurologists to advise families on what to expect from surgery.

An important question now is not whether epilepsy surgery works in selected TSC patients, but how soon it should be performed in order to rescue children from a lifetime disability. From this point of view, optimizing the timing of surgery will be fundamental.

In TSC, seizures persist after surgery because residual epileptogenic cortex was left, due to its proximity to eloquent cortex, or because a distant independent focus was not addressed. Recent data suggest that a selected group of TSC patients may benefit from a multistage invasive monitoring and a more aggressive surgical approach (Romanelli et al. 2002). Converging information between video-EEG monitoring and extracranial localization with MRI fusioning can improve our ability to select candidates who could benefit from surgical treatment.

There is little doubt that the treatment of TSC will benefit from the present and future research on the molecular mechanisms involved in the pathogenesis of this devastating disease. This progress will enable child neurologists to provide better care for patients affected with tuberous sclerosis.

Even before the molecular picture of TSC is completed, the application of powerful molecular biology tools to the investigation of tuberin and hamartin physiological functions will, it is hoped, lead to the identification of targets for an effective treatment. Furthermore, current research in gene manipulation and the use of inhibiting factors will probably help control several different forms of benign and malignant tumoral growth, and could offer new hope for a better quality of life for patients.

REFERENCES

Aicher LD, Campbell JS, Yeung RS (2001) Tuberin phosphorylation regulates its interaction with hamartin. Two proteins involved in tuberous sclerosis. *J Biol Chem* 276: 21017–21.

Bolton PF, Park RJ, Higgins JN, Griffiths PD, Pickles A (2002) Neuroepileptic determinants of autism spectrum disorders in tuberous sclerosis complex. *Brain* 125: 1247–55.

Curatolo P, Verdecchia M, Bombardieri R (2002) Tuberous sclerosis complex: a review of neurological aspects. *Eur J Ped Neurol* 6: 15–23.

Dan HC, Sun M, Yang L, Feldman RI, Sui XM, Ou CC, Nellist M, Yeung RS, Halley DJ, Nicosia SV, Pledger WJ, Cheng JQ (2002) Phosphatidylinositol 3-kinase/Akt pathway regulates tuberous sclerosis tumor suppressor complex by phosphorylation of tuberin. *J Biol Chem* 277: 35364–70.

Di Michele F, Verdecchia M, Dorofeeva M, Bernardi G, Curatolo P (2003) Gaba(A) receptor active steroids are altered in epileptic patients with tuberous sclerosis. *J Neurol Neurosurg Psychiatry* 74: 667–70.

Goncharova EA, Goncharov DA, Eszterhas A, Hunter DS, Glassberg MK, Yeung RS, Walker CL, Noonan D, Kwiatkowski DJ, Chou MM, Panettieri RA Jr, Krymskaya VP (2002) Tuberin regulates p70 S6 kinase activation and ribosomal protein S6 phosphorylation. A role for the TSC2 tumor suppressor gene in pulmonary lymphangioleiomyomatosis (LAM). *J Biol Chem* 277: 30958–67.

Inoki K, Li Y, Zhu T, Wu J, Guan KL (2002) TSC2 is phosphorylated and inhibited by Akt and suppresses mTOR signalling. *Nat Cell Biol* 4: 648–57.

Lou D, Griffith N, Noonan DJ (2001) The tuberous sclerosis 2 gene product can localize to nuclei in a phosphorylation-dependent manner. *Mol Cell Biol Res Commun* 4: 374–80.

Lucarelli P, Palminiello S, Bottini N, De Luca D, Elia M, Fiumara A, Curatolo P (2003) Association study of autistic disorder and chromosome 16p. *Am J Med Genet* 119A: 242–6.

Manning BD, Tee AR, Logsdon MN, Blenis J, Cantley LC (2002) Identification of the tuberous sclerosis complex-2 tumor suppressor gene product tuberin as a target of the phosphoinositide 3-kinase/akt pathway. *Mol Cell* 10: 151–62.

Nellist M, Verhaaf B, Goedbloed MA, Reuser AJ, van den Ouweland AM, Halley DJ (2001) TSC2 missense mutations inhibit tuberin phosphorylation and prevent formation of the tuberin-hamartin complex. *Hum Mol Genet* 10: 2889–98.

Nellist M, Goedbloed MA, de Winter C, Verhaaf B, Jankie A, Reuser AJ, van den Ouweland AM, van der Sluijs P, Halley DJ (2002) Identification and characterization of the interaction between tuberin and 14-3-3zeta. *J Biol Chem* 277: 39417–24.

Potter CJ, Huang H, Xu T (2001) Drosophila TSC1 functions with TSC2 to antagonize insulin signaling in regulating cell growth, cell proliferation, and organ size. *Cell* 105: 357–68.

Potter CJ, Pedraza LG, Xu T (2002) Akt regulates growth by directly phosphorylating TSC2. *Nat Cell Biol* 4: 658–65.

Romanelli P, Najjar S, Weiner H, Devinsky O (2002) Epilepsy surgery in tuberous sclerosis: multistage procedures with bilateral or multilobar foci. *J Child Neurol* 17: 689–92.

Tee AR, Fingar DC, Manning BD, Kwiatkowski DJ, Cantley LC, Blenis J (2002) Tuberous sclerosis complex-1 and -2 gene products function together to inhibit mammalian target of rapamycin (mTOR)-mediated downstream signaling. *Proc Natl Acad Sci USA* 99: 13571–6.

INDEX

Note: TSC refers to 'tuberous sclerosis complex'. Page numbers in *italics* refer to figures and tables.